STATE OF THE ART IN
DIGITAL MAMMOGRAPHIC
IMAGE ANALYSIS

SERIES IN MACHINE PERCEPTION AND ARTIFICIAL INTELLIGENCE

Editors: **H. Bunke** (Univ. Bern, Switzerland)
P. S. P. Wang (Northeastern Univ., USA)

Vol. 1: Pattern Recognition and Image Analysis: Selected Papers from the IVth Spanish Symposium
(Eds. *N. Pérez de la Blanca, A. Sanfeliu and E. Vidal*)

Vol. 2: Theory and Applications of Image Analysis: Selected Papers from the 7th Scandinavian Conference on Image Analysis
(Eds. *P. Johansen and S. Olsen*)

Vol. 3: Neural Networks in Vision and Pattern Recognition
(Eds. *J. Skrzypek and W. Karplus*)

Vol. 4: Parallel Image Processing
(Eds. *A. Saoudi, M. Nivat and P. S. P. Wang*)

Vol. 5: Advances in Structural and Syntactic Pattern Recognition: Proceedings of the International Workshop on Structural and Syntactic Pattern Recognition
(Ed. *H. Bunke*)

Vol. 6: Active Robot Vision: Camera Heads, Model Based Navigation and Reactive Control
(Eds. *H. I. Christensen, K. W. Bowyer and H. Bunke*)

Vol. 7: Advances in Pattern Recognition Systems Using Neural Network Technologies
(Eds. *I. Guyon and P. S. P. Wang*)

Vol. 8: Thinning Methodologies for Pattern Recognition
(Eds. *C. Y. Suen and P. S. P. Wang*)

Vol. 9: State of the Art in Digital Mammographic Image Analysis
(Eds. *K. W. Bowyer and S. Astley*)

Vol. 11: Experimental Environments for Computer Vision and Image Processing
(Eds. *H. I. Christensen and J. L. Crowley*)

Forthcoming

Vol. 10: Generic Object Recognition Using Form and Function
(Eds. *K. W. Bowyer and L. Stark*)

Series in Machine Perception and Artificial Intelligence – Vol. 9

STATE OF THE ART IN
DIGITAL MAMMOGRAPHIC
IMAGE ANALYSIS

Edited by

K W Bowyer

Department of Computer Science
and Engineering
University of South Florida
Tampa, Florida, USA

S Astley

Department of Medical Biophysics
University of Manchester
Manchester, UK

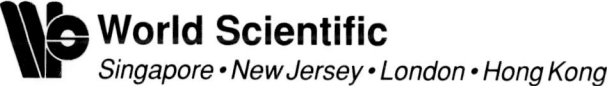

World Scientific

Singapore • New Jersey • London • Hong Kong

Published by

World Scientific Publishing Co. Pte. Ltd.
P O Box 128, Farrer Road, Singapore 9128
USA office: Suite 1B, 1060 Main Street, River Edge, NJ 07661
UK office: 73 Lynton Mead, Totteridge, London N20 8DH

**STATE OF THE ART IN
DIGITAL MAMMOGRAPHIC IMAGE ANALYSIS**

Copyright © 1994 by World Scientific Publishing Co. Pte. Ltd.

All rights reserved. This book, or parts thereof, may not be reproduced in any form or by any means, electronic or mechanical, including photocopying, recording or any information storage and retrieval system now known or to be invented, without written permission from the Publisher.

For photocopying of material in this volume, please pay a copying fee through the Copyright Clearance Center, Inc., 27 Congress Street, Salem, MA 01970, USA.

ISBN: 981-02-1509-6

Printed in Singapore by Utopia Press.

EDITOR'S INTRODUCTION

The interpretation of medical images is one of the most technically challenging applications of computer vision, largely because of the high degree of variability associated with both normal and abnormal appearances. This special issue focuses on one particularly important problem; the detection of breast cancer in X-ray mammograms. Throughout the western world, where around one in twelve women suffer from breast cancer at some time in their lives, screening programmes based on mammography have been instituted. (Unlike our western Europe counterparts, the U.S.A. does not yet have any national screening program – KB.) Such programmes aim to increase the effectiveness of treatment by identifying sufferers before any tumour becomes palpable. When detected late, the disease carries a high risk of mortality.

Mammographic images are notoriously difficult to interpret. The human breast varies considerably in composition, giving mammographic appearances ranging from relative uniformity to complex patterns of bright streaks or blobs. In screening programmes, the vast majority of images are unequivocally normal, but each image must be carefully searched for any sign of abnormality. Significant features may be small or subtle; malignant microcalcifications, for example, can be detected when they are only a tenth of a millimetre across. There is a considerable body of evidence to suggest that radiologists find the task of interpretation difficult; indeed, in many centers films are studied by two radiologists in an attempt to reduce error rates. Computers could be used to aid the process in a variety of ways, from detecting and prompting specific signs of abnormality to distinguishing between benign and malignant tumours. In recent years there has been rapid progress in computer-aided mammography, with the widespread and serious nature of the problem providing a powerful motivation for those engaged in the research. This progress is reflected in the variety and high standard of the papers in this volume.

This book is the end result of the efforts and considerations of many people. Dmitry Goldgof and Raj Archarya, the co-chairs of the *1993 SPIE Biomedical Image Processing Conference*, were kind enough to allow a substantial portion of the program of their meeting to be filled with papers related to mammographic image analysis. This portion of the meeting informally became the *First International Workshop on Mammographic Image Analysis*, with a total of 28 papers contributed by 25 different research groups in seven different countries around the world. Following the indulgence shown by Dmitry Goldgof and Raj Acharya, Horst Bunke was kind enough to allow a special issue of the International Journal of Pattern Recognition and Artificial Intelligence devoted to selected papers from this meeting. A total of sixteen papers were initially submitted for possible publication in the special issue. The reviewing of most of these papers was handled jointly by Sue Astley in the U.K. and Kevin Bowyer in the U.S. (The reviewing of papers from the University of Manchester group was handled by Prof. Bowyer in the U.S. and the reviewing of papers from the University of South Florida group was handled by Prof. Astley in the U.K.) Based on the reviewers' comments, nine contributed papers were eventually selected to appear in the IJPRAI special issue. Limitations on the space available forced us to omit some papers which merited wider dissemination. Thus the publisher agreed to bring out this book. The book contains an additional five papers not in the special issue, including some which were not originally submitted to the special issue but were solicited by the editors after the presentations at the *1993 SPIE Biomedical Image Processing Conference*.

The papers in this book touch on a variety of different subtopics in mammographic image analysis.

The paper by Astley and co-workers describes a number of experiments performed in Manchester with the aim of identifying the problems, tools, and methods of presenting results that will be of the most value to the radiologist. Results are summarized for detection of microcalcifications, masses, spiculated (stellate) lesions and asymmetry. A comparison is given of radiologist performance (ROC curves) working with and without the benefit of prompting by automated image analysis.

The paper by Magnin and co-workers concentrates on data compression techniques for use in creating a mammography database. The basic method is *Discrete Cosine Transform* (DCT) of block subimages followed by Huffman encoding of the DCT coefficients. The claim is that compression ratios of up to 30 can be achieved without the radiologist being able to discriminate between the original and the compressed/reconstructed image. This paper also describes "SENOBASE", a database available on CD that contains 400 commented digitized mammograms.

The paper by Aghdasi and co-workers deals with deconvolution and image smoothing filters for mammograms images. The authors point out that the literature specific to mammogram images has generally just considered smoothing and enhancement techniques and not also deconvolution techniques.

The paper by Hajnal and co-workers deals with a proposed procedure to automatically separate the flow of images through a screening program into "fatty" and "dense" categories, with the motivation being that the more difficult images to read could be given to a more experienced reader or allocated more time.

The paper by Nishikawa and co-workers gives an overview of the work done by the University of Chicago group, which has an established history of pioneering work in mammographic image analysis. This paper discusses approaches to detection of clustered microcalcifications, detection of breast masses and classification of breast masses. Performance results are presented as ROC curves.

The paper by Barman, Granlund and Haglund proposes a framework for *wavelets* oriented analysis of mammograms. (Several papers related to the use of wavelets techniques were presented at the workshop.) The authors explain the wavelets approach and present some results for detection of clusters of microcalcifications. Results are given as performance points; that is, Receiver Operating Characteristic (ROC) curves are not generated for the technique.

The paper by Karssemeijer brings together and updates his various previous results in the area of mammographic image analysis. One element of his approach is an algorithm to rescale mammogram images so that noise levels are equal at all intensities. Another part is a *Markov random field* model applied to detect clusters of microcalcifications. Results are given as FROC curves, using a test set of 40 images and a training set of 25 images.

The paper by Chitre, Dhawan and Moskowitz describes a method for classifying microcalcifications into benign and malignant categories. The approach does not require image segmentation; an already (hand) segmented cluster of microcalcifications is classified as either benign or malignant. *Second-order histogram* statistics are extracted and used for classification by a neural network.

Shen, Rangayyan and Desautels have also tackled the detection and classification of microcalcifications. In their paper they describe a detection method based on *multi-tolerance region growing*. A variety of shape measures are computed, and a neural network is employed for classification of detected microcalcifications into benign and malignant categories. Classification rates are presented for a range of different classifiers.

The detection of microcalcifications has also been addressed by Woods and co-workers. Candidate microcalcifications are segmented on the basis of local brightness, and classified into microcalcification and non-calcification categories. Several features were evaluated, and the most powerful were used to compare classifiers both for the detection of individual microcalcifications and for the detection of clusters. Results are given as ROC curves for linear and quadratic classifiers, a binary decision tree, several different neural networks and a k nearest neighbor method.

The paper by Brzakovic and Neskovic develops an approach to mammographic image analysis called *fuzzy pyramid linking*. The technique can be applied to the detection of both microcalcifications and masses. The "pyramid" data structure reflects an explicit multiresolution analysis of the image. The "fuzzy" part indicates that classification is done by carrying through a "degree of membership" until a final step when the result is "crispened" and a decision made. The linking in the pyramid gives some adaptive local flavor to the processing. Performance is given as point results (no ROC curves).

The paper by Parker and co-workers concentrates on development of a classifier to distinguish between comedo and non-comedo *Ductal Carcinoma In Situ*. Calcifications are hand-labelled in a set of images. A large number of possible features are considered for use with a general k nearest neighbor classifier. Results are given in the form of ROC curves.

Miller and Astley present results of a method to detect abnormalities by assessing the degree of asymmetry between left and right breasts. They first segment the breast images on the basis of texture to identify non-fat regions, and then compare shape, grey-level and topological properties of these regions to identify potential abnormalities. Results of the segmentation procedure (ROC curves), and of classification of mammogram pairs both into normal and abnormal categories and into specific abnormality groups, are shown.

The paper by Kegelmeyer focuses on development of an approach for automated detection of stellate lesions. Rather than segmenting regions of the image and then computing properties of the segmented regions, as the other papers do, Kegelmeyer computes properties for a window around every pixel to find "stellate-ness" for each pixel and then groups pixels with high stellateness. The features used to measure stellate-ness are *Laws' texture energy measures* and the *analysis of locally oriented edges* (ALOE) measure developed by Kegelmeyer. A binary decision tree is used as the classifier and results are presented as ROC curves.

Lastly, the paper by Etta Pisano and Faina Shtern is a special treat. Doctors Pisano and Shtern give us a perspective on this field of research from the point of view of the practicing M.D. who reads mammogram studies in a clinical setting. We are fortunate that they have been willing to take the time to consider the work in this area and give us the benefit of their experience and insight.

We would like to extend our sincere thanks to all of the people who contributed to making this special issue happen. We hope that the readers will find the papers interesting and that some readers will even be stimulated to begin research work in this very important area.

Finally, we are pleased to announce the *Second International Workshop on Mammographic Image Analysis*, which will be held at the Royal York Hotel in York, England, from 10th to 12th July 1994. Further information can be obtained from Prof. Alastair Gale, the Applied Vision Research Unit, University of Derby, Derby DE3 5GX; Fax: +44 332 514323; email: a.gale@uk.ac.derby.

KEVIN BOWYER
University of South Florida
Tampa, Florida

SUE ASTLEY
University of Manchester
Manchester, England

CONTENTS

Editor's Introduction — v

Automation in Mammography: Computer Vision and Human Perception — 1
    S. Astley, I. Hutt, S. Adamson, P. Miller, P. Rose, C. Boggis,
    C. Taylor, T. Valentine, J. Davies, and J. Armstrong

Image Database and Dedicated Coding Algorithm for Digital Mammography — 26
    I. E. Magnin, A. Baskurt, D. Vray, O. Baudin, and A. Brémond

Restoration of Mammographic Images in the Presence of Signal-Dependent Noise — 42
    F. Aghdasi, R. K. Ward, and B. Palcic

Classifying Mammograms by Density: Sorting for Screening — 64
    S. Hajnal, P. Taylor, M.-H. Dilhuydy, and B. Barreau

Computer-Aided Detection and Diagnosis of Masses and Clustered Microcalcifications From Digital Mammograms — 82
    R. M. Nishikawa, M. L. Giger, K. Doi, C. J. Vyborny, and R. A. Schmidt

Mammogram Screening Using Multiresolution-Based Image Segmentation — 103
    D. Brzakovic and M. Neskovic

Feature Extraction for Computer-Aided Analysis of Mammograms — 128
    H. Bårman, G. Granlund, and L. Haglund

Adaptive Noise Equalization and Recognition of Microcalcification Clusters in Mammograms — 148
    N. Karssemeijer

Artificial Neural Network Based Classification of Mammographic
Microcalcifications Using Image Structure Features   167
    Y. Chitre, A. P. Dhawan, and M. Moskowitz

Detection and Classification of Mammographic Calcifications   198
    Liang Shen, R. M. Rangayyan, and J. E. Leo Desautels

Comparative Evaluation of Pattern Recognition Techniques for
Detection of Microcalcifications in Mammography   213
    K. S. Woods, J. L. Solka, C. E. Priebe,
    W. Philip Kegelmeyer, Jr., C. C. Doss, and K. W. Bowyer

Digital Mammography: Image Analysis and Automatic
Classification of Calcifications in Ductal Carcinoma *in situ*   232
    J. Parker, D. R. Dance, D. H. Davies, L. J. Yeoman,
    M. J. Michell, and S. Humphreys

Automated Detection of Breast Asymmetry Using Anatomical
Features   247
    P. Miller and S. Astley

Evaluation of Stellate Lesion Detection in a Standard
Mammogram Data Set   262
    W. Philip Kegelmeyer, Jr.

Image Processing and Computer Aided Diagnosis in Digital
Mammography "A Radiologist's Perspective"   280
    E. D. Pisano and F. Shtern

STATE OF THE ART IN
DIGITAL MAMMOGRAPHIC
IMAGE ANALYSIS

AUTOMATION IN MAMMOGRAPHY:
COMPUTER VISION AND HUMAN PERCEPTION

Sue Astley*, Ian Hutt*, Stephen Adamson†, Peter Miller*,
Peter Rose*, Caroline Boggis‡, Chris Taylor*, Tim Valentine†,
Jack Davies* and Janette Armstrong*

*Departments of *Medical Biophysics and †Psychology, University of Manchester, Oxford Road, Manchester M13 9PT, UK, ‡The North West Regional Training Centre for Breast Screening, Withington Hospital, Nell Lane, Manchester, and *The Wolfson Breast Pathology Unit, Southmead Hospital, Bristol.*

ABSTRACT

Mammographic screening programmes generate large numbers of highly variable, complex images, most of which are unequivocally normal. When present, abnormalities may be small or subtle. Two processes critical to the success of screening programmes are the perception of potential abnormalities and the subsequent analysis of each detected lesion to determine its clinical significance. The consequences of errors are costly, and in many screening centres, films are read by two radiologists in an attempt to reduce errors. The prime objective of our research is to improve the accuracy of the detection and analysis of breast lesions by providing radiologists with computer–aided digital image analysis tools. In this paper we focus on the detection and analysis of mammographic microcalcifications.

We describe a philosophy of research aimed at generating useful computer–based aids for radiologists. Firstly, it is necessary to accurately identify specific tasks which are difficult for the human observer. Having correctly identified a problem, appropriate computer vision methods must be developed and their performance evaluated. It is then important to determine effective ways of using such methods to aid radiologists, and it is essential to prove that the effect on radiologists' performance is entirely beneficial.

We present results of experiments to determine factors affecting radiologists' perception of microcalcifications, and to investigate the effects of attention–cueing on detection performance. Our results show that radiologists' performance can be significantly improved with the use of prompts generated from automatically-detected microcalcification clusters.

We describe a new method for the delineation of mammographic abnormalities based on the analysis of multiple high quality X–ray projections of excised lesions. Biopsy specimens are secured inside a rigid tetrahedron, the edges of which provide a reference frame to which the locations of features can be related. A three–dimensional representation of an abnormality can be formed and rotated to resemble its appearance in the original mammogram.

1. INTRODUCTION

There is now unequivocal evidence that the mortality from breast cancer can be reduced by mammographic screening[18]; consequently, a number of organised screening programmes based on X-ray examination of the breasts (mammography) have been instituted. For example in Britain, all women between the ages of 50 and 65 are invited to join a national programme which currently involves single-view medio-lateral oblique mammography once every three years. At present, this programme generates over 1.5 million mammograms per year, most of which are interpreted at a small number of specialised centres distributed around the country[22].

In the UK, screening mammograms are carefully searched for any signs of abnormality by experienced breast radiologists, who are expected to maintain their level of expertise by interpreting at least 6,000 mammograms every year[38]. Despite a strong emphasis on training, practice and experience, radiologists still find mammographic interpretation demanding; both normal and abnormal appearances are highly variable and often complex, and clinically important lesions may be small or subtle. There is a significant level of intra- and inter-observer variability[19], and in many centres mammograms are read independently by two radiologists in an attempt to reduce errors.

Radiologists look for three major classes of mammographic abnormality; discrete abnormalities, diffuse changes, and alterations between successive films of the same breast[18]. Discrete abnormalities include clusters of microcalcifications, local opacities, and localised distortion of the normal structure of the breast. Diffuse changes may manifest themselves as asymmetry between right and left breast images, or as widespread calcification.

A process central to mammographic interpretation is the perception of potential abnormalities. Individual particles of microcalcification as small as 0.1mm can be detected mammographically, although they are only considered to be clinically significant if they appear in clusters of three or more particles[42]. Invasive tumours must be detected before they exceed about 1cm in diameter if screening is to be successful[18]. The problem of perception is compounded by the fact that abnormalities are relatively infrequent; in the British programme, less than 1.5% of women screened have mammographic abnormalities considered sufficiently suspicious to warrant biopsy[17].

Another critical aspect of mammographic interpretation is the analysis of each potential abnormality to determine its clinical significance. Analysis is more likely to be a problem for relatively inexperienced interpreters, or those working in smaller practices, who may not have come across sufficient examples of different lesion types to be able to reliably distinguish them from one another. In the UK approximately two benign lesions are biopsied for every one malignant lesion[17]; clearly, it would be advantageous to reduce this ratio, provided no genuine malignancies would then be missed.

Computer-based image processing and analysis tools are now commonplace in radiology departments; for example, windowing facilities are routinely used to interactively change the appearance of CT images, and echocardiographers regularly make measurements of ventricular volumes by indicating key points on the images with a cursor. Benefits of computer-based techniques such as these include the ability to make accurate, objective, reproducible measurements.

We are investigating the application of computer vision techniques to mammography, with the aim of improving the accuracy of interpretation. Although we would ideally like to construct a system in which all forms of abnormality are automatically detected and classified, the current state of the art in mammographic image analysis renders this a long-term goal. We are therefore developing computer-based aids which will be useful in their own right, but will also eventually contribute to a completely automated system. We have considered a number of possible modes of assistance: enhancement, in which abnormalities are made more conspicuous by enhancing diagnostically significant features and suppressing insignificant features; prompting, in which image features related to abnormalities are detected automatically and then used to draw the observer's attention to suspicious locations; and analysis, in which properties of potentially abnormal regions are extracted to determine whether or not the abnormality is genuine, and to allow classification, where appropriate.

In this paper, we selectively examine the state of the art both in the automated detection and analysis of mammographic abnormalities, and in the application of these methods in a clinical environment. We then describe our own strategy for developing practical, realistic, computer-based aids for radiologists engaged in mammographic interpretation. This is viewed in the context of a functional description of a system which might realistically be of benefit to radiologists in the short term. We identify the gaps in our knowledge which prevent us from constructing such a system immediately, and those experiments essential to a thorough investigation of feasibility. We describe our own attempts at answering some of these questions, focusing on the detection and analysis of microcalcifications.

2. BACKGROUND

Much of the published research in automated mammographic interpretation has focussed on the detection of microcalcifications. Microcalcifications are a natural place to start research in this field; they are one of the earliest signs of breast cancer and, although small, they are easy to describe and relatively easy to distinguish from normal breast structures.

Several apparently successful techniques for detecting microcalcifications have been described in the literature[9,12,25 etc.], though none have yet been tested thoroughly. Most methods apply a sequence of progressively more sophisticated operations to an image to generate and refine a set of candidate abnormalities. The properties of these candidates are then measured, and pre-determined thresholds decide which candidates merit further investigation. A major problem with this type of approach is that any errors in the earlier stages of the detection process are propagated through to later stages. Karrsemeijer has described a probabilistic approach which overcomes this difficulty by generating separate parametric images to represent local shape and contrast, and by incorporating continuity and clustering constraints in an iterative scheme[25]. His method is theoretically attractive, but computationally expensive. Our own approach to detecting microcalcifications, which we discuss later in this paper, is also based on Bayesian statistics[2]. Bourrely and Muller have demonstrated the use of a neural network to discriminate mammographic microcalcifications from normal background structures[4]. Their results are promising, with relatively low false negative rates, although the high degree of background variability results in a large proportion of image regions remaining unclassified by the network.

The automated classification of microcalcifications has also been investigated with moderate success by researchers aiming to identify characteristic properties of benign and malignant individual calcifications and calcification clusters [e.g. 21,30]. There is general agreement that one of the most salient properties in discriminating benign from malignant clusters is the number of particles in close proximity. Lanyi[30] has performed extensive studies of the shapes of clusters of microcalcifications. His results suggest that the discrimination between benign and malignant lesions can be greatly improved by evaluating both the shapes of individual microcalcifications and the configurations of clusters. A significant drawback of his approach is that the apparent shape of a cluster will change with X-ray projection.

Automated tumour detection has been less widely researched and produced less impressive results, partly because of the wide variability in tumour appearance, and the visual similarity of some tumours to normal structures in dense and fatty-glandular breasts. Approaches range from a comparison of left and right breast images[20,31,35] to indirect detection by searching for radiating patterns of lines characteristic of spiculation and architectural distortion[3,26]. To date, few researchers have attempted a thorough assessment of performance.

Giger[20], Kimme[27], Hoyer[23] and Semmlow[39] have used asymmetry between left and right breasts as an initial cue. These researchers all failed to deal satisfactorily with the problem of differences in size and shape of the two breasts; Hoyer and Kimme applied arbitrary partitioning to obtain approximate correspondence, whilst Giger matched the breast boundaries as far as possible and then performed a direct subtraction, ignoring any potential abnormalities close to the skinline. Our strategy for the detection of asymmetry is based on the comparison of regions of similar composition, detected by texture analysis[35,36]. Alternative approaches to lesion detection have been proposed by Lai[29], Brzakovic[5] and Kegelmeyer[26]. Lai's computationally expensive method involved template matching at a range of resolutions, and Brzakovic's method was based on a multi-resolution analysis of image texture; neither produced clinically acceptable error rates. Kegelmeyer has investigated the detection of spiculated lesions by the analysis of locally oriented edges and by texture analysis; his initial results, using a limited test set of five images, are encouraging. We have also performed preliminary experiments on the detection of spiculated lesions, using a technique based on the Hough transform to detect characteristic properties of radiating linear structures[3]. Our method performs well for relatively uniform parenchymal patterns, although an extensive evaluation has not yet been performed.

Radiographic enhancement has been described by a number of authors[8,13,11,16 etc.], although few have attempted to assess the clinical impact of such techniques. Enhancement falls into two broad categories; general improvement of image appearance[11,16], and enhancement of specific features associated with disease. For example, Chan[8] employed an unsharp-mask filter to selectively enhance microcalcification–like features and found that this led to improvements in radiologists' detection performance when compared to their performance viewing the unprocessed digital image, although the best results were still obtained using the original, undigitised image. Dhawan[13] investigated a range of contrast enhancement procedures based on optimal adaptive neighbourhood processing. Unfortunately, his results were not presented to any radiologists to determine whether the procedures actually led to improvements in the detectability of clinically significant structures. We are currently performing a series of experiments designed to test the effect of enhancement of lines, edges and small peaks on radiologists' perception of subtle mammographic abnormalities. Our enhancement operator is Dixon's line detector[14]; it is applied to a gaussian pyramidal representation of the mammogram[6]. These experiments use 156 normal and abnormal mammograms, each presented in the original form, as an unenhanced digital image printed on film, and in an enhanced form also printed on film. Results of the full experiments are not yet available, but an initial feasibility study has indicated that use of Dixon's operator might partially overcome the degradation in performance noted when radiologists are required to make diagnoses from digital images.

Another application of computer vision methods in mammography is the analysis of parenchymal patterns. Based on the premise that breast patterns may be related to the natural risk of a woman developing breast cancer, a number of researchers have attempted, with varying degrees of success, to automatically classify patterns into those designated by Wolfe[44] as being clinically significant. The identification and analysis of glandular patterns is also useful from a dosimetry standpoint, since the risk incurred by screening depends partly on the glandular composition of each woman's breasts. Although Magnin's analysis of textural features did not appear to yield any effective way of discriminating between parenchymal pattern types[34], Caldwell's method, based on fractal analysis, did demonstrate a classification agreement between the system and a group of radiologists that was only slightly lower than the agreement between the radiologists[7]. Similarly, Shadagopan attempted to quantify duct patterns and obtained a good correlation between the computer's calculations and the measurements made by a human observer, although the data set used in this study was limited[41].

It has been reported that significant levels of intra– and inter–observer variability exist in mammography[19]. False positives can be determined by studying screening centre audit data such as the ratio of benign to malignant lesions biopsied. False negatives (cancers missed due to observer error) can be identified by studying the so called interval cancers found in the more mature screening programmes. In a study of interval cancers over during twelve years of the Nijmegen programme[37] it was found that 26% of these cancers were actually missed at the previous screening examination because of technical or observer error. This is about half of the number of genuine interval cancers, that is, cancers arising within the two year screening interval. It was found that, of all cancers detected at screens other than the initial screen, approximately 20% could, in retrospect, be detected in a previous mammogram.

Kundel and Nodine have studied the search behaviour of radiologists scanning for small lung abnormalities in chest X-rays[28], a task analogous to the detection of small abnormalities in mammograms. They observed that the scanning patterns employed by these radiologists were neither systematic nor complete, and that the pattern of fixations could be influenced by the provision of specific clinical information regarding the patient prior to the presentation of the film. Kundel and Nodine also investigated the types of errors made by radiologists during the film reading process; their results suggest that around half of the errors were due to an insufficient level of attention being directed towards the location of the abnormality. A small but important literature is devoted to assessing the effect of computer-based tools on the performance of human interpreters. Experimental evidence suggests that prompting can improve human detection performance in highly controlled visual search tasks, by directing observers' attention towards targets[43]; this has been investigated to a limited extent in relation to the perception of mammographic abnormalities[10]. In this paper we describe results of experiments which provide independent confirmation that prompting can indeed be beneficial in improving radiologists' detection of subtle mammographic abnormalities.

3. A FRAMEWORK FOR ASSISTANCE

To date, research into computer-based mammographic interpretation has been performed in a largely uncoordinated manner. Good progress has been made in some areas, whilst potentially successful methods have still not been found for the more difficult, subjective manifestations of abnormality. Few methods have been rigorously tested, and proven to be of clinically acceptable standard. Here we describe a framework in which both new and existing computer-based mammographic interpretation tools could be placed; we then modify this description to a more immediately realistic level.

Ideally, our system would perform the following functions:
- performance monitoring
- image acquisition from digitised film images and from digital radiography systems
- data compression
- image display and manipulation
- image restoration
- image enhancement
- pre-screening
- prompting
- analysis and classification
- on-line assistance
- reporting
- teaching and research

The digitisation system for acquiring mammograms from film should be flexible and relatively fast, producing high resolution, high quality images. It should support automatic input of films, possibly reading bar-codes to obtain film identification and patient data. Rapid, loss-free data compression will be essential to enable effective transmission, storage and retrieval of images. Quality control is vital for successful mass screening programmes; our system should monitor factors such as patient positioning, image quality, and interpretation standards, with the aim of identifying and correcting any problems at an early stage. Remedial action to correct defects or distortions due to the imaging and acquisition process can also be taken, to minimise the number of repeat mammograms required.

A variety of hard-copy and soft-copy display mechanisms and image manipulation tools should be provided to allow control over both the appearance of the image and the nature of the display. We assume that the system will be used primarily by radiographers and radiologists, so it must have a simple, adaptable user interface that can be tailored to individual user's requirements. In addition to standard functions such as contrast enhancement, windowing, pan and zoom, more application-specific display tools can be provided. For example, one method of facilitating the comparison of right and left breast images would be to horizontally reverse one of the pair and then register and rapidly toggle between the two images. A similar technique without reversal could assist the assessment of subsequent examinations of the same breast. Similarly, enhancement of image features specifically associated with signs of abnormality might aid the perception process.

Ideally, we would like our system to perform pre-screening, that is, to automatically categorize mammograms into groups such as 'definitely normal', 'definitely abnormal', 'equivocal', and 'technical failure'. This requires reliable detection of all manifestations of mammographic abnormality, since one cannot classify a mammogram as 'definitely normal' without eliminating the possibility that it contains any abnormality. Clearly, this is a much more difficult task than assigning a film to one of the other three categories. However, if our system is able to detect specific types of abnormality, it can be used to 'prompt' radiologists by indicating to them any locations deemed to be suspicious. There are two main requirements for the development of a prompting system; at least one method for detecting suspicious regions, and the ability to present the information to the radiologist in a way which will be helpful.

Once an abnormality has been detected either by human or machine, it must be analysed to determine its clinical significance and, if possible, to make a tentative diagnosis. There are many facets to analysis, including the extraction of quantitative descriptions of radiological properties such as size, shape and density, and comparison with models of known lesion types. Such models incorporate prior knowledge of lesion properties and of the radiological process, and can in part be generated from example lesions. Our system may also provide more specific analytical assistance including: lesion measurements, to enable the accurate assessment of the efficacy of treatment; estimates of the risk associated with screening an individual, based on measurements of the amount of parenchymal tissue; delineation of abnormalities for the planning of further investigation and treatment; and assistance with relating features in multiple X-ray projections of the same breast. A library of example lesions and other abnormal features can also be made available to refresh radiologists' memory of less common abnormalities.

Such a system will inevitably lead to the establishment of a database not only of images, but of image and lesion features, and of radiologists' annotations. Each new proven example of an abnormality can be added to the database, and incorporated into the appropriate statistical models to improve model reliability in capturing individual parameters and their variability. The database will be invaluable both for research and teaching purposes. The system will itself be a useful training aid for mammographic interpreters given the provision of suitably structured access to the database of images, experienced radiologists' annotations and comments, and pathological information about each case.

A final important stage in the interpretation of mammograms is reporting. There are considerable advantages in using a computer-based system for this purpose; to date, most reports incorporate a highly stylized sketch diagram on which the radiologist can indicate the location of any abnormality. With digital images, it will be possible to produce a diagram based on a reduced version of the original mammogram accurately annotated by the radiologist. Such a diagram will provide detailed, accurate information for those involved in treating any abnormalities detected.

Having described the functionality of an ideal computer-based mammographic interpretation system, we now consider how such a system might be realised in practice, bearing in mind both technical issues and other important factors such as cost-effectiveness and time-scale for development. From our analysis of the state of the art in computer-based mammographic image analysis, we can clearly see that the production of a comprehensive system such as that described above is infeasible at the present time. The most significant difficulty lies with automated pre-screening, since reliable methods for the detection of *all* mammographic signs of abnormality have not yet been developed. Another major problem lies in the engineering of the system; the handling of large numbers of X-ray films, digitisation to sufficiently high quality at reasonable speed and cost, and dealing with copious quantities of digital data.

A more realistic target in the short term would be a system to aid radiologists by providing basic functions such as image restoration, image manipulation and display tools, the automatic detection of a limited range of specific types of abnormality, prompting of these abnormalities, and analysis. Such a system could be implemented incrementally, with further functionality added as it becomes available. Problems still exist in system engineering terms, but we are no longer faced with the daunting task of finding and validating a method for every possible abnormal appearance. In practice, the system could be used to detect abnormalities and generate prompts overnight; in the day-time, radiologists could use it interactively for image enhancement, prompting, analysis and reporting.

4. DETERMINING FEASIBILITY : THE MANCHESTER APPROACH

Although considerable progress has been made by ourselves and others developing computer-based mammographic analysis methods, a number of important issues are outstanding. Firstly, we must question our motivation for developing particular methods. Are we actually focussing our attention on areas where human interpreters need assistance? Secondly, we need to know how well our methods must perform to provide useful assistance. For example, if a detection method is to be used as a basis for prompt generation, we must establish the effects of different types of prompting error on radiologists' performance. Thirdly, we must be aware of possible side-effects. For example, if we prompt observers with the locations of one type of automatically detected abnormality, we must determine any effect these prompts might have on the observers' detection of other signs of abnormality. These issues can be resolved by performing experiments to investigate the behaviour of experienced human interpreters.

In this section, we describe progress which we have made in Manchester towards investigating the feasibility of computer-aided mammographic interpretation. Our general strategy is as follows:

- find out what detection and analysis tasks are problematic for radiologists
- establish a framework for measuring performance
- develop computer-based methods for detection and analysis
- find out how these methods can be used effectively

We now address each of these areas in turn.

4.1 Identify problematic tasks

Two important requirements for effective breast screening are accurate, consistent detection and analysis of mammographic abnormalities, and the efficient use of human experts' time. Both of these areas can be addressed using computer vision methods; we must therefore determine the precise nature of problems encountered by human interpreters, and target our research appropriately.

More specifically, we must identify aspects of mammogram interpretation which are:
- perceptually difficult
- analytically difficult
- tedious
- time-consuming

Signs of abnormality which are difficult to perceive are natural candidates for computer-based enhancement, detection and feature extraction. Both normal and abnormal features can pose analytical problems; they may be subjective or ill-defined, highly variable, complex or rare. It may thus be difficult for radiologists to learn their characteristic patterns and to achieve accurate, consistent assessment. Tasks which are tedious are more likely to give rise to inconsistent performance, whilst those which are relatively easy but time-consuming are expensive in radiologists' time.

In many cases it is easy to suggest plausible candidates for these types of tasks. Microcalcifications are small, and may have poor contrast (i.e. are perceptually difficult). Asymmetry and subtle distortions of breast architecture are analytically difficult, being variable, ill-defined and subjective. The screening process as a whole can be tedious and time-consuming, as the vast majority of films are unequivocally normal. However, these suggestions are based mainly on intuition and on knowledge of the visual task. A more correct approach is to examine 'missed' abnormalities, that is, interval cancers and inconsistencies which come to light in double reading, and to relate radiological diagnoses to pathological data. Experiments with human observers and carefully controlled visual stimuli can be used to confirm or refute hypotheses about which tasks are problematic, and why.

One such hypothesis is that the density and complexity of the glandular pattern will influence the ability of radiologists to detect subtle features; if this is indeed the case, we can target our assistance at those types of image which cause the most problems. We have performed experiments to test this hypothesis in the case of microcalcification clusters, using synthetic abnormalities superimposed on digitised normal mammograms[1]. These images, and a selection of normals, were presented briefly to observers who were required to detect and localise any abnormalities.

Our data comprised a set of 15 normal mammograms, classified by an experienced breast radiologist into three categories; fatty-homogeneous, fatty-glandular, and dense-homogeneous. A 6.5cm square region of each image was digitised to an effective pixel size of 0.3mm, with 8 bit grey resolution. The mammograms were magnified by a factor of five to ensure that the natural size relationship between microcalcifications and normal structures was maintained, since the minimum size of the synthetic microcalcifications was determined by the spatial resolution of the viewing device (a high resolution computer screen). In each case, the region digitised was selected to cover the area of the mammogram in which microcalcifications are most likely to arise. No obvious orienting features such as the skin-line or the pectoral muscle were included. The image set was expanded to a total of 60 images by image duplication. Images were randomly allocated to normal and abnormal groups of equal size. One third of all the images were rotated by 90° clockwise and one third by 90° anti-clockwise to produce a greater diversity of appearance.

Artificial clusters of microcalcifications were generated graphically, using the following constraints:
- 3 to 8 particles per cluster
- 1 to 5 pixels per particle
- particle grey level values in top 21.5% of range

Within these constraints, the assignment of particle shapes, sizes and grey levels was random. The number of pixels in each cluster and the locations of individual particles within a bounding box 25 pixels in diameter were also assigned randomly. Each image was partitioned into nine square response regions. Each cluster was placed manually in a realistic location on an 'abnormal' image, avoiding the boundaries between response regions. A training data set was produced in a similar fashion, using different mammograms to produce fifteen images with which subjects could familiarise themselves with the protocol. Our five observers were all experienced breast radiologists.

Observers were repeatedly presented with the following sequence of images: a response grid with the cursor positioned at the centre to provide a fixation point (1 second); the normal or abnormal mammogram (2, 5 or 8 seconds); the response grid, in which the observer was required to mark the location of any cluster (unlimited). The images were randomised, and divided into three blocks, corresponding to the three mammogram presentation times. Each observer was assigned a block order with either decreasing or increasing presentation time, since true counterbalancing could not be achieved with just five observers.

Observers were instructed to indicate their responses using one of the following criteria; a cluster is definitely present, a cluster is probably present, a cluster is possibly present, or the image contains a suspicious region. Our results showed that the criterion used had no significant effect on performance. We believe that, despite our written request, the observers did not actually adopt different criteria, since there was no powerful incentive for them to do so.

The variation of presentation rate between two and eight seconds also had little effect on performance, although a trend was observed in P(TP), the probability of detecting a genuine cluster. At two seconds the mean over the five observers was 0.69, rising to 0.78 at five seconds and 0.90 at eight seconds. More surprisingly, in these experiments no significant relationship was found between background type and missed clusters (false negatives). Possible reasons for this are discussed later.

Initially, we found that detection performance was related to cluster location. In particular, there was a significant relationship between missed clusters and their locations in the images (F–observed = 3.30, F–critical = 3.13 at $P < 0.01$, df = 8). We identified a number of factors which might have contributed to this effect. In particular, the limited size of our data set, the relationship between its members, and the manual selection of 'realistic' locations rather than entirely random cluster placement, could all be problematic. For example, realistic cluster locations are most likely to reside within the gland, and in a predominantly fatty image with a limited glandular component, the number of such locations will be small. We used only five images of each glandular type; if the glandular regions in these images were biased towards particular squares, rotation to produce additional images would increase the effect of the bias. However, an analysis of false negatives (missed clusters) shows that approximately one third of the total number of missed clusters were missed by three or more of the radiologists, suggesting that these errors might have been caused by physical properties of the stimulus. When these are excluded from the location analysis, no significant relationship between cluster location and missed clusters is found.

In order to investigate the effects of local stimulus properties on detection, true positive locations were defined where all the radiologists correctly located a cluster, false positives where any radiologist mis–classified a normal region, and false negatives where clusters were missed by more than three observers. The mean grey level standard deviation was measured in 25 pixel square regions corresponding to each of these cases, and to representative normal regions. It was found to have a value of 7.4 in normal background regions, 10.6 in regions where spurious detections were made, 12.8 for missed clusters, and 13.9 for correctly detected clusters. In the false negative cases (missed clusters) it seems likely that genuine clusters were masked by the natural variation of the surrounding structures. A measure of contrast defined by the difference in mean grey levels between calcification and non-calcification pixels, scaled by the standard deviation, was used to investigate any further difference between those clusters which radiologists were able to detect, and those which they failed to detect. There was indeed a significant difference in contrast between the two (T-observed = 3.20, T-critical = 2.80 at $P<0.01$), with the true positives having higher contrast. In addition, we found that the grey level standard deviations of regions surrounding correctly identified clusters were significantly lower (T-observed = 3.35, T-critical = 3.11 at $P<0.01$) than those of regions surrounding missed clusters, again implying a masking effect.

In summary, clusters were successfully detected by observers when the surrounding background was relatively uniform, and where the cluster had high contrast. Clusters were missed when the surrounding tissue was non-uniform, and where the cluster had low contrast with its surroundings. This suggests that developing methods to classify images into radiologist-defined glandular pattern categories is unlikely to meet with success, whereas measuring local image properties may be a valid mechanism to guide search for microcalcifications.

4.2 Establish a framework for measuring performance

A major problem for those developing computer-based interpretation tools lies in the difficulty in demonstrating that methods work to an acceptable standard of performance. In this section we describe the various aspects of this problem, and suggest some possible solutions.

One of the first difficulties we encounter is the selection of data for our experiments. If our techniques are to be used for breast screening, we should ideally select data which is representative of that generated by screening programmes. Screening data has two important properties; firstly, the vast majority of films are normal, and secondly, abnormalities are often small or subtle. It is generally necessary to bias the data set to include multiple examples of an abnormality; however, a pitfall of many researchers is that methods tend to be evaluated using only normal films and films showing the type of abnormality the method is tuned to detect. We rarely see what effect a spiculated lesion, for example, might have on the performance of a method for detecting microcalcifications. In addition, any bias of data sets should be declared prior to any psychological experiments, so the results are not influenced by radiologists' prior expectation of the number and type of abnormalities likely to be present.

The size and subtlety of screen-detected lesions is less likely to be problematic, since some relatively advanced lesions can be expected in the first round of screening.

However, data sets should reflect the probable bias to small, subtle abnormalities. The exception to this rule is in the selection of data for preliminary and exploratory experiments, such as those investigating the effects of image enhancement. In this case it is valuable to include both subtle and 'ball-park' examples in the data set. It is also important to ensure that the natural variability both of lesion and background appearances is captured in the data set. We have adopted a matrix approach to selecting examples; the matrix has dimensions representing glandular pattern (predominantly fatty, mixed fatty-glandular, predominantly glandular), abnormality type (no abnormality, calcification, well-defined lesion, ill-defined lesion, spiculated lesion, asymmetry, architectural distortion), and diagnosis type (benign, equivocal, malignant). In this matrix, subtlety is represented in the third dimension, in which lesions of known pathology that are difficult to classify radiologically are placed in the equivocal group.

Another important issue is how to accurately identify and delineate normal and abnormal structures visualised in mammograms. This is essential for both training and test purposes. The most reliable source of evidence about a given region in a mammogram is pathological investigation; this is rarely practical, and while it may be appropriate for characterising a specific pathology such as fibroadenoma, it is clearly inappropriate for radiological *signs* of abnormality such as asymmetry. The problem can be circumvented to a limited extent by the use of synthetic or partially synthetic mammographic images, or of specimen X-rays. Fully synthetic images can either be created digitally using graphical techniques, or by imaging and/or digitising a synthetic object such as a radiographic phantom. Partially synthetic images can be created by combining synthetic abnormalities with real backgrounds, or vice versa. A synthetic abnormality can be created digitally by drawing lesion-like features into a digital image, or by extracting relevant image features from a real image. Films of normal and abnormal structures can also be physically superimposed prior to digitisation. In addition, it is possible to generate a synthetic abnormality prior to the imaging stage, by creating a lesion-like object and either embedding it within a mastectomy specimen or X-raying it alone. Purely synthetic images, including X-rays of mammographic phantoms and digitally created target-background pairs, are really only valuable in the early stages of developing and validating techniques.

We have approached this problem of establishing the ground truth in two ways, using pathologically proven examples, and radiological consensus. Both approaches have their drawbacks. We have used only biopsy-proven examples for developing detection and analysis methods for microcalcifications; however, it can be argued that this biases our data set towards difficult and obviously malignant examples, and away from those clusters which are perhaps very small, or obviously benign. In most of our work, we have chosen to use radiological consensus to define the ground truth, since this allows the identification of normal structures such as the gland disc, and it is based on mammographic appearance, that is, the appearance of those images we are attempting to interpret. Our consensus is generally obtained from independent annotations marked with a fine pen on registered acetate overlays. These are digitised, and may then be edited by the annotating radiologist. The simplest form of consensus involves using only regions agreed upon by all of the annotating radiologists. This method has the advantage of eliminating spurious annotations, and the disadvantage that many subtle abnormalities will be excluded from analysis. A more sophisticated approach is to assign probabilities to regions depending on the number of radiologists in agreement about their status. A significant problem with the consensus approach has arisen in our work on breast asymmetry, where two radiologists were asked to delineate the glandular disc in a set of mammograms[36]; this is a difficult, subjective task, and there were distinct variations in outline between the two sets of annotations. Our experiments were intended to compare the *shapes* of the left and right glandular discs; a simple combination of the two sets of annotations was thus inappropriate, as it generated features unrelated to the underlying structures. We eventually elected to use both sets of annotations independently.

It is important to determine the standard of performance at which we are aiming. It is likely that all our methods will be subject to error, so we must determine what error rates will be clinically acceptable. Acceptable levels of performance are dependent upon the task in hand; a pre-screening system is likely to have more stringent requirements than a prompting system, but both may ultimately achieve a similar cancer detection rate. We can determine acceptable standards for both prompting and classification systems by investigating the effects of different error rates on radiologists' performance using the systems. That said, it is unlikely that any system which cannot either perform at least as well as an expert radiologist, improve a less experienced observer's performance to that of an expert radiologist, or improve an expert radiologists' performance (perhaps reducing the necessity for double reading), will find clinical acceptance. Further issues include the degree of accuracy of any measurements required either for human purposes (such as assessment of therapy, and treatment planning) or for subsequent machine analysis and classification. This will also have a bearing on the required spatial resolution for analysis. For classification systems, the effect of errors both in diagnosis and in probability estimation must also be analysed.

Once the appropriate performance goal has been determined, extensive evaluation is essential if methods are to be accepted for clinical use. Receiver operating characteristic (ROC) analysis, supported by substantial trials on carefully selected data sets appear to be the methods of choice. Problems involve knowledge of the ground truth about the images used for evaluation (discussed above) and recruitment of sufficient experts both to provide opinions about the original films, and to participate in evaluation studies. It is also important to look carefully at the cases where automated methods fail, to assess the significance of such errors, and to identify any side-effects. For example, some methods for enhancing linear structure also have a broadening effect on peaks, which could make microcalcifications appear larger and less suspicious[14]. Technical assessment using ROC analysis should precede large scale evaluation by radiologists, both to avoid unnecessary exposure of experts to the test data set, and to maintain goodwill and optimism in the radiological community.

4.3 Develop computer-based methods for detection and analysis

We have developed computer-based methods for the detection of three major signs of mammographic abnormality; microcalcifications, asymmetry and spiculated lesions. There are a number of areas of similarity in our approach to detecting these different signs, including the use of radiologists' annotations to provide the ground truth for training and testing, training by example, the use of probabilistic methods, and the combination of evidence to increase detection performance. The work on analysis described in this paper is described in relation to clusters of microcalcifications, but the approach is also suitable for other forms of abnormality.

Detection of microcalcifications

Our approach to the detection of microcalcifications is based on grey-level mathematical morphology[40]. Previously we have described a method by which cues for microcalcifications were generated by applying a morphological inner-edge detector (an eroded image subtracted from the original) and the top hat transformation[3]. This latter operator was formed by eroding the original image until all microcalcification-sized objects disappeared, and then dilating by the same amount to restore the background. All structuring elements used were approximately circular. Radiologists were asked to identify the locations of over 900 individual microcalcifications in a set of twenty image patches, thus identifying regions which were known to contain microcalcifications, and regions which were known to represent normal background. This enabled us to gather statistical distributions of both on- and off-target responses by our cue generators, which we then used to create images representing the likelihood of the presence of microcalcification at each image point, based on prior knowledge of the response of the cue generators. Using Bayesian statistics, we can combine evidence from different cue generators. Our results were presented as ROC curves; there was no overlap between training and test data, as a leave-one-out methodology was employed. These results demonstrated that the systematic combination of evidence can lead to improvements in detection performance[2].

We expressed our results in terms of individual microcalcifications detected rather than clusters detected, since it is a simple step to apply thresholds and clustering rules once individual particles have been identified correctly. A consequence of this was that our test set comprised a large number of very subtle particles, identified by radiologists studying both the original mammogram and a magnified digital version. Other published work focuses on the detection of clusters; most clusters of microcalcifications comprise both subtle and more readily detectable particles, so it is possible to achieve good cluster detection rates, whilst not actually detecting very subtle individual particles. We achieved a true positive pixel classification rate of over 97%, with a false positive rate of less than 2%.

Our method had a number of drawbacks, some of which we have since addressed. Firstly, we had problems training and testing our system, because of the difficulty in establishing a 'gold standard', that is, in determining exactly what each image contains. Our approach involved annotations made by an experienced radiologists who was instructed to "mark all calcifications". When we analysed our results in depth, we found our results degraded by mis-identifications in our training and test data. Initially, all annotations were made on registered acetate overlays, with subsequent revision on a computer monitor. This method can be improved by using multiple radiologists to annotate the images, allowing either the exclusion of regions of disagreement from subsequent analysis, or the assignment of probabilities based either on degree of confidence in the annotations or on number of radiologists in agreement. Another problem with our method arose because the top hat transformation as described above will detect all image peaks smaller than the defined maximum size. Study of the combined cue images has shown that many such peaks are below the size of genuine microcalcifications in our images, so we are now investigating pre-processing with a median filter or a single pass of erosion followed by dilation ('closing').

Detection of spiculated lesions

We have performed preliminary studies evaluating a method for detecting spiculated lesions by identifying characteristic patterns of co-radial lines[3]. This method is based on the Hough transform, and was tested on a set of twenty mammograms digitised with an effective pixel size of 0.2mm. A neighbourhood of equivalent diameter 2cm was defined, which determined the maximum diameter of any spiculated lesion detectable by the method. Neighbourhood size was limited by an assumption that only one spiculated lesion would reside in each such neighbourhood. All mammograms were pre-processed with Dixon's line operator[14]. The neighbourhood was then systematically moved across each mammogram, with an overlap of 25% in width and height, selected as a compromise between execution time and sensitivity. At each position of the neighbourhood, the image was transformed in such a way that co-radial lines become co-linear points in transform space[15].

The transform space can be represented as a grey level image. If there exists a single pattern of co-radial lines in the current neighbourhood of the line-enhanced original image, it will appear in the transformed image as a bright line. The gradient and intercept of this line define the centre of the co-radial pattern in the original image. We can thus detect the strongest co-radial pattern in the current neighbourhood by fitting a line to the data in the transform space, and we can then estimate the likelihood of the detected pattern representing a stellate lesion by measuring various properties of the line.

We have made three measures in transform space, after performing a least-squares line fit to the data. The first measure, the linear correlation co-efficient, characterises the degree of organisation of any lines in the enhanced original image. The second measure, designed to characterise the amount of line information related to the strongest pattern, is defined as the total number of 'votes' in a corridor along the fitted line. The third measure gives the degree of spread of lines around the focus of a detected co-radial pattern, by examining the distribution of evidence along the fitted line. All three measures were transformed back into the original image space, with values written at the detected foci. We thus produced three intrinsic images, each characterising a different property. The data from the three images was again combined using a Bayesian approach[2].

Our results are encouraging, particularly for fatty breasts in which all the lesions in our data set were correctly identified. The experiments must, however, be regarded as very preliminary, with such restricted data for training and testing. Training was particularly problematic; attempts to model the distributions of measure responses failed, and we were forced to use smoothed versions of the raw distributions, which gave rise to inaccurate probability assignments.

Detection of asymmetry

Asymmetry between contra-lateral breast images is an important indicator of breast disease. However, it is difficult to detect asymmetry automatically, as radiologists appear to use a sophisticated analysis procedure incorporating radiological, anatomical and pathological knowledge. We have performed experiments to elucidate the type and degree of asymmetry considered significant by radiologists. Results of experiments in which radiologists were shown only the boundaries of non-fatty regions in mammograms indicate that, in addition to densities, radiologists may use shape, size, location or topology of such regions in their assessment, as they were able to achieve approximately 70% accuracy in discriminating significant asymmetries from benign asymmetries and normal mammograms[36].

Our approach to the detection of asymmetry between left and right breast images attempts to utilise this result. We first segment each breast into regions of like tissue type[35]; this enables both an analysis of the shapes of individual regions, and direct comparison of similar breast structures. Our best segmentation results to date, using one of Laws' texture energy measurements[32], achieve over 80% agreement with radiologists. The second stage of our approach involves measuring and comparing shape and grey-level properties of the detected regions. A variety of methods have been investigated, with the best classification accuracy of nearly 87% being obtained from a statistical combination of measures. One difficulty with shape measurement, however, is the fact that many simple shape measures are rotationally invariant; this does not fit well with our knowledge of breast anatomy.

Registration and normalisation remain areas of difficulty for comparing contra-lateral breasts and for comparing successive examinations of the same breast. Further psychological experiments are required to determine, for example, whether the absolute size of the non-fatty region is more significant than the size relative to the breast in which it is sited, and to what degree a difference in size between the two breasts affects radiologists' judgements about asymmetry. The results will have important implications for automated analysis. For those methods which require registration, we have elected to avoid distortion-based methods, on the grounds that they are likely to modify significant image structure.

Analysis of microcalcification clusters

We are investigating a new, low cost approach to the identification and delineation of mammographic abnormalities for training and test purposes. Although our methods are described in terms of clusters of microcalcifications, the overall strategy is also applicable to other localised abnormalities. For this work we have elected to use X-rays of excised lesions. Whilst we realise the importance of working with the images we are ultimately intending to interpret, the use of images of excised abnormalities has a number of advantages including superior image quality, reduced obscuration by overlying tissue, known pathology, and the freedom to experiment with imaging parameters. Such images provide a valuable half-way-house between the analysis of images of synthetic lesions and of images of lesions within patients' breasts.

Our method extracts morphologic descriptions of excised clusters of microcalcification from multiple X-ray views. A specimen of tissue containing a cluster is chilled to increase its rigidity, and secured inside a small cardboard Tetrahedron edged with fuse wire. The edges of the Tetrahedron provide a reference frame so that, when the Tetrahedron is X-rayed lying on each of its faces, features in the four resulting images can be related. At present we are working with three types of specimen providing images of varying degrees of difficulty: X-rays of fragments of lead embedded in normal breast tissue from a reduction mammoplasty; acetate overlays of X-rays of genuine microcalcification clusters; and X-rays of genuine microcalcification clusters.

The first stage of our method involves segmenting the images. This is performed semi-automatically, using histogram-based thresholding to extract particle pixels from digitised acetates, and a line detection algorithm[14] to extract the fuse wire triangle at the base of the Tetrahedron in the current view. Microcalcifications are identified manually in the X-rays of genuine clusters, as our automated detection method is insufficiently specific. The accurate identification of the reference frame is crucial. Any spurious lines are eliminated by a process of edge-linking, and by the constraint that the three lines we are seeking should have 60° angular separation. Straight lines are fitted to the resulting data, and the centre of gravity of the triangle can then be identified. Any spurious particles are removed automatically on the basis of size, or manually. The procedure is repeated for all four views.

The boundary of each detected particle is stored as a list of real co-ordinate pairs. An error vector, normal to the local boundary curve, is associated with each point; this allows compensation for tissue mobility, inaccurate Tetrahedron construction and the imaging and detection processes. The approach used for identifying common features in different views is based on the 'auxiliary line' method described by MacKay[33]. This method uses the fact that an object which appears as a single point in one X-ray projection could appear anywhere along a line in another projection. The gradient and intercept of the line depend on the relative projections. In our case, we have an object which appears as a core region (a calcification particle) surrounded by an error region defined by the error vectors. In a second view, the object will appear on a band, of which the limits are defined by the extremities of the particle in the first view. The band, which we call the 'auxiliary band', is surrounded by an auxiliary error region defined by the limits of the error region in the first view. For each microcalcification in the first view, we seek a match along the appropriate auxiliary band in the other three views. In some cases the match is unambiguous; there is only one calcification within the auxiliary band. In other cases, there may be multiple candidates; these are resolved by seeking confirmation from other projections, and by matching basic properties such as total density.

To date, we have successfully matched 'calcifications' from the images of lead shot embedded in real breast tissue, and from acetate overlays of clusters containing up to approximately thirty particles. Clearly, in the latter case, we have neither particle shape nor density to aid the matching process. A significant difficulty with both the acetate images and with the specimen X-rays is the problem of missing data. In many cases, we found particles identified (or identifiable) in only one projection, either because of superposition of tissue, superposition of particles, or because the particle was very small, but elongated and could only be distinguished when it was aligned perpendicularly to the X-ray plane.

The potential uses of this technique include three-dimensional classification of cluster shapes to validate the two-dimensional approach of Lanyi[30], and the extraction of detailed, quantitative descriptions of the radiological appearance of abnormalities with known pathology, from high quality images. Once a high-resolution, three-dimensional representation of an abnormality has been formed, it can be rotated to resemble the appearance in the original mammogram, allowing more accurate identification of normal and abnormal structures for training and test purposes.

4.4 Find out how these methods can be used effectively

We have described a number of computer-based methods for the detection and analysis of breast abnormalities, but we have not yet addressed the issue of how such methods might be used to improve performance in clinical practice. Since pre-screening is some distance away, we have focussed our efforts on prompting, in which we indicate the locations of automatically-detected suspicious regions to radiologists. As indicated earlier, we believe that there are many unanswered questions associated with prompting. We have started to investigate these areas by studying the effects of prompting radiologists with the locations of clusters of microcalcifications detected using a method based on that described above[24].

Our subjects, five experienced breast radiologists, were asked to locate microcalcification clusters in digital images presented with and without prompts. Our data set consisted of a set of 30 mammograms, half of which were normal and half of which had been classified as abnormal on the basis of a single microcalcification cluster. From each of these mammograms, a central 15cm square region was extracted and digitised. The resulting digital image was 1024x1024 pixels in size, and had a spatial of 0.15mm pixel^{-1}, with 8 bit grey resolution. In each case, the digitised region was selected to include as much of the breast tissue as possible; in abnormal images, the microcalcification cluster was always present in the digitised region. The digital images were displayed on a sun SPARC workstation with a pixel size of 0.3mm.

Each of the 30 images was processed by an automatic cluster detection system based on the method described earlier. For each region identified as a potential cluster by the system, a prompt was generated. Prompts took the form of open red circles, 100 pixels in diameter, superimposed on the digital image. The images were then presented, in both processed and unprocessed forms, to each of the radiologists. The order of the 60 presentations was randomised differently for each subject, with the constraint that two occurrences of the same image were separated by at least 20 presentations.

Prior to the experimental session, each subject was given a standardised set of verbal instructions and 6 practice images with which to familiarise themselves with the task and the equipment. The practice images included examples of each of the experimental conditions but did not include any images that were used in the main experiment. The verbal instructions contained the following information: the number of presentations; the requirements of the task; the ratio of normal/abnormal images; the ratio of processed/unprocessed images; the approximate accuracy of the prompt generation algorithm.

For each presentation, the subjects were required to study the image, identify any potential clusters and mark their locations by means of a cursor controlled by a mouse. After marking each suspicious location, the subjects were required to indicate their confidence that the marked location represented a cluster by means of the following five point scale: definitely a cluster; probably a cluster; possibly a cluster; possibly not a cluster; probably not a cluster. A sixth scale point, 'definitely not a cluster', was represented by a 'next image' option, which the subjects could select without making a location judgement if they believed that there were no clusters in the image. The subjects were asked to keep their interpretations of the confidence levels consistent throughout the experiment, and to try to use the whole scale.

The subjects were able to make as many location judgements as they thought appropriate on any given image, with each location judgement followed by a confidence judgement. Once the subjects had finished making location and confidence judgements, or if they wished to make no such judgement, they were able to move on to the next presentation by selecting 'next image' with the mouse. This allowed the subjects to control the time spent studying each image, which reflects the normal film screening environment better than a fixed presentation time. In addition, the study time was recorded for further analysis. In those presentations where prompts were available, they were briefly displayed for 200msec when the image first appeared. This should have served to direct the attention of the subjects to the prompted region and alert them to the availability of the prompts, while minimising the effect of the prompts as distractors. After this initial brief presentation, the subjects were allowed to toggle the prompts on and off as they desired.

The performance data from each subject were recorded and processed by means of receiver operating characteristic (ROC) analysis. The detection sensitivity of the radiologists, in terms of the signal detection measure d', was observed to be significantly higher than that of the automated detection system, both when the radiologists were prompted, ($t_{obs} = 13.22$, $p < 0.0005$), and when they were unaided, ($t_{obs} = 3.33$, $p < 0.025$). Figure 1 shows the composite ROC curves for the subjects in both the prompted and unprompted conditions. The most important result of our study is that the detection performance of the radiologists was significantly higher when the images were presented with prompts than when they were unprocessed, ($t_{obs}=3.47$, $p<0.025$). Our results are consistent with the findings of Chan, who suggested that an observer working in conjunction with a computer-aided diagnosis (CAD) system is more effective than either the observer or the CAD system working alone.

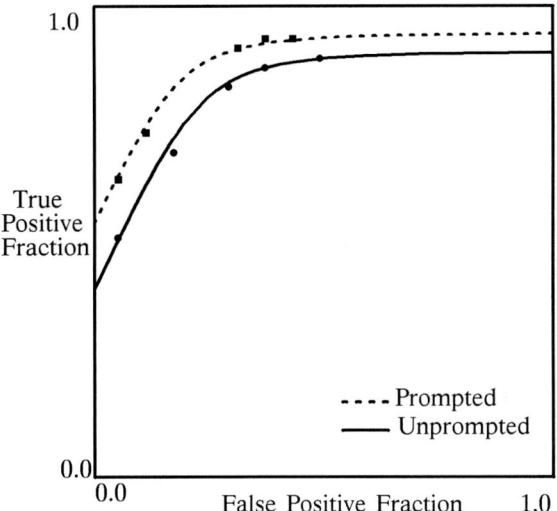

Figure 1. ROC curves showing improvements in radiologists' detection of microcalcification clusters using prompting compared with their performance without prompts.

Having determined that prompting had a significant effect on detection performance, we analysed the ways in which prompts were used by the subjects. Prompts were available on 26 of the 60 images, and after the initial brief display, subjects were able to switch them on and off as desired. Therefore there was a distinction between the initial passive display and any subsequent active use of the prompts. Overall, active use was made of the prompts in 34% of the cases where they were available, with individual subjects varying between 15% and 69%. The cases in which prompts were most frequently used, that is, those images on which two or more subjects made active use of the prompts, generally corresponded to those cases in which more than one prompt was displayed. In 13 of the 15 images with more than one associated prompt, the prompts were actively used by more than one subject, while active use by two or more subjects occurred in only 2 of the 11 images that had only a single associated prompt. The correlation between the number of prompts associated with an image and the number of subjects who actively used the prompts on that image was calculated to be 0.61. The generation of multiple prompts is a likely result of any CAD system. Our results show one possible consequence of having multiple prompts associated with an image; the need to examine the prompt information in more detail. It seems as though, as would be expected, a single prompt acts to cue attention, directing it towards the prompted region, in which case a single brief presentation is sufficient. However, when multiple prompts are presented, the indivisibility of attention requires that each be checked in turn. It is possible that the need to check each prompt in sequence may impose artificial constraints on the natural search pattern of the observer, requiring a greater level of cognitive processing and consequently an increase in the time required to study the image.

An analysis of the study time per image revealed that the radiologists took significantly longer to examine the processed images than the unprocessed images, ($t_{obs} = 2.64$, $p < 0.025$). However, the subjects were not aware that their study times were being recorded during the experiment and were therefore not under any pressure to respond rapidly. This may make the study time data less reliable than the accuracy data.

Our results have demonstrated that a prompt generation system with a moderate false-positive rate be of some benefit to the radiologist screening for clustered microcalcifications, at least in an experimental setting. There are a number of issues that still need to be addressed before prompting could be effectively implemented in a clinical environment and we are currently undertaking experiments to investigate the effects of varying the accuracy of the prompt generation system, and the effect of prompting on the detection of non-prompted abnormalities.

5. CONCLUDING REMARKS

Considerable effort has been invested in developing methods for automatically detecting mammographic signs of breast disease. The greatest success has been in the detection of microcalcifications, which are relatively well-defined and thus amenable to detection using conventional computer vision methods. We have described a framework into which such methods could be placed. Five important areas which require attention before such a system can be realised are; identifying the most appropriate targets for assistance, determining performance standards for different tasks, defining a mechanism for demonstrating clinical acceptability, developing new techniques for the automatic detection and analysis of signs of abnormality, and determining the effects of computer-based aids on human performance.

We have described progress in Manchester towards these goals. In particular, we have described: experiments to investigate the factors which affect radiologists' ability to detect microcalcifications; methods for detecting microcalcifications, spiculated lesions and asymmetry; a new approach to extracting quantitative descriptions of mammographic abnormalities from biopsy specimens; and a demonstration that computer-generated prompts can significantly improve radiologists' performance in detecting microcalcification clusters.

ACKNOWLEDGEMENTS

This research has been funded primarily by the Cancer Research Campaign, with additional support from the Science and Engineering Research Council, the Wolfson Breast Pathology Unit and IBM. We are grateful to Prof Alastair Gale of the University of Derby for many helpful discussions, and to the radiologists, radiographers and physicists who have given their time to assist with our experiments.

REFERENCES

1. S. J. Adamson "Perceptual recognition of breast cancers." *MSc Thesis, University of Manchester*, 1992.
2. S. M. Astley and C. J. Taylor "Combining cues for mammographic abnormalities." *Proc. 1st British Machine Vision Conference*, pp. 253–258, 1990.
3. S. M. Astley, C. J. Taylor, C. R. M. Boggis, D. L. Asbury, M. Wilson "Cue generation and combination for mammographic screening." Chapter 13 of *Visual Search II*, ed. D. Brogan, Taylor and Francis, London, 1992.
4. C. Bourrely and S. Muller "Detection of microcalcifications in mammographic images." *Neurocomputing (NATO ASI Series, Vol. F68)* eds. F. Fogelman Soulie and J. Herault, Springer Verlag, Berlin 1990.
5. D. Brzakovic, X. M. Luo and P. Brzakovic "An approach to automated detection of tumours in mammograms" *IEEE MI-9*, Vol. 3, pp. 232 – 241, 1990.
6. P. J. Burt "The pyramid as a structure for efficient computation." *Multiresolution image processing and analysis*, ed. A. Rosenfeld, pp. 6–36, Springer–Verlag, 1984.
7. C. B. Caldwell et al "Characterisation of mammographic parenchymal pattern by fractal dimension." *Physics in Medicine and Biology*, Vol. 35, No. 2, pp. 235–247, 1990.
8. H–P. Chan et al "Evaluation of unsharp mask filtering for the detection of subtle mammographic microcalcifications." *Proc. SPIE International Society of Optical Engineers (USA)*, Vol. 626, Pt. 1, pp. 347–348, 1986.
9. H–P. Chan et al "Computer–aided detection of microcalcifications in mammograms." *Investigative Radiology*, Vol. 23, No 9, pp. 664–671, 1988.
10. H–P. Chan et al "Improvement in radiologists' detection of clustered microcalcifications in mammograms: the potential of computer aided diagnosis." *Investigative Radiology*, Vol. 25, pp. 1102–1110, 1990.
11. A. R. Cowen et al "The computer enhancement of digital grey–scale fluorography images." *British Journal of Radiology* Vol. 61, pp. 492–500, 1988.
12. D. H. Davies and D. R. Dance "Automatic computer detection of clustered microcalcifications in digital mammograms." *Physics in Medicine and Biology*, Vol. 35, No. 8, pp. 1111–1118, 1990.
13. A. P. Dhawan and E. Le Royer "Mammographic feature enhancement by computerized image processing." *Computer Methods and Programs in Biomedicine*, Vol. 27, pp. 23–35, 1988.
14. R. N. Dixon and C. J. Taylor "Automated asbestos fibre counting." Chapter 4 of *Machine Aided Image Analysis*, ed. W. E. Gardner, Institute of Physics Conference Series No. 4, 1979.

15. T. P. Ellison "Detection of Stellate Lesions in Mammograms" *MSc. Thesis*, University of Manchester 1989.
16. M. Flynn et al "Replication of diagnostic radiographs using a film scanning/printing system." *SPIE Medical Imaging IV: Image Capture and Display*, Vol. 1232, pp. 88–96, 1990.
17. A. P. M. Forrest "Screening for breast cancer: the UK scene." *British Journal of Radiology*, Vol. 62, pp. 695–704, 1989.
18. A. P. M. Forrest and R. J. Aitken "Mammography screening for breast cancer." *Annual Reviews of Medicine*, Vol. 41, pp. 117–132, 1990.
19. A. G. Gale, G. E. Walker, E. J. Roebuck and B. S. Worthington "The quest for accuracy, consistency and uniformity of performance in mammographic screening: the systematic imperative." *British Journal of Radiology* Vol. 62, S10, 1989.
20. M. L. Giger et al "Image features of mammographic masses used in the development of computerized schemes." *SCAR 90: Computer Applications to Assist Radiology.* eds. R. Arenson and R. M. Friedenberg, 1990.
21. R. Gilles, F. Bouvet–Lefebvre, J. Masselot and E. Kahn "Characterisation of benign clustered microcalcifications with a new image analysis method" *Proceedings of Computer Assisted Radiology*, 1991.
22. HMSO *Breast Cancer Screening (the Forrest Report)*, Her Majesty's Stationery Office, London, 1986.
23. A. Hoyer and W. Spiesberger "Computerized mammogram processing."*Philips Technical Review* Vol. 38, Part 11/12, pp. 347–355, 1978/79.
24. I. W. Hutt "The effects of prompting on the detection of microcalcification clusters in digital mammograms." *MSc Thesis, University of Manchester,* 1992.
25. N. Karssemeijer "A stochastic method for the automated detection of microcalcifications in digital mammograms." *Proc. XIIth Conference on Information Processing in Medical Imaging, Wye College, Kent,* 1991.
26. W. P. Kegelmeyer "Computer detection of stellate lesions in mammograms" *SPIE Biomedical Image Processing and Three–Dimensional Microscopy*, Vol. 1660, 1992.
27. C. Kimme, B. J. O'Loughlin, J. Sklansky "Automatic detection of suspicious abnormalities in breast radiographs."*Data Structures, Computer Graphics and Pattern Recognition*, ed. Klinger, pp. 427–447, Academic Press, New York, 1975.
28. H. L. Kundel and C. F. Nodine "Studies of eye movements and visual search in radiology"In: *Eye movements and the higher psychological function* ed. J. A. W. Senders, D. Fisher and R. Monty, Hillsdale NJ, Lawrence Earlbaum Associates, 1978.
29. S. M. Lai, X. Li and W. F. Bischof "Automated detection of breast tumours" *Computer Vision and Shape Recognition*, eds. A. Krzyzkak, T. Kasvand and C. Y. Suen, World Scientific Series in Computer Science, Vol. 14, pp. 115–132, World Scientific, Singapore, 1989.
30. Lanyi M. "Morphological analysis of microcalcifications." In: *Early Breast Cancer*, ed J. Zander and J. Baltzer, Springer–Verlag, Berlin, 1985.
31. T–K. Lau and W. Bischof "Automated detection of breast tumors using the asymmetry approach." *Computers and Biomedical Research*, Vol. 24, pp. 273–295, 1991.

32. K. I. Laws "Textured image segmentation" *Image Processing Institute Report,* No. 940, University of Southern California, Los Angeles, 1980.
33. S. A. MacKay, M. J. Potel and J. M. Rubin "Graphics methods for tracking three-dimensional heart wall motion." *Computers and Biomedical Research,* Vol. 15, pp. 455–473, 1982.
34. I. E. Magnin, F. Cluzeau, C. L. Odet "Mammographic texture analysis: an evaluation of risk for developing breast cancer." *Optical Engineering,* Vol. 25(6), pp. 780–784, 1986.
35. P. I. Miller and S. M. Astley "Classification of breast tissue by texture analysis." *Image and Vision Computing,* Vol. 10, No. 5, pp. 277–282, 1992.
36. P. I. Miller and S. M. Astley "Detection of Breast Asymmetry Using Anatomical Features" *Proceedings of SPIE Biomedical Image Processing IV, San Jose,* 1993
37. P. H. M. Peeters, A. L. M. Verbeek, J. H. C. L. Hendriks, R. Holland, M. Mravunac and G. P. Vooijs "The occurrence of interval cancers in the Nijmegen screening programme." *British Journal of Cancer* Vol. 59, pp. 929 – 932, 1989.
38. The Pritchard Committee "Guidelines on the establishment of a quality assurance system for the radiological aspects of mammography used for breast screening." *UK Radiation Advisory Committee: Subcommittee on Quality Assurance,* 1988.
39. J. L. Semmlow, A. Shadagopan, L. V. Ackerman, W. Hand and F. S. Alcorn, "A fully automated system for screening xeromammograms." *Computers and Biomedical Research* Vol. 13, pp. 350–362, 1980.
40. J. Serra *Image Analysis and Mathematical Morphology,* Academic Press, London, 1982.
41. A. Shadagopan, F. S. Alcorn, J. L. Semmlow, L. V. Ackerman "Computerized quantification of breast duct patterns." *Radiology,* Vol. 143, pp. 675–678, 1982.
42. E. A. Sickles "Mammographic evaluation of breast calcifications" *Radiology* Vol. 160, pp. 289–293, 1986.
43. A. Treisman "Preattentive processing in vision." *Computer Vision, Graphics and Image Processing,* Vol. 31, pp. 156–177, 1988.
44. J. N. Wolfe "Risk for breast cancer development determined by mammographic parenchymal pattern." *Cancer,* Vol. 37, pp. 2486–2492, 1976.

IMAGE DATABASE AND DEDICATED CODING ALGORITHM FOR DIGITAL MAMMOGRAPHY

I.E. Magnin[1], A. Baskurt[1], D. Vray[1], O. Baudin[1], A. Brémond[2]

1. National Institute of Applied Sciences, INSA 502, URA CNRS 1216 affiliated to INSERM, 69621 Villeurbanne cedex France.
2. Gynaecological clinic, Ed. Herriot Hospital, 69003 Lyon Cedex, France.

1. Introduction

X-ray mammography is the most efficient tool now available to detect a breast cancer early. The accuracy of breast radiographs allows the examination of a small number of radiological features that are valuable in discriminating between malignant and benign diseases. We consider the problem of building a reference image database, named SENOBASE [1], containing a series of 400 documented digitized mammograms, for which the disease has already been clearly established and confirmed. Because of the volume of important clinical data associated with series of images, they cannot be stored in their original format, compression before storage is necessary. In medical imaging, image storage and archiving constraints have led researchers to develop efficient data compression methods. Recent work in picture coding has significantly increased both coding rates and the quality of the decoded images [2-7]. However, few image data compression techniques available in the medical field have reasonable coding rates (more than 8).

This work aims to perform data compression of x-ray images of the breast. Among medical images, mammograms present particularly low contrast. Because the breast contains water, fat, conjunctive and epithelial tissues for which x-ray absorption coefficients are very similar, the contrast within the image is poor, making the visual and quantitative discrimination between the components of the breast difficult. This is not the case for most of the other medical x-ray images (except perhaps for the chest) in which the bone structure provides a naturally high contrast. When natural contrast is not high, in angiography for example, a contrast material is injected before x-ray examination to opacify the vascular network. The proposed data compression method intends to preserve the main features of these images.

In section 2, we detail the structure of normal and pathological mammograms and propose an optimal sampling of these images in section 3. The image database SENOBASE is described in section 4. After a brief recall concerning image coding transforms in section 5, we develop the proposed adaptive coding method in section 6. Comments and results are presented in section 7.

2. Mammographic Features

We consider the problem of building an image database and then of using a data compression method on those mammograms. To be successful, the sampling step and, in a second time, the coding and decoding steps applied to each mammogram, must maintain unchanged, the meaningful features contained within each image. Our interest involves opacities and calcifications [8-11] which are the most common lesions in mammography. In addition, the main features used to discriminate between malignant and benign lesions are given.

2.1. Opacities

Two types of opacities are distinguished according to their shape. Nodular opacities have a rounded shape and stellate opacities have a radiological appearance like a "star" with spicules.

A nodular opacity is a benign lesion if its shape is rounded and smooth and its contour is sharp and well defined. It is a malignant lesion if its shape, rather than smooth, presents small spicules in the periphery or if its contour is not sharp all around the lesion but is blurred, even on a small portion.

A stellate opacity is always a malignant lesion. It generally has irregular, often blurred, contours with more or less long spicules.

2.2. Calcifications

We distinguish calcifications, which sizes over 400 µm, from microcalcifications, whose size can decrease to zero.

Calcifications derive from the deposit of calcium within the breast. They have a rather large size and can be found, for example, either isolated with a rounded shape or grouped along a vessel. Calcifications are generally benign and can be easily detected on a mammogram because of their high constrast.

Microcalcifications can be separated in two types [11] :

Type I microcalcifications can be observed in benign breast lesions only or in lobular carcinomas *in situ*. They are never seen in intraductal carcinoma or in infiltrating carcinoma. They have a crystalline nature and the crystals are made up of weddellite. Type I microcalcifications are the result of the precipitation of crystals in breast microcysts. Their radiological appearance (magnifications 3 to 5) is rounded, sometimes like discs, whereas their microscopic shape is sharp, with regular contours separated from each other or grouped together in an organized fashion either in a line or forming a bee's nest.

Type II microcalcifications are noncrystalline in nature and can be observed in benign lesions but are always present in infiltrating carcinomas. They consist of different types of calcium phosphate. Type II microcalcifications are made of a calcium deposit, generally in necrotic intra-ductal carcinoma. Their radiological shape (magnification 3 to 5) is often oblong or branched out, whereas their microscopic shape is irregular with angular and ill-defined contours. They are separated or grouped in a random fashion.

Microcalcifications are, therefore, an excellent marker of breast lesions but they cannot be divided into benign or malignant types.

3. Optimal Sampling of Mammograms

It is obvious that nowadays, film is the most accurate support for mammograms. Direct digital mammography is not yet available and the question we have to answer now is the following : what is the right size of pixel to be used to digitize a mammogram ? Is it 200 µm, 100 µm, 50 µm or why not 10 µm ? the corresponding amount of data goes from 10^6 to 4.10^8 pixels for one film area with a size of 20 x 20 cm^2. The answer is not trivial and mainly depends on the context. A pixel size of 200 µm seems to be small enough to preserve the main visual features of the parenchyma and the edge characteristics (shape or blur) of a large opacity (more than 0,5 cm in diameter). A pixel size of 100 µm would be prefered to detect microcalcifications [8-10], isolated or in cluster, larger than 70 µm in diameter. However, this sampling rate is not sufficient to provide the shape of individual microcalcifications [11]. This shape, elongated or roughly circular, is a main feature discriminating malignant from benign lesions.

This short overview of the sampling problem suggests that a rather low sampling rate could be enough for most of the mammogram area and that a high sampling rate should be prefered in the pathological regions of interest. This is the way the image database SENOBASE has been built, including low sampling rates (around 280 µm) for whole mammograms and rather high sampling rates (around 40 µm) for pathological regions of interest such as cluster of microcalcifications.

4. Senobase

SENOBASE is an image database containing 400 documented digitized mammograms. Each image is described, commented and labelled following the World Health Organisation (WHO) classification (figure 1).

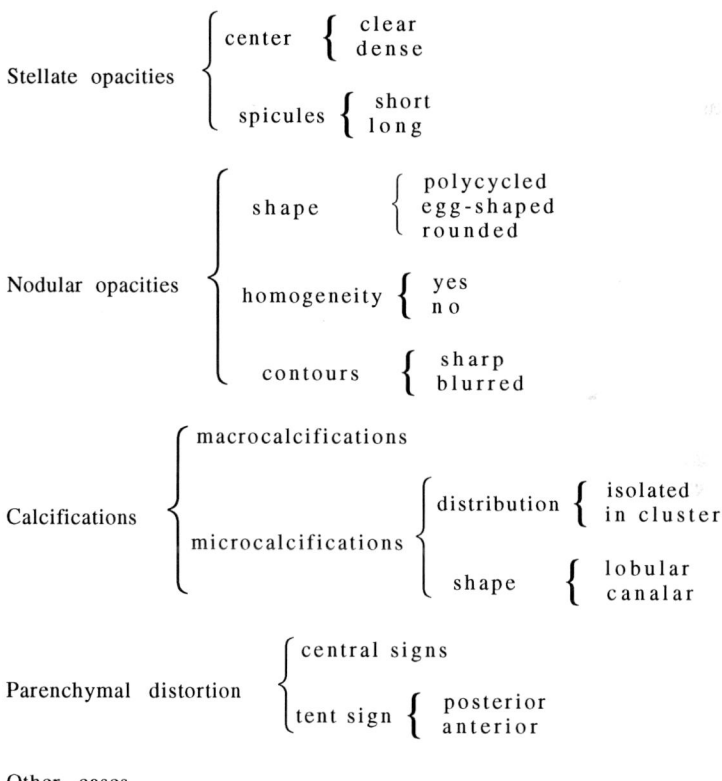

Figure 1 : Mammographic pathological features usually encountered in breast pathology.

It is associated with a file of text giving a complete description of lesion, diagnosis and corresponding desease. Images are classified according to the scheme given in figure 1. At each label corresponds a set of visually slightly different mammograms corresponding to various diagnoses. The amount of images is large enough to allow a continuous evolution from one label to another one. For example, the set of images containing a *nodular rounded lesion* having an *homogeneous radiological density* and *blurred edges* may differ in blur and contrast. A file of text, including a complete description of lesion and diagnosis is given for each case.

Three access modes are available :

(i) *"Characteristics"* access mode. For example, it is possible to ask for a *Nodular lesion* or more precisely for a *Nodular lesion with homogenous radiological density and blurred edges*. At this level, several reference images exist and can be displayed sequentially .
(ii) *"Disease"* access mode . The user can ask for *galactophoric in situ carcinoma* or *medullary carcinoma* and SENOBASE displays a series of mammograms demonstrating the so-called deseases.
(iii) *"Sequential"* access mode . It is possible to visualize images of the database like an image dictionary.

SENOBASE can be easily up-dated using SENOFAC software that provides the user the key words necessary for describing any mammogram. The database is available on conventional CD-ROM.

5. Transform Image Coding

In 2D data compression, we can generally distinguish two levels of coding :

(i) Elimination of redundancies : the information is conserved and the transformation is reversible, but limited in terms of coding rate.
(ii) Coding with loss of information : in this case, one accepts a controlled loss of information while trying to conserve useful features. The transformation is nonreversible but the coding rate can reach high values.

Coding methods using transforms [2-6] are powerful. They can usually be used either as reversible transformations with low coding rates or as nonreversible transformations with a particular efficiency, even with high coding rates (0,5 bit/pixel ; 1 bit/pixel). They are widely used, although their implementation is complex compared to methods working in the image domain such as predictive methods (Differential Pulse-Code Modulation DPCM) or run-length coding. Among these, the Discrete Cosine Transform [5,12,13] (DCT), is distinguished by its performance properties (efficiency for redundancy reduction, real coefficients, reversible transform, and easy implementation using fast algorithms). It is defined as

$$X(k, \ell) = \frac{4C(k)C(\ell)}{N^2} \sum_{i=0}^{N-1} \sum_{j=0}^{N-1} x(i,j) \cos\left(\frac{(2i+1)k\pi}{2N}\right) \cos\left(\frac{(2j+1)\ell\pi}{2N}\right) \quad (1)$$

for $k = 0, 1, ..., N-1$ and $\ell = 0, 1, ..., N-1$, with $C(0) = 1/\sqrt{2}$ and $C(k) = 1$ for $k = 1, 2, ..., N-1$, where $x(i,j)$ is the value of the pixel with spatial coordinates (i,j) and $X(k,\ell)$ is the DCT coefficient with spatial frequency coordinates (k,ℓ).

The image is usually divided into subimages, or blocks of size NxN. Each block is computed separately using the DCT. The block size is chosen according to the local correlation properties of the image. Quantization and coding of the transform domain can change and can be adapted to the structure of the image. Two types of existing methods are the zonal and threshold methods. In zonal methods, a predetermined region of interest is selected in the DCT domain and the coefficients belonging to this area are systematically retained, whatever their amplitude . This region of interest is the same for all the blocks of the encoded image. In threshold methods, a predetermined threshold is selected and all the DCT coefficients that are greater than this threshold are retained. The threshold can be the same for all the blocks of the encoded image or specific to each block, according to a given criterion. In this case, the selected coefficients can be quantized and coded using different techniques, such as a uniform quantizer or fixed- or variable-length codes.

6. Adaptive Coding Method for Mammograms

The low contrast of the mammograms to be coded is related to the choice of the coding scheme, and the data compression method must be able to retain the main characteristics of these images. In this context, we propose the DCT for coding each block of each mammogram separately, with a self-adaptive threshold, automatically computed by the algorithm[12,13]. The mammogram is subdivided into a series of subimages. The DCT of each subimage is computed and a set of thresholds, related to each subimage, is then automatically determined. Each threshold is used for the selection of the DCT coefficients of the corresponding subimage. The algorithm is decomposed into three steps.

6.1. Thresholding

The threshold is obtained by defining an upper limit E_T for the sum of the energy E of DCT discarded coefficients. This energy represents the mean-square-error computed on the discarded coefficients. The value of E_T can be chosen in accordance with the mean value of the energy of the subimages. For each block of size NxN, the algorithm used for thresholding is as follows :

(i) The DCT coefficient of lowest amplitude in absolute value, different from zero, is selected :

$$X_m (k, \ell) = \min \{| X(k, \ell) | / X (k, \ell) \neq 0\} \quad (2)$$

for $k = 0, ..., N-1$ and $\ell = 0, ..., N-1$.

(ii) The energy of this minimum $E_m = X_m^2 (k, \ell)$ is added to the cumulated energy E, provided by the previously selected DCT coefficients

$$E = E + E_m. \quad (3)$$

(iii) If $E < E_T$, then set $X_m (k, \ell)=0$ and go back to step (i).
If $E \geq E_T$, stop. All the DCT coefficients different from zero are retained and the threshold value T of this block corresponds to the current minimum value $X_m (k, \ell)$.

We observe that the obtained threshold value as well as the location of the retained coefficients change from block to block, depending on the DCT activity. To optimize the final coding rate, both the location of the selected DCT coefficients and their amplitude are coded.

6.2. Coding the Location of the DCT

For each block, the location of the selected coefficients is coded using a quadtree representation [5].

$$T_M(k,\ell) = 1 \text{ if } |X(k,\ell)| > T \quad (4)$$
$$= 0 \text{ elsewhere,}$$

Where $X(k,\ell)$ is a DCT domain coefficient and T the threshold determined in section 6.1. The binary matrix T_M is divided into four subblocks. A subblock is empty if there are only 0's in it; otherwise, it is mixed. This approach does not consider the subblock full of 1's, and supposes that the 1 values are a minority in T_M matrices. Therefore, one bit is sufficient to code one subblock. The division goes on until it reaches the pixel size. Each subblock (node of the quadtree) is then coded. A binary vector is created by joining all the node codes, beginning with the root from top to bottom, and for each subblock size from left to right, the binary vector is then coded with a run-length coding[7] :

- the 0 runs are coded using a fixed length code M
- each 1 value is replaced with the Huffman code corresponding to the amplitude of this coefficient (see next section).

6.3. Coding the Amplitude of the DCT

The selected DCT coefficients $X(k,\ell)$ are replaced by the nearest integer values $X_q(k,\ell)$, such that :

$$X_q(k,\ell) = \text{trunc } (X(k,\ell) + \text{sign } [X(k,\ell)] * 0,5) \quad (5)$$

with
$$\begin{cases} * \text{ sign } [X(k,\ell)] \begin{array}{l} = +1 \text{ if } X(k,\ell) \geq 0 \\ = -1 \text{ if } X(k,\ell) < 0 \end{array} \\ * \text{ trunc } (.): \text{ gives the integer part.} \end{cases}$$

Using the probability density of the DCT coefficients amplitude computed from a representative set of mammograms (figure 2), we determine a table of Huffman codes. The Huffman codes (table I) depend on the probability of occurrence of the various amplitudes. The higher the probability is, the shorter the associated code will be.

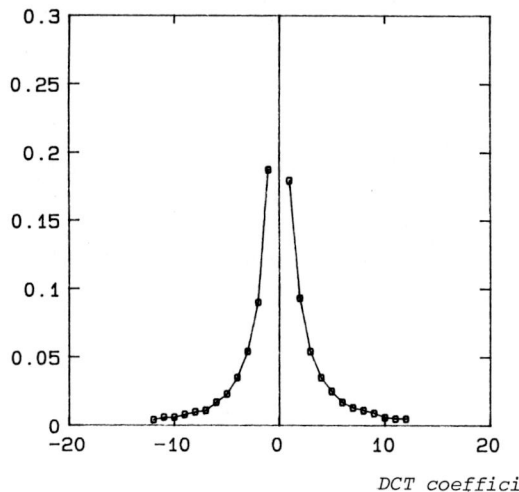

Figure 2 : Probability density function of the amplitude of the DCT coefficients computed from a set of mammograms.

6.4. Properties of the Whole Coding Scheme

Let us summarize the reasons that led us to develop this coding scheme:
(i)   The block approach provides a true local adaptability.
(ii) The thresholding takes into account all the low- and high-frequency coefficients of the DCT spectral domain, if these coefficients are of high values. In fact, an isolated microcalcification has high-frequency information that must be retained after the thresholding process.
(iii) Choosing the same distorsion (sum of the energy of the discarded coefficients) for all the blocks of an image, allows standardizing the coding error on this image.
(iv) Using a table of Huffman codes leads to approaching the actual entropy of each block.
(v)   The quadtree and the run-length coding of the threshold mask are necessary to minimize this overhead information to keep a reasonable global coding rate.
(vi) This coding scheme is with loss of information, allowing high coding rates with a known and controlled distorsion rate, as discussed.

Amplitude of DCT coefficients	Probabilities	Huffman codes
P_1	0.299	00
-1	0.131	011
+1	0.126	101
P_2	0.067	0101
+2	0.065	1000
-2	0.063	1001
+3	0.038	1110
-3	0.038	1111
+4	0.025	11001
-4	0.025	11010
+5	0.017	010001
-5	0.016	010010
+6	0.012	110110
-6	0.012	110111
+7	0.009	0100001
-7	0.008	1100000
+8	0.008	1100001
-8	0.007	1100010
+9	0.006	1100011
-9	0.006	01000000
+10	0.004	01001110
-10	0.004	01001111
+11	0.004	01001100
-11	0.004	01001101
+12	0.003	010000010
-12	0.003	010000011

Table I : Huffman codes corresponding to the probability density function of the amplitude of the DCT given in figure 2.

7. Results and Discussion

A selection of three digital images of 512 x 512 pixels quantized on 8 bits composed of breast parenchyma with a cluster of microcalcifications (figure3), a stellate opacity (figure 4) and a set of cysts (figure 5) is presented here. Figure 3 presents a mammogram (512 x 512 x 8) with a resolution of 100 microns. This image shows a set of microcalcifications in cluster. The description of this image provided in SENOBASE is the following : *"Clearly visible canalar microcalcifications in cluster. The "branched" aspect of some of them is typical of a malignant lesion. It is an infiltrating canalar carcinoma"* and the corresponding disease and diagnosis, confirmed by a biopsy and an anatomopathological exam are : ***disease*** : canalar carcinoma, ***diagnosis*** : infiltrating canalar carcinoma.

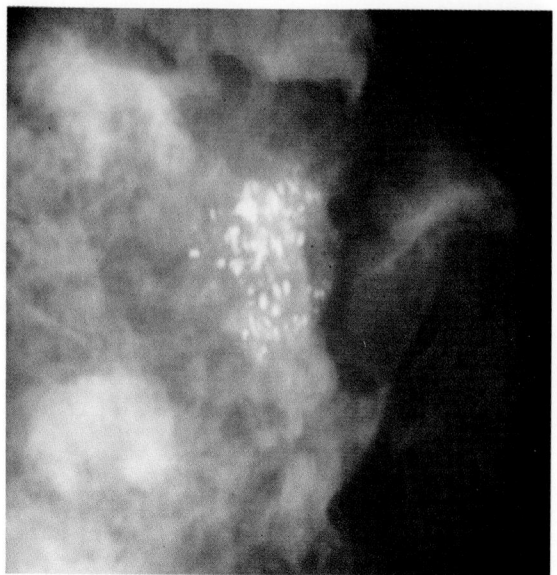

Figure 3 : Mammogram (512 x 512) pixels quantized on 8 bits, containing a cluster of microcalcifications

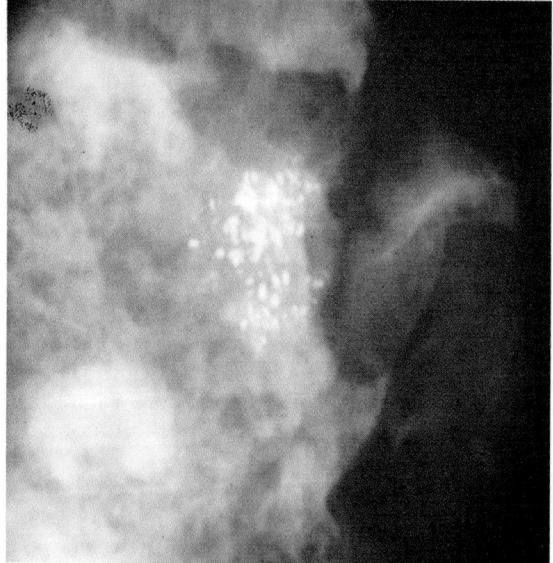

Figure 4 : Image presented in fig. 3 after coding with a compression rate of 19.

The image after coding and decoding steps is given in figure 4. The visual aspect is good and the pertinent features as the "branched" aspect of the microcalcifications is well preserved. The mean image compression rate is 19 and the signal to noise ratio (SNR) is 46.7 dB.
The SNR is calculated using the following relation :

$$SNR = 10 \log_{10} \frac{255^2}{\frac{1}{512^2} \sum_{i=0}^{N-1} \sum_{j=0}^{N-1} e^2} \qquad (6)$$

where the error e is the algebraic difference between the original image and the coded/decoded one. A more interesting information is given in figure 5 where the local compression rate, corresponding to each block, is visualized.

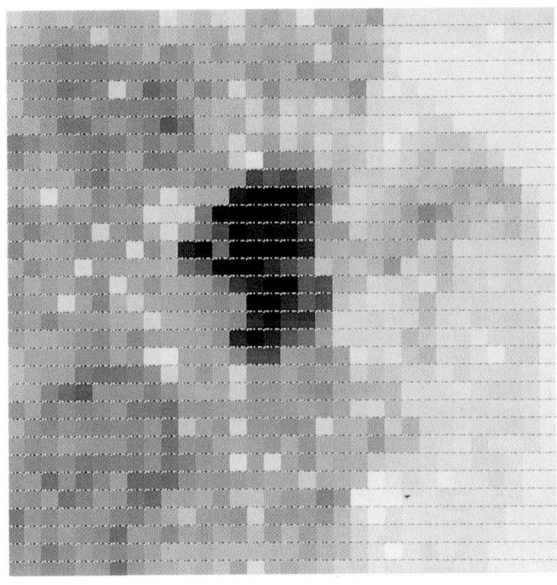

Figure 5 : Local compression rates automatically provided by the algorithm. Their value ranges from 10 (black) inside the region of interest to 114 (white) outside.

The highest compression rate, reached in the background region of the image, is 114 (in white), whereas the lowest compression rate, exactly in the region of interest, is 10 (in black). This property is of main interest because it both preserves well the basic features essential for diagnosis, within the ROI while providing particularly high compression rates outer this region. This adaptive approach guarantees a global reasonable compression rate of the image [1].

Another example is given in Figure 6a with the radiograph of a stellate opacity. It is a typical malignant lesion that contains a series of canalar microcalcifications, uneasy to see because of the local low contrast, and that are also in favor of a malignant disease. The description associated to this image in SENOBASE is : *"Stellate opacity with short but sharp spicules. Some typical elongated microcalcifications are also present. It is an infiltrating canalar carcinoma"* and the corresponding disease and diagnosis confirmed by complementary examinations are : ***disease*** : *canalar carcinoma,* ***diagnosis*** : *infiltrating canalar carcinoma.*

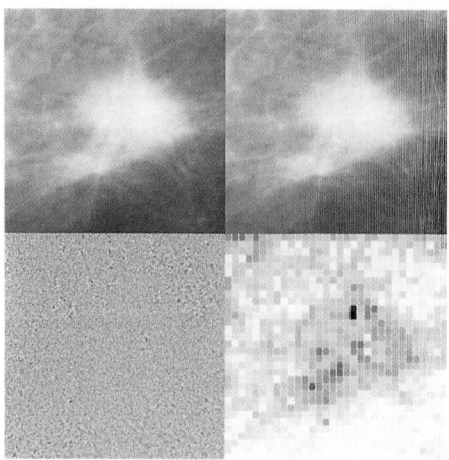

Figure 6 : a. Stellate opacity with short spicules. b. Image a after coding with a compression rate of 19.15. c. Noise corresponding to the information lost by the coding procedure. d. Local compression rates automatically provided by the algorithm. Their value ranges from 10 (black) inside the region of interest to 114 (white) outside.

After coding and decoding, the visual aspect remains very good (figure 6b) and the noise is well distributed all over the image (Figure 6c). The local compression rate is minimum (10) in the region of interest, and maximum (114) in the parenchyma. Here also, the coding process is well adapted to the content of the image (Fig. 6c). The pertinent features, essential for the diagnosis, which are the presence of *spicules* indicating a stellate malignant lesion and the series of *elongated* microcalcifications within the opacity, remain obvious. The mean compression rate is 19 leading to 0.42 bits per pixel. The signal to noise ratio is 45.6 dB with a mean grey level error of 0.99.

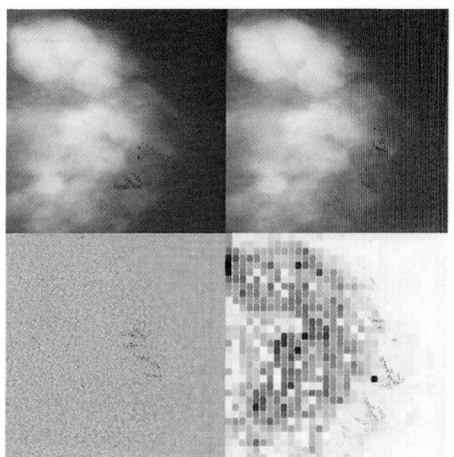

Figure 7 : a. Mammogram containing a large set of cysts. b. Image a after coding with a compression rate of 19. c. Noise corresponding to the information lost by the coding procedure. d. Local compression rates automatically provided by the algorithm. Their value ranges from 10 (black) inside the region of interest to 114 (white) outside.

Figure 7a is a mammogram containing *"a large set of cysts close together. Their individual visual analysis is difficult. The parenchyma is locally pressed back by the cysts"*. The mean coding rate is 19 and the local compression rate varies from 10 (black) to 114 (white) (figure 7d). We notice the homogeneity of the residual noise (Figure 7c) and the very good visual quality of the coded/decoded image (figure 7b).

A series of images (nodular opacities, stellate opacities, and microcalcifications) has already been coded and decoded afterwards. The same visual quality as the three previous examples is obtained, in every case, for a mean coding rate of 22. The whole image data base is currently being coded for detailed visual examination by the expert.

7. Results - Discussions

We have presented a reference image database, SENOBASE, containing a set of 400 commented digitized mammograms with the description of pathology, desease and diagnosis. This database is available on a CD ROM including the original digitized mammograms (without any compression). An adaptive coding method dedicated to x-ray mammograms has been described. An experience involving two experts showed that for a compression ratio up to 30, the experts never succeeded in discriminating the original images from the other when simultaneously displayed on the TV screen. This result is very encouraging and demonstrates that medical image compression is no more unrealistic even in such a difficult field as mammography. Further studies will be necessary to statistically evaluate the fiability of such a coding method for various compression rates, in the field of mammography.

9. References

1. I.E. Magnin, O. Baudin, A. Baskurt, D. Vray and A. Brémond, *Int. Conf. IST/SPIE* ,**1905**,(1993).
2. A.K. Jain, *Proceedings of the IEEE*, **69**, n° 3, (1981) p. 349-389.
3. P.A. Wintz, *Proceedings of the IEEE*, **60**, n° 7, (1972) p. 809-820.
4. N. Ahmed, T. Natarajan and K.R. Ras, *IEEE Trans. on Computers*, C-**23**, (1974), p. 90-93.
5. A. Baskurt and R. Goutte, *ICASSP-89*, Scotland,(1989) p.755-756.
6. A.N. Netravali, J.O. Lim, Picture coding : a review, *Proceedings of the IEEE*, **68**, n° 3, (1980), p. 366-406.
7. T.S. Huang and O.J. Tretiak, *Gorden and Breach*, New-York,(1972) p. 221-266.
8. B.W. Fam, S.L. Olson, P.F. Winter, F.J. Scholz, *Radiology*, **169** (1988) p. 333-337.
9. H.P. Chan et al., *Invest. Radiol.*, **22** (1987) p. 581-589.
10. D.H. Davies, D.R. Dance, C.H. Jones, *Int. Conf. SPIE, Med. Im. III*, Newport Beach, **1092**, (1989),

11. I.E. Magnin, M. El Alaoui, A. Brémond, *Int. Conf. SPIE, Sciences and Eng. of Medical Imaging,* **1137** (1989) p. 170-175.
12. A. Baskurt, I. Magnin, A. Brémond and P.Y. Charvet, *Int. Conf. SPIE Medical imaging V*, San Jose, **1653** (1991) p. 219-227.
13. A. Baskurt, I.E. Magnin and R. Goutte, *Opt. Eng.,* **31,** n°9 (1992) p. 1922-1928.

RESTORATION OF MAMMOGRAPHIC IMAGES IN THE PRESENCE OF SIGNAL-DEPENDENT NOISE

F.Aghdasi[1,3], R.K.Ward[1] and B.Palcic[2,3]

1- Dept. of Electrical Eng. University of British Columbia (UBC)
2- Depts. of Physics and Pathology, UBC
3- Cancer Imaging, B.C. Cancer Agency
601 W. 10th Ave, Vancouver, BC, Canada V5Z 1L3

ABSTRACT

Previous efforts in improvement of appearance of digitized mammograms have concentrated on using image enhancement techniques. In this work we propose the application of image restoration.

We considered a non-stationary image model and signal-dependent noise of photonic and film-grain origins. Both the camera blur and the MTF of the screen-film combination were considered. The camera noise was minimized through averaging and background subtraction. The signal-dependent nature of the radiographic noise was modeled by a linear shift-invariant system and the relative strengths of various noise sources were compared.

We developed and implemented two locally adaptive image smoothing filters to improve the signal to noise ratio of digitized mammogram images. To minimize the effects of the system blur a deconvolution filter was then applied in conjunction with these smoothing filters resulting in better visualization of image details.

The deconvolution filter was based on the Minimum Mean Squared Error (MMSE) criteria, while the smoothing filters utilize the Baysian and the Wiener criteria. Of the two smoothing filters the Baysian estimator was found to outperform the adaptive Wiener filter. The filters were implemented in a real time processing environment using our mammographic image acquisition and analysis system.

1. Introduction

Breast cancer is a leading cause of cancer deaths among women. For women in the developed countries, it is also the most frequently diagnosed cancer. Nearly 10 percent of all women in North America will develop breast cancer during their lifetime [1]. Breast cancer therefore is a major health threat to women of epidemic proportions.

Early detection is the most promising method of management of this disease. It has been well documented that by screening post menopausal women using X-ray mammography, the mortality rate can be reduced significantly [2]. Of equal importance is the fact that detecting the cancer at carcinoma *in situ* stage, when treatment with minimal surgery followed by ionizing radiation is still possible, results in a much higher quality of life for the patient.

More breast cancers are now detected in earlier stages as a result of greater participation of women in screening programs. The majority of early carcinomas of the breast are indicated by the presence of one or more clusters of microcalcifications on a mammogram. Detection of subtle, small, and low contrast microcalcifications, is therefore gaining increased significance.

From correlated pathologic-radiologic studies it has been shown that the smallest microcalcifications are not visible on the mammogram. A larger number of microcalcifications can normally be detected on magnification mammography and on biopsy specimen radiography than on screening or diagnostic mammography. For this reason mammography usually underestimates the extent of a lesion. This problem is particularly significant when multifocality is involved and satellite carcinoma cells are present in the vicinity of the primary tumor [3].

Two factors contribute to this phenomenon namely the observation system noise and the system blur. These factors are discussed at length in section 2 below.

Image restoration is a mathematical process in which operations are performed on an observed image so as to estimate the original object that would be observed if no degradations were present in the image formation system used. Basically the procedure is to model the image degradation effects of the system and then find and perform appropriate operations to 'undo' these degrading effects. Thus in order to effectively design a digital image restoration procedure it is necessary first to quantify or characterize the image degradation effects of the physical imaging system, the image digitizer, and the image display. Due to the statistical nature of the degradations, ideal restoration is not possible. However, some degree of improvement may be feasible. We seek such improvements in the X-ray imaging of the female breast.

Several researchers have attempted recently to apply image enhancement algorithms to digitized mammograms [4-10]. These techniques either employ global manipulation of grey levels or locally adapt such manipulations to image features. In one approach a linear combination of smoothed images and a non-linear contrast transformation is used to obtain enhancement [4]. Alternatively a global estimate of the background breast structure is employed to bring out pathologic abnormalities [5]. Image neighborhoods are selected that are locally adapted to the spatial extent of image features. In this way enhancement techniques such as contrast manipulation, histogram equalization, etc. respond to the local image detail [6-9]. Finally a non-linear mapping is used to encode the image grey levels in an attempt to equalize the system noise which is signal dependent [10].

While image enhancement techniques have their own advantages they do not consider the process of image degradation in the derivation of algorithms. We have already noted that the most subtle signs of abnormality are not visible in the raw mammogram or in its digitized version because of the noise and blur in the image. These are due to the X-ray machine, the screen-film detector and the camera and the digitizing equipment. We postulate that if the characteristics of the noise and the different blur functions are known or obtained then these effects may be removed or reduced by image restoration techniques. The restored image may then be directly viewed on the monitor, subjected to further image enhancement or processed for automated diagnosis.

The objective of this study was to compare the effectiveness of appropriate estimation algorithms to reduce the noise and to apply appropriate restoration algorithms to compensate for the system blur in the presence of the noise. We have already reported an algorithm for the automatic detection and segmentation of microcalcifications from the background of a normal breast parenchymal pattern [11]. The present study is a natural extension of the previous work and seeks to facilitate the detection of microcalcifications at the earliest stage of their formation. In section 2 we characterize the image formation system and derive an image observation model in section 3. In section 4 different image restoration procedures are discussed and designed so as to minimize or reduce the effects of the different blurs and noise degradations.

2. Image Formation System

In order to find the image degradation model, the different components of the image formation system are first examined. The system degradations are considered to originate from the cascade of two imaging systems as shown in Fig. 1. Firstly there is the X-ray (screen-film) image formation system which has a non-uniform frequency response and whose Modulation Transfer Function (MTF) is specified by the manufacturer. The X-ray system is followed by the digitizing optoelectronic camera. We have developed a digitizing camera based on a large area Charge Coupled Device (CCD) and have reported a procedure for determining its Optical Transfer Function (OTF)[12]. We will first consider these two systems separately and then in section 3 we combine them to formulate an overall image formation model.

2.1. The X-ray Screen-Film Imaging System

Radiographic images suffer from a number of degradations which are inherent in

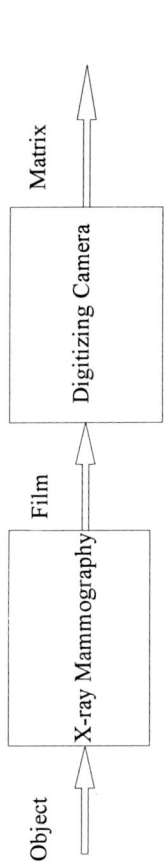

Fig. 1. Formation of digitized mammogram images

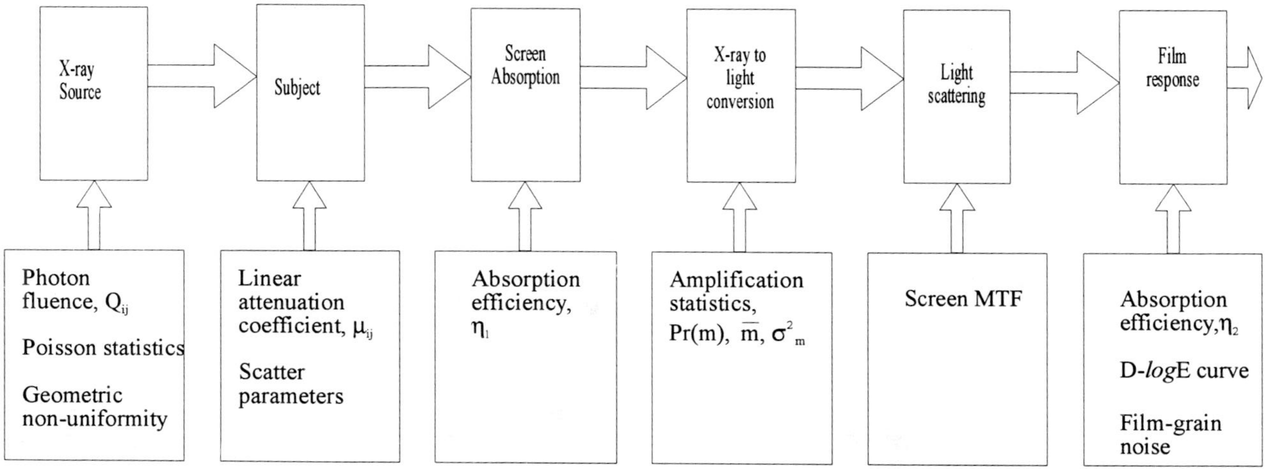

Fig. 2 The radiographic image formation model

the image formation system. These degradations may be broadly divided into four categories. These are due to a) the X-ray source; b) the geometry of imaging; c) the beam scattering by the subject; and d) the image detection and display components. The illumination received at the screen is non-uniform due to the X-ray source and the geometry of the imaging. The largest amount of exposure is received along the central beam, with the quantum fluence decreasing proportional to $cos^3\theta$, where θ is the angle of inclination from the normal [13]. This effect is modulated by the 'heel' effect of the anode. Additionally, the focal spot on the anode of the X-ray tube has a finite size creating penumbral shadows in the image. The extent of this shadow depends on the object-film distance, and it affects the spatial resolution limit of the image. It is also this effect that limits the extent of useful magnification views to about two times only [14]. We could model this effect by a two-dimensional convolution of the point spread function corresponding to the effective focal spot aperture with the image.

The X-ray scatter in the breast reduces the contrast of the image. This is a major source of degradation. Breast compression devices and vibrating anti-scatter grids are intended to reduce this effect. Nevertheless X-ray scatter remains a major limitation. The overall effect of these limitations can be partially evaluated practically by comparing a pre-operative mammogram of a patient who has undergone biopsy, with the specimen radiograph. In specimen radiography the object-film distance is reduced and much of the breast mass responsible for beam scatter is absent. Additionally higher doses are employed leading to better contrast and reduced input quantum noise. The specimen is also centrally located reducing the effects of geometrical distortions.

The screen-film combination as a detector has been studied extensively [15]. The intensifying fluorescent screen absorbs the X-ray photons and radiates many more photons in the visible range of wavelengths which expose the film. The X-ray absorption and re-radiation efficiency of the screen as well as the photon absorption efficiency of the film contribute to the overall contrast for a given dose to the patient. The amplification and scattering mechanisms of the screen are stochastic in nature. Rabbani [16] has shown that the uncorrelated component of the quantum noise passes through the screen unaltered while the correlated component is filtered by the system contrast transfer function. The scattering process can be modeled by a two-dimensional linear convolution operation and forms the major component of the screen film Modulation Transfer Function (MTF). For contrast below 6%, the system noise is the limiting factor in the visibility of the image details whereas the system MTF has little effect on it [17]. For higher contrasts however the MTF contributes significantly to these limitations. This fact indicates that in digitized mammograms restoring the image from the effects of the system MTF may result in better visualization of smaller objects.

Finally the response of the film to the incident photons is non-linear. This non-linearity is described by the $D-\log E$ characteristic curve. Although this is commonly written as $D = \gamma \log E + \beta$ we note that both γ and β are functions of the exposure level E. The contrast transfer function of the screen-film combination is both a function of exposure (due to the characteristic curve) and frequency (due to MTF).

The process of X-ray image formation is also associated with noise which is generated by four sources. These noise sources are: a) the quantum noise due to the discrete nature of the X-ray photons; b) the screen mottle due to the stochastic nature of amplifications and scattering; c) the screen structure noise due to its inhomogeneous phosphor coating; and d) the film grain noise of the emulsion coating. The screen structure noise is generally considered to contribute less than 2% to the overall noise [15].

We provide a block diagram of radiographic image formation in Fig. 2. The effect of focal spot size is modeled by convolution with its aperture function, and that of the X-ray scatter is represented as an effective low pass filter. The effects due to $\cos^3 \theta$ term are quiet small since for typical geometries involved θ is less than $5°$. In Fig. 2, X-ray quantum fluence Q_{ij} contains spatial non-uniformities due to the geometry of imaging and the inherent photon noise which has a Poisson distribution. We use the Kodak Ortho-M film together with a Kodak Min-R screen. The densitometric data, MTF, and other parameters of this screen-film combination have been reported by Bunch [15]. Details of this model are further described in section 3.

2.2 The CCD Camera

In addition to the X-ray, the digitizing camera also blurs the image. The finite size of each pixel gives the aperture function and provides the theoretical limit to the MTF of the camera. The lens contribution to the blur can at best be limited to the diffraction properties of the optical components employed. We use a two-dimensional CCD (Kodak KAF 1400) with 100% fill factor and 1035 x 1320 square pixels of 6.8 μm per side. This gives an MTF of the form '$sinc(\omega_x)sinc(\omega_y)$'. This function is multiplied by the MTF of the lens. We used a Nikon Nikkor 55 mm lens which, for the best focus conditions has a minimum MTF of 0.6 at the Nyquest sampling frequency of our sensor. The experimental measurement of the camera MTF was reported earlier [18].

The MTFs of the camera and that of the screen-film are shown in the same plot in Fig. 3. The spatial frequency axis refers to the frequency content of images formed on the film and on the CCD planes, respectively. When comparing these two MTFs we note that these two curves should refer to the same imaging plane. If the geometry of imaging and the focal length of the lens are chosen such that a 'life size' image is formed at the CCD then the two MTF curves are directly comparable. Under these

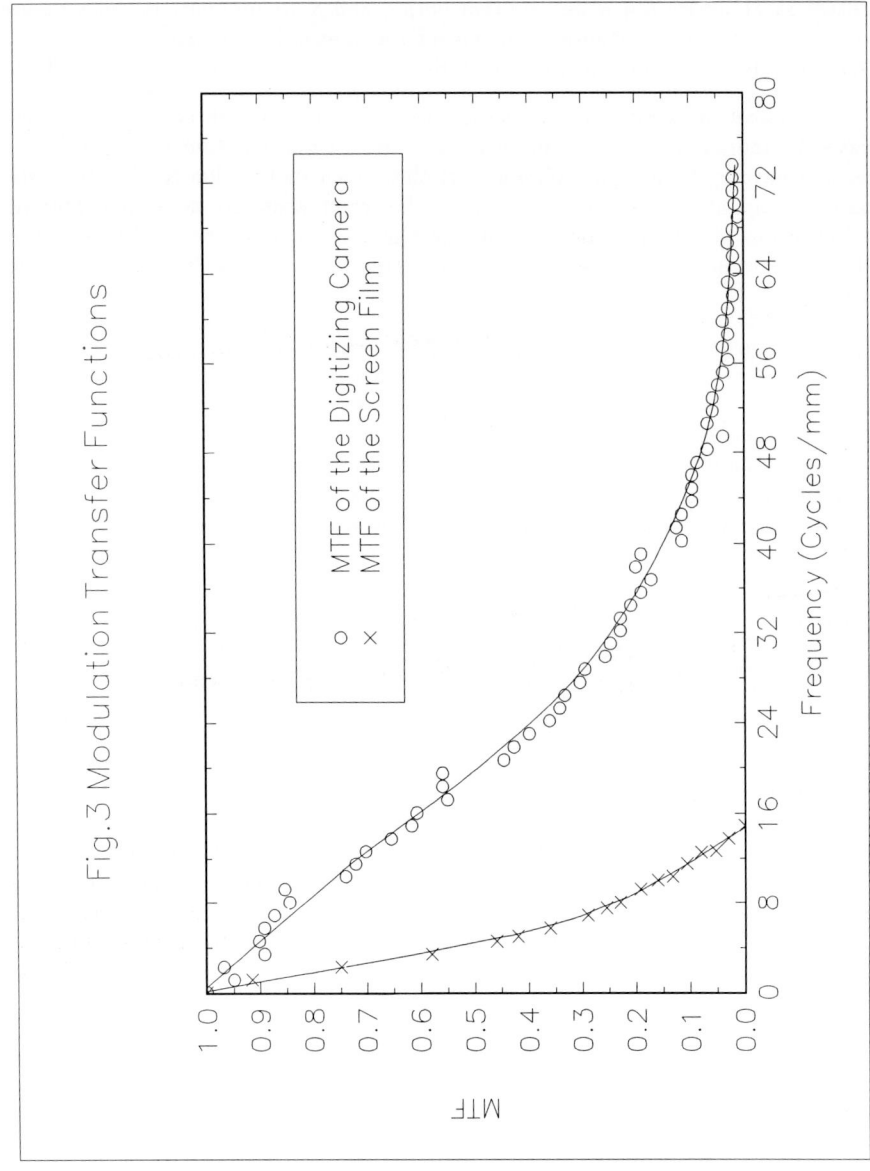

Fig.3 Modulation Transfer Functions

conditions we note that the screen-film combination (and not the digitizing camera) is the limiting factor in spatial resolution. The field of view is now restricted to the area of the CCD, i.e. a mere 7 mm x 9 mm. As we increase the field of view the effective camera MTF referred to the object (mammogram) plane deteriorates.

In addition to the noise present on the developed film the digitizing system adds another noise element. This noise element is due to the following four sources: a) the illumination source; b) the lens; c) the CCD and its associated amplifier; and d) the analogue to digital converter. Fig. 4 gives a block diagram of the CCD image formation from the mammogram. We combine these four sources and divide the overall noise present in the data into two types, the fixed pattern noise such as the optical shading of the light source and the aberrations of the lens, and the random noise of optical and electronic origin. The fixed pattern noise can generally be corrected by image calibration, while the random component of the camera noise may be reduced using averaging [18]. The final calibrated image therefore will contain a small amount of observation noise, which is due to the camera and uncorrelated to the image, and a more significant radiographic noise which is signal-dependent.

3. Image Observation Model

It is customary in image restoration literature to consider the image observation model to be linear. In a commonly used model the observed image, g, is considered to be the result of linear convolution of the latent image, f, with a blur function, h, and addition of independent, zero-mean, white, Gaussian noise. While this model has the advantage of mathematical tractability, it is an over simplification of the actual situation.

We have previously employed this model and have shown that improvement in the appearance of digitized mammographic images is possible [17]. In particular the blur and noise contributed by the digitizing camera can be modeled in this form. The X-ray image formation however, can not be modeled in this way. Specifically radiographic noise is strongly signal-dependent and the film density vs. log exposure characteristic curve introduces non-linearity in the convolution term.

We formulated an image observation model for the X-ray system as shown in Fig. 5. In this model the weakening of off-axis rays may be compensated for by a pointwise normalization of each pixel value by the $\cos^3 \theta$ term. The input is Q_{ij}, the number of X-ray quanta received at the screen per pixel, and the output is g_{ij}, the observed optical density of each pixel. We have included three sources of blur in this model: $h_{focalspot}$, $h_{scatter}$, and h_{screen}. There are also three scaling factors: $\bar{m}$ is the mean screen amplification ratio; and η_1 and η_2 are the absorption efficiencies of the screen and the film respectively. The three noise sources represent n_1, the correlated

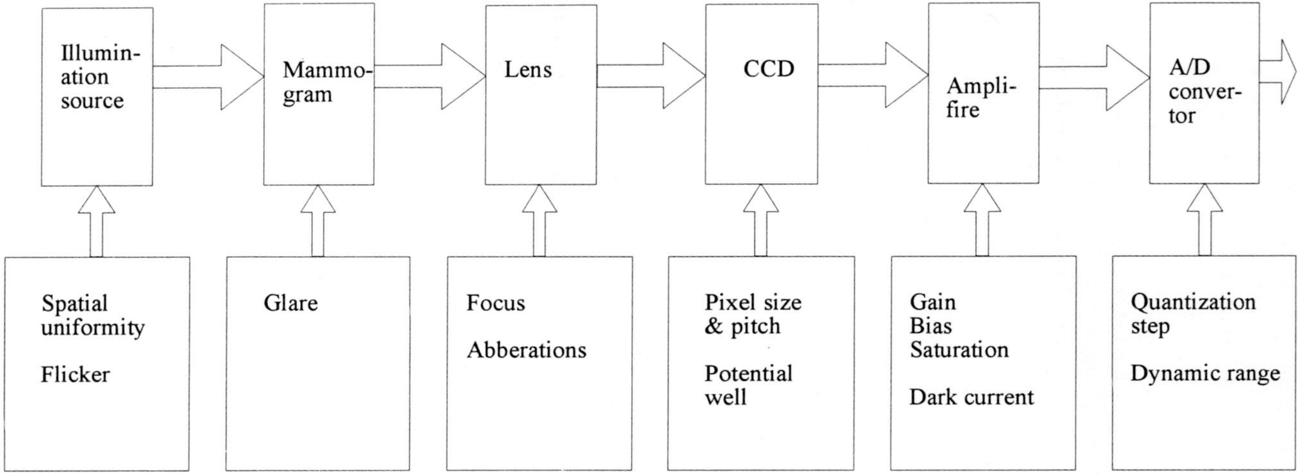

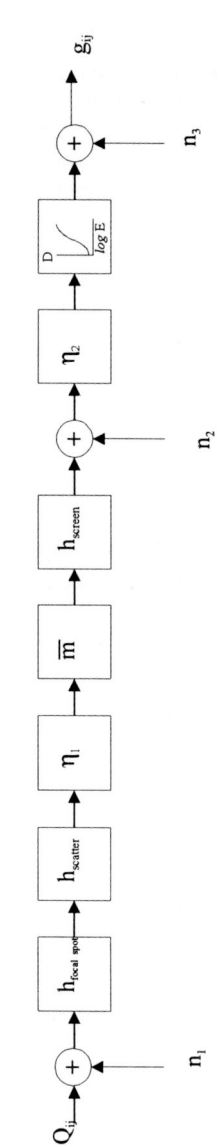

Fig. 4. The digitizing camera image formation model

Fig. 5. A model of radiographic image formation

and n_2, the uncorrelated components of the input quantum noise, and n_3, the associated film-grain noise.

This model may be simplified by making the following observations. The scalar factors may be taken out of the system block diagram and reflected at the input. The blur due to the focal spot size is a function of the relative distance of the lesion of interest and the screen. This is of course not known *a priori* and for the cases where the object of interest is in contact with the screen there are no blur contributions from the focal spot. Finally we assume that the X-ray scatter in the subject is largely absorbed by the vibrating grid.

Based on these consideration a simplified version of the above model is given in Fig. 6. In this model we have ignored the effects of the weakening of the off-axis rays, the focal spot size and the X-ray scatter in the subject.

In Fig. 6 the 'ideal' image f_{ij} is the number of light quanta, q_{ij}, absorbed by the film in each pixel (i, j)

$$f_{ij} = q_{ij} = \eta \bar{m} Q_{ij} \qquad (1)$$

where Q_{ij} is the number of X-ray quanta received at the screen per pixel, $\bar{m}$ is the mean screen amplification ratio, and $\eta = \eta_1 \eta_2$, i.e. the combined absorption efficiencies of the screen-film combination. Note that in Fig. 6 the images f, f_1, and f_2 are in the exposure domain while f_3 and g are in the optical density domain. Γ is the non-linear, $D - \log E$, characteristic function of the film.

The noise sources in Fig. 6 n_1, n_2, and n_3 are zero-mean additive signal-dependent white noise sources uncorrelated with each other. The effects of the scalar factors of Fig. 5 are now incorporated in the magnitudes of these sources. Specifically, n_2 is the uncorrelated component of the Poisson noise of the X-ray source and is generated as in Fig. 7.

$$n_2 = \sqrt{f} \cdot n' \qquad (2)$$

where n' is a zero-mean unit-variance Gaussian random variable. f' is a random variable with Poisson probability distribution whose expected value is f. The noise component n_1 is the amplified noise due to the screen amplification fluctuations:

$$n_1 = k_1 \sqrt{f} n' \qquad (3)$$

It is generated according to the block diagram of Fig. 8. The gain factor is

$$k_1 = \sqrt{\bar{m} \left(1 + \frac{\epsilon}{\bar{m}}\right)} \qquad (4)$$

where ϵ is the excess Poisson noise. The film-grain noise is represented by n_3:

$$n_3 = k_3 f_3^\beta n' \qquad (5)$$

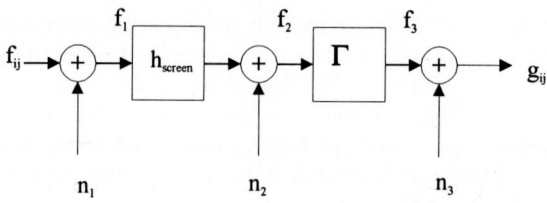

Fig. 6. A simplified model of radiographic image formation

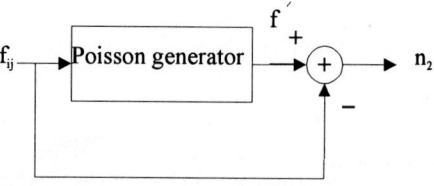

Fig. 7. Generation of the noise source n_2

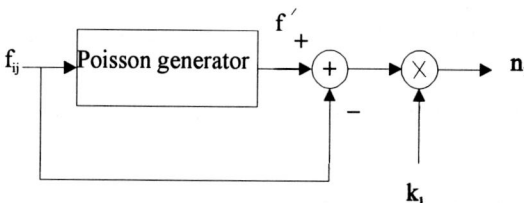

Fig. 8. Generation of the noise source n_1

and

$$k_3 = \frac{1}{\Delta}\sqrt{a \cdot \log_{10} e} \qquad (6)$$

where a is the average film-grain area, and Δ is the sampling interval, i.e. the pixel size. For optimally exposed film β is taken to be 0.5.

From Fig. 6 we can write the following image observation equations

$$\begin{aligned} g &= \Gamma\left[h_{sf} * (f + n_1) + n_2\right] + n_3 & (7) \\ &= \Gamma\left[h_{sf} * f + (h_{sf} * n_1 + n_2)\right] + n_3 & (8) \end{aligned}$$

where h_{sf} is the point spread function of the screen-film and $*$ signifies linear convolution. Using the constant parameters for our screen film combination ($\eta = 0.58$, $\bar{m} = 284$, $\epsilon = 112$, and MTF and densitometric data as published in [5]) we note that n_2 is at least two orders of magnitude smaller than either n_1 or n_3. The latter two quantities are of comparable magnitudes. We will therefore ignore n_2 from now on and write:

$$g = \Gamma\left[h_{sf} * (f + n_1)\right] + n_3 \qquad (9)$$

The problem of film non-linearity may be handled in any one of the following three ways: i) the function Γ may be explicitly incorporated in the restoration filter; ii) the processing may be done in the exposure domain where a linear relationship exists; or iii) a small-signal model may be used to derive a linear equation. Since mammographic images are of very low contrast we will use the small-signal analysis assumption. If a linear approximation to the above non-linear equation is made then

$$\begin{aligned} g &\simeq h_{sf} * f + n_4 & (10) \\ n_4 &= h_{sf} * n_1 + n_3 & (11) \end{aligned}$$

where all variables are now in the density domain and the appropriate conversion constants are incorporated in them. n_4 is now the total radiographic noise.

This relation can be combined with the linear convolution model of digitization by the CCD camera. We therefore consider that first the 'ideal' image, $f(i,j)$, is blurred by the system impulse response, $h(i,j)$, and a small amount of uncorrelated camera observation noise, $n_c(i,j)$ is added to it to produce the blurred image $f_b(i,j)$. Subsequently the signal-dependent radiographic noise $n_4(i,j)$ is added to it, which results in the final observed image $g(i,j)$:

$$\begin{aligned} f_b(i,j) &= h(i,j) * f(i,j) + n_c(i,j) & (12) \\ g(i,j) &= f_b(i,j) + n_4(i,j) & (13) \end{aligned}$$

The system impulse response h is due to the combined effect of the camera and the screen-film system, i.e.:

$$h(i,j) = h_{sf}(i,j) * h_c(i,j) \qquad (14)$$

Note that the additive noise model above is not restrictive since any multiplicative noise can be reformulated as additive signal-dependent noise. We consider n_c to be a white noise field with zero-mean Gaussian distribution.

4. Image Restoration

We will use the image formation model of equations (12) and (13). According to this model the observed image was formed in two steps. The latent image f, was first blurred (with the addition of n_c) to form f_b, and then contaminated by signal-dependent noise n_4. We therefore divide the restoration problem into two steps. In the first step we apply smoothing techniques using local statistics to 'clean-up' the image from the signal-dependent noise n_4. In the second step we apply a classical Wiener filter to deblur the image from the combined effects of the system's Modulation Transfer Function and the noise n_c. The following two criteria of optimality were used in the first step in deriving two smoothing filters: the minimum mean squared error (MMSE), and the maximum *a posteriori* (MAP) joint probability.

The required image smoothing may be achieved using either the global image or the local image approach. In the first approach the image is assumed to be a stationary random process. In [18] a Wiener smoothing filter is employed, assuming the system noise is a white Gaussian process independent of the image grey levels. This is a non-adaptive global approach in which the MMSE criterion of optimality is applied over the whole image.

In this paper, we study the more realistic of the two approaches (i.e. the one which uses local processing). We postulate that the breast image is non-stationary due to the presence of structure in the parenchymal pattern. This is particularly true of mammograms containing microcalcifications or masses. Additionally the blur process is a local operation and therefore it is reasonable to expect that the restoration should also be performed locally.

The grey level histogram of a complete mammogram is commonly not Gaussian. If we subtract the local mean from each pixel however, the resulting image grey levels have a nearly normal distribution. Therefore in this work we consider the image model to be Gaussian with non-stationary mean and non-stationary variance (NMNV).

4.1 Local adaptive Wiener smoothing filter

For the NMNV model [19] the image is considered to be Gaussian only locally in small neighborhoods. Using the MMSE criterion locally will lead to an adaptive local linear minimum mean square error (LLMMSE) filter. The estimated pixel value $\hat{f}$ [20] is:

$$\hat{f}_b = \bar{g} + \frac{\sigma_g^2 - \sigma_{n4}^2}{\sigma_g^2}(g - \bar{g}) \tag{15}$$

where $\bar{g}$ and σ_g^2 are the local mean and variance of the observed image, and σ_{n4}^2 is the noise variance. The required local statistics are estimated from the observed image and *a priori* knowledge about the image is not required.

The noise power is first estimated for each pixel and this knowledge is used to calculate a new estimate of the signal according to eqn. (15). If the noise power is negligibly small (i.e. $\sigma_g^2 >> \sigma_{n4}^2$) then the estimated pixel value is very close to its observed value. At the other extreme if all of the observed power is due to noise (i.e. $\sigma_g^2 \simeq \sigma_{n4}^2$) then the best estimate of the signal is the local average.

The noise power is estimated from a knowledge of the noise model. The total radiographic noise n_4 is the sum of the film-grain noise, n_3 and the noise due to the quantum mottle. The noise power σ_{n4}^2 can therefore be readily estimated for each pixel.

For the quantum mottle n_1, we observe that the underlying noise process is due to the discrete nature of the X-ray photons and therefore has a Poisson probability distribution. The grey level $f_b(i,j)$ for the pixel (i,j) is related to the number of photons I(i,j) incident on it. The grey level has a code value between zero and 255 which is a linear quantization of the film density $D(i,j)$, and the film density is a known function of the exposure. Therefore the number of incident photons can be calculated for each pixel. Since the mean and variance of a Poisson distribution are equal, the exposure value will directly determine the noise power σ_{n1}^2.

Finally, since the two components of the radiographic noise are independent of each other the combined noise power σ_{n4}^2 can be obtained as

$$\sigma_{n4}^2 = \sigma_{n1}^2 \mid MTF \mid^2 + \sigma_{n3}^2 \tag{16}$$

4.2 Baysian smoothing filter

The maximum *a posteriori* (MAP) filter for the above case of the non-stationary mean and non-stationary variance (NMNV) image model and Poisson noise has the form [21]:

$$\hat{f}_b = \frac{(\bar{g} - \sigma_{f_b}^2) + \sqrt{(\bar{g} - \sigma_{f_b}^2)^2 + 4\sigma_{f_b}^2 \cdot g}}{2} \quad (17)$$

where the average power of the blurred image $\sigma_{f_b}^2$ is obtained from the observed image

$$\sigma_{f_b}^2 = max[(\sigma_g^2 - \bar{g}), 0]. \quad (18)$$

4.3. The Deconvolution Filter

After the application of one of the above smoothing filters, the resultant image $\hat{f}_b$ is an estimate of the blurred image f_b (eqn. 13). A modified Wiener restoration filter was selected to obtain $\hat{f}$, an estimate of the ideal image:

$$\hat{F}(\omega_x, \omega_y) = H_r(\omega_x, \omega_y) \cdot F_b(\omega_x, \omega_y) \quad (19)$$

$$H_r(\omega_x, \omega_y) = \frac{H^*(\omega_x, \omega_y)}{|H(\omega_x, \omega_y)|^2 + \alpha} \quad (20)$$

where $\hat{F}(\omega_x, \omega_y)$, $F_b(\omega_x, \omega_y)$, and $H(\omega_x, \omega_y)$ are Fourier Transforms of $\hat{f}$, f_b, and h respectively, and * is the complex conjugation. H_r is the reconstruction filter in the frequency domain and α is a measure of the noise to signal power ratio.

5. Results

We have examined some 400 mammograms and associated radiographs from patients who have undergone breast biopsy at British Columbia Cancer Agency's Vancouver Clinic. From among these mammograms, 70 images containing clusters of microcalcifications were selected. The calcifications varied in appearance from clearly benign to highly suspicious for malignancy. These images formed the data base for testing the effects of our algorithms.

These images were digitized with a Xillix Micro Imager 1400 digitizing camera. This detector uses a two-dimensional CCD array (Kodak KAF-1400) to capture 1320 x 1035 pixels with square sensor elements of 6.8 μm per side. Up to six frames per second can be acquired with variable integration times. The CCD output is digitized to 10 bits, 8 of which can be displayed at any one time on a high resolution (1280 x 1024 pixels) monitor. The X-ray film to camera distance was arranged to give a sampling interval of 100 μm. Selected regions of some mammograms were also digitized with sampling intervals of 12 μm.

The fixed pattern noise (such as optical shading due to non-uniform illumination) was measured and subsequently the digitized images were corrected for this effect. The random element of digitization noise was also reduced by averaging multiple frames.

We implemented both the LLMMSE filter (eqn. 15) and the MAP filter (eqn. 17), followed by the deconvolution filter (eqn. 20). We note that the application of these filters may or may not be required depending on our operating conditions (such as the sampling interval) and also depending on the application in mind. For example in any reading of a mammogram where attention to fine spatial and photometric details is not required, image deconvolution will not be necessary. An example of this is when mammograms of the left and right breast of the same woman are being examined for the detection of bilateral asymmetry. In such cases large pixel sizes (e.g. 200 μm per side) may be used which leads to smaller, and therefore more manageable images. The radiographic noise will also be smaller in these images obviating the need for image smoothing.

We evaluated each of the above three filters individually and also as combinations. The two smoothing filters may be used individually in cases where radiographic noise is judged to be the limiting factor in interpreting the films. The deconvolution filter may be employed alone in cases where the image blur is the principal consideration and only a small amount of uncorrelated noise is present. This would be the case when a relatively large sampling interval (i.e. pixel size) is utilized. The cascade of adaptive smoothing and deblurring filters should be applied in cases where both radiographic noise and image blur are present.

To examine the effect of the deblurring filter we digitized the image of a test phantom as shown in Fig. 9. The object was placed at a distance from the camera such that the ideal optical image formed at the CCD plane contained substantial energy at frequencies near the limit of the resolution capability of the camera. A blurred image was obtained in this way while the camera was maintained at its best focus setting. A fixed noise to signal ratio (NSR) is assumed in the design of the Wiener filter. The value of this constant was adjusted empirically to obtain the best restored image, as judged visually. The filter takes the form of a sharpening high pass filter and assists in better visualization of image details.

To compare the performance of the deconvolution filter with enhancement filters we include the effects of two high pass filters shown in Figure 9. Both of these filters are 3x3 convolutional filters with the following mask values:

$$sharp1 = \begin{bmatrix} 0 & -1 & 0 \\ -1 & 5 & -1 \\ 0 & -1 & 0 \end{bmatrix} ; sharp2 = \begin{bmatrix} -1 & -1 & -1 \\ -1 & 9 & -1 \\ -1 & -1 & -1 \end{bmatrix}$$

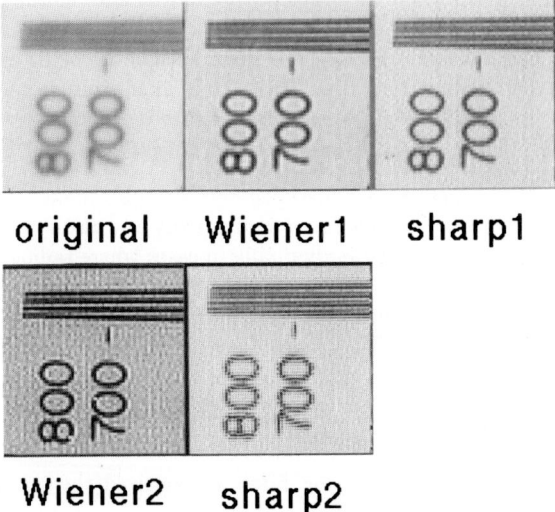

Fig. 9. A portion of a standard test phantom imaged at a far distance near the resolution limit of the camera. Results of restoration by the two Wiener filters: Wiener1 with NSR=.01 & Wiener2 with NSR=.001, and enhancement by 3x3 convolutional masks sharp1 & sharp2 as defined in the text.

These edge sharpening filters were implemented in the spatial domain and therefore were computationally faster and more economical for the storage requirements. The Wiener filter with NSR=.001 produces the sharpest image in which the four separate lines at the top half of the image are clearly distinguished.

We have chosen visual assessment of processed images to determine image quality. Various quantitative measures, such as MMSE have also been proposed in the literature. Calculation of MMSE however requires knowledge of the ideal image and may be performed using simulated degradations.

To evaluate the effectiveness of each one of the two smoothing filters we considered a portion of a digitized mammogram containing a cluster of microcalcifications suspicious of malignancy. Radiographic noise was then added to this image. Although this will exaggerate the total amount of noise present in a mammogram it enables us to assess, more readily, the performance of the smoothing filters. It also represents a mammogram obtained under less than the ideal imaging conditions. A 5x5 square window was used to calculate local statistics. The performance factor P for each filter is defined as the square root of the ratio of average noise power before smoothing ϵ_1^2, to the average noise power after smoothing ϵ_2^2 [21]:

$$\epsilon_1^2 = \frac{1}{N} \sum_i \sum_j (f_b(i,j) - g(i,j))^2 \qquad (21)$$

$$\epsilon_2^2 = \frac{1}{N} \sum_i \sum_j \left(f_b(i,j) - \hat{f}_b(i,j)\right)^2 \qquad (22)$$

$$P = \frac{\epsilon_1}{\epsilon_2} \qquad (23)$$

Table 1 shows the advantages of our noise compensation procedure and gives a summary of the performance factor for each filter. The extent of the noise was controlled by a constant multiplier factor, λ, in these experiments. The cases of λ = 1, 0.5, & 0 correspond to 'severe', 'moderate', and no noise respectively.

Finally to examine the effect of the combined operation we processed 30 images from our data base. Following smoothing, each smoothed image was deblurred by the Wiener filter. In this implementation, we again considered the signal to noise ratio to be a constant independent of the spatial frequency of the image. We used a signal to noise power ratio of 20 in the deconvolution filter.

The images were displayed on a high resolution (1024 x 1280 pixels, colour) monitor, and a radiologist and an image processing engineer reviewed the images. In all cases the processed images were sharper and revealed greater amounts of image detail. Generally the noise content of the images were also increased. This, however

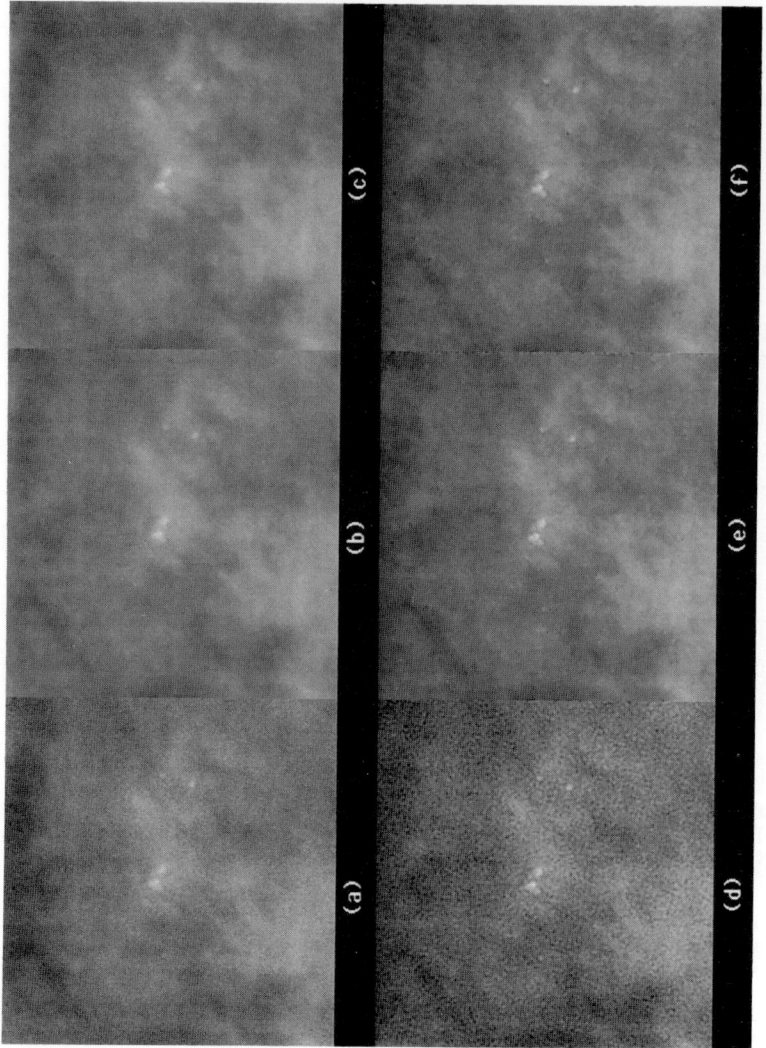

Fig.10 (a) observed image, (b) smoothed by LLMSE filter, (c) smoothed by MAP filter, (d,e,f), result of Wiener deconvolution of images (a,b,c), respectively.

Table 1: Filter performance factors

	Moderate Noise	Severe Noise
LLMMSE	1.63	1.47
MAP	1.76	1.63

did not interfere with identification of microcalcification clusters. The opinion of the reviewers were that application of these processing steps normally assisted in better visualization of image detail.

Fig. 10 presents a typical image at various processing stages. Here the mammogram contains 'real' (i.e. not simulated) radiographic noise. The results of the deconvolution both before and after smoothing of the mammograms are shown. Fig. 10a is the observed noisy and blurred mammogram, and Fig. 10d is the restoration of it using the Wiener filter but without any prior smoothing. The amplification of the noise obscures much of the detail of this image. Fig. 10b is the result of processing the image of Fig. 10a with the LLMMSE smoothing filter, and Fig. 10e is its restoration using the Wiener filter. Clearly the image detail has been sharpened without any significant gain in the noise. Fig. 10c is the result of smoothing of Fig. 10a with the MAP filter, and Fig. 10f is the deblurring of Fig. 10c with the Wiener filter. The beneficial effects of these noise smoothing and detail sharpening filters are clearly visible. The visual appearance of these images are consistent with the measured values of the filter performance factors. Since the MAP filter shows higher performance factors, this filter was implemented as part of our real-time mammographic image acquisition and analysis system.

6. Conclusions

Radiographic images suffer from both signal-dependent noise and system blur. We have designed and implemented locally adaptive smoothing filters to reduce the effect of the noise. The smoothed images are then subjected to a deblurring algorithm to reduce the effects of system blur. The resulting images improve the visibility of subtle signs of abnormality and may help in the earlier detection of breast cancer.

7. Acknowledgments

This work has been supported in part by a Canadian Commonwealth Scholarship, and a grant from British Columbia Science Council.

8. References

[1] L.W.Bassett and R.H.G.Gold, <u>Breast Cancer Detection</u>, Grune & Stratton, 1987.

[2] M.Moskowitz, "Mammography to screen asymptomatic women for breast cancer" American J. Roentgenology vol.143, pp.457- 459, Sept. 1984.

[3] R.Holland, S.H.J.Veling, M.Mravunac and J.H.C.L.Hendriks "Histologic Multifocality of Tis, T1-2 Breast Carcinomas", Cancer Vol.56 pp.979-990, September 1985.

[4] P.G.Tahoces, J.Correa, M.Souto, C.Gonzalez, L.Gomez, and J.J.Vidal *"Enhancement of Chest and Breast Radiographs by Automatic Spatial Filtering"*, IEEE Trans. Med. Image., Vol. 10, No. 3, pp. 330-335. Sept. 1991.

[5] S.Yabashi, M.Hata, K.Kubo, and T.Ishikawa, *"Image Processing for Recognition of Tumor on Mammography"*, Proceedings of the 1989 International Symposium on noise and clutter rejection in radars and imaging sensors, Japan, Nov. 1989.

[6] R.Gordon, and R.M.Rangayyan, *"Feature enhancement of film mammograms using fixed and adaptive neighborhoods"*, Applied Optics, Vol. 23 No. 4, pp. 560-564, 15 Feb. 1984.

[7] A.P.Dhawan, G.Buelloni, and R.Gordon *"Enhancement of Mammographic Features by Optimal Adaptive Neighborhood Image Processing"*, IEEE Trans. Med. Image., Vol. 5, No. 1, pp. 8-15, March 1986.

[8] A.P.Dhawan and E.L.Royer, *"Mammographic Feature Enhancement by Computerized Image Processing"*, Computer Methods and Programs in Bio- medicine, Vol. 27, pp. 23-35, 1988.

[9] W.M.Morrow, R.M.Rangayyan, and J.E.L.Desautels *"Feature Adaptive Enhancement and Analysis of High-Resolution Digitized Mammograms"*, Proc. Annual Int. Conf. of IEEE Eng. in Med. and Biol. Vol. 12, No. 1, pp.165-166, 1990.

[10] N.Karssemeijer and L.V.Erning, *"Iso-Precision Scaling of Digitized Mammograms to Facilitate Image Analysis"*, Proceedings SPIE Vol. 1445, pp. 166-177, Image Processing, 1991.

[11] F.Aghdasi, R.K.Ward, and B.Palcic *"Detection and Segmentation of Microcalcifications in Mammographic Image Analysis"*, Proceedings of the Fourth Canadian Conference on Electrical and Computer Engineering, Quebec city, Quebec, Vol. 2, pp. 63.1.1-3, Sep. 25-27, 1991.

[12] F.Aghdasi and B.Palcic, *"A Large Area CCD Camera for Mammographic Image Acquisition"*, Proceedings of the Annual International Conference of the IEEE Engineering in Medicine and Biology Society, Vol. 13, Part 1, pp.243-4, 1991.
[13] A.G.Haus, Ed., The Physics of Medical Imaging, 1979.
[14] D.R.Jacobson and C.R.Wilson, *"Focal Spot Size, Magnification and Sharpness in Mammography"*, Med. Phys., Vol. 19, No. 3, pp. 832, May/June 1992.
[15] P.C.Bunch, *"Detective Quantum Efficiency of Selected Mammographic Screen-film Combinations"*, SPIE Vol.1090, Medical Imaging III: Image Formation, 1989.
[16] M.Rabbani and R.Shaw, *"Detective Quantum Efficiency of Imaging Systems with Amplifying and Scattering Mechanisms"*, J. of Optical Soc. of America, Vol. 4, pp.495, May 1987.
[17] J.W.Motz and M.Danos, *Quantum Noise-Limited Images in Screen-Film Systems"*, SPIE Vol. 347, Application of Optical Instrumentation in Medicine X, pp. 62-66, 1982.
[18] F.Aghdasi, R.K.Ward and B.Palcic, *"Restoration of Mammographic Images Acquired by a New Fast Digitization System"*, Proceedings of SPIE/IS&T Symposium on Electronic Imaging: Science and Technology, SanJose, Ca., Image Processing Algorithms and Techniques III, SPIE Vol. 1657, pp.256-67, 1992.
[19] B.R.Hunt and T.M.Cannon, *"Nonstationary assumptions for Gaussian models of images"*, IEEE Trans. Syst., Man, Cybern., Vol. 6, pp. 876-881, 1976.
[20] D.T.Kuan, A.A.Sawchuk, T.C.Strand, and P.Chavel, *"Adaptive noise smoothing filter for images with signal dependent noise,"* IEEE Trans. Pattern Anal. Machine Intell., Vol. 7, pp. 165-177, 1985.
[21] M.Rabbani, *"Baysian filtering of Poisson Noise Using Local Statistics"*, IEEE Trans. Acous. Speech & Sig. Proc., Vol 36, No. 6, June 1988.

Classifying mammograms by density: sorting for screening

S. Hajnal,[†] P. Taylor,[†] M.-H. Dilhuydy,[‡] B. Barreau [‡]

† Advanced Computation Laboratory, Imperial Cancer Research Fund, 61 Lincoln's Inn Fields, London WC2A 3PX, UK

‡ Fondation Bergonié, 180 rue de Saint-Genès, 33076 Bordeaux Cedex, France

Abstract

We are investigating techniques for automatically sorting mammograms according to whether the breast tissue is fatty or dense. The hypothesis is that areas of dense tissue are a major factor in making certain mammograms harder for both radiologists and computers to interpret. Being able to identify dense mammograms automatically would enable expert radiologists to use their time and skills more efficiently, since only the difficult mammograms would be examined by the most experienced readers. Concentrating on the easier, fatty mammograms might make the computer-aided detection of abnormalities more tractable.

A number of local statistical and texture measures have been applied to manually selected patches from digitised mammograms. One of the measures (local skewness in tiles) gives a good separation between fatty and dense patches. A method of automatic patch placement has been devised and a fully automatic procedure for sorting mammograms is therefore possible.

1. Background

There has been some literature on the computer analysis of mammograms since 1967 [27]. Research in this area has recently been stimulated both by the advent of direct digital mammography and by the adoption of mammography as a mass screening technique. The UK National Breast Screening Programme has led to over 1.7 million screenings in the first two full years [20]. Mammographic screening is a controversial subject [10,26], but if there are to be screening programmes the quality of the screening is of paramount importance, and we believe that work in computerised image analysis could help to guarantee that quality.

Mammograms show differences in tissue density: dense tissue is more opaque to X-rays than fat. Thus dense tissue and ducts in the breast, and many abnormalities as well, show up as patterns of light structures against darker fat. Most of the work on computer analysis of mammograms has concentrated on the detection of small abnormalities, specifically microcalcifications [5,6,8]. There has, however, been some work on the analysis of parenchymal patterns.[1] These patterns have been investigated for two main reasons. Firstly, asymmetry in patterns of density between the breasts is one of the signs for which radiologists routinely check when examining mammograms [4] and the automated detection of such asymmetries has been the goal of some research [14]. Secondly, Wolfe [28] has proposed a grading of parenchymal patterns into four classes, held to be indicative of the risk of developing breast cancer. Although this system and its relationship to risk is not universally accepted and has been widely discussed in the literature [25], there have been attempts to classify mammograms according to the Wolfe grades automatically, and to produce more objective measures of parenchymal patterns [3,12,22,18].

Our project involves looking at dense tissue for a slightly different purpose. We believe that a method of sorting mammograms automatically according to whether the breast tissue is fatty or dense could have advantages, independent of possible correlations with risk. The hypothesis is that areas of dense tissue are a major factor in determining whether a mammogram will be difficult for radiologists to read. However, only about 20% of women in the screening age-group, (50-64 years of age in the UK) have dense breasts.[2] Merely being able to identify this subgroup automatically might allow expert radiologists to use their time and skills more efficiently, since the more difficult mammograms could be examined by the more experienced readers.

It is also plausible that the presence of such tissue makes the computer-aided detection of abnormalities more difficult. The classification would allow techniques for computer-aided detection of abnormalities to be developed specifically for fatty images: the class in which they are likely to be more successful. We envisage a system which sorts mammograms into two classes: those which are fatty and contain nothing suspicious and those which are dense and/or suspicious. This separation would be beneficial since the attentions of senior radiologists could be directed to the latter class.

There is another potential longer-term advantage. Density is related to, but not entirely correlated with, age [29]. Screening has not been shown to be effective in women under 50, partly because the majority of younger women have dense breasts. The fatty/dense distinction may provide a criterion complementary to that of age in the planning of screening programmes and procedures.

2. The Fatty/Dense Distinction

The hypothesis that density is a major factor in determining difficulty is supported by work which has been done on improving image quality for dense breasts [15] and by

---

1. The definition of 'parenchyma' suggests that this term should refer to the functional parts of an organ, as opposed to supporting tissue, or 'stroma'. However, other authors seem to use the term 'parenchymal pattern' to refer to any mammographically visible structure in the breast.
2. It is difficult to establish a precise figure for this proportion. The figure given is based on the experience of senior radiologists and seems plausible given both the published frequencies of Wolfe's classes P2 and DY [29,23] and a similar estimate quoted by Law [15].

studies of the reliability of mammography in these cases [9]. Reviewing work in automated tumour detection, Astley [1] suggests "the visual similarity of some tumours to normal structures in dense and fatty-glandular breasts" as a reason why this area has been less widely researched and produced less impressive results than the detection of microcalcifications. Kimme-Smith [13] found that dense films required a different digitisation method in order to be acceptable for screen viewing by radiologists.

The proposal is to classify mammograms into two categories: 'fatty' and 'dense', where 'dense' mammograms have sufficient dense tissue to make them relatively difficult to read. We have investigated whether radiologists can make this distinction reliably, in order to provide a 'gold standard' for assessing computerised sorting methods [24]. Two radiologists independently classified 103 pairs of mammograms. The radiologists agreed on the classification of 97 pairs. Kappa (a measure of agreement between two observers) is 0.88 for these data. Guidelines on the interpretation of this statistic [2] suggest that this indicates a very high level of agreement.

It might have been expected that the images would form a continuum from fatty to dense, and that any individual's classifications would be based on an arbitrary setting of a threshold on this continuum. Perhaps because this simple classification task was based on terms used by the radiologists themselves, there was, in practice, near unanimity.

3. Related Work

In this section we give a brief summary of other work in the computerised assessment of mammographic tissue patterns, and relate it to the approach taken in this paper. There are a small number of reports dealing with two related tasks: classification by Wolfe grades [3,12,22,18] and segmentation of glandular tissue [19]. One of these [22] will not be discussed, since it deals specifically with the identification of ducts, which seems less relevant to the current task.

The appearance of glandular tissue in mammograms is very variable. Texture, rather than intensity, is used as the means of classification for breast tissue in the reported work. There are a very large number of texture analysis techniques [7,11,21]. They can be broadly divided into structural and statistical methods. Structural approaches to texture analysis involve the explicit identification of primitive texture elements. This is possible for some classes of regular or man-made textures. While the identification of structure in mammograms is clearly of primary importance for interpretation, breast tissue is not composed of identifiable primitive elements, and no use of structural texture methods has been reported in this field. (Note that morphological granulometry, reported by Miller [19], measures predominant texture scale and is thus statistical, despite using 'structuring elements'.)

Statistical methods for texture analysis can be further subdivided (following [21]) into those using features derived from operators (e.g. Laws' texture energy), from statistical tests (such as grey-level spatial co-occurrence) from the transform domain, and from models (including fractal models). A full review of these methods would be inappropriate here (see references above), but it is interesting to note that the small number of papers in the mammography area include techniques from at least three categories.

Magnin et al. [18] use both first and second order grey-level statistics. They calculate four global image parameters (dynamic range, variance, skewness and kurtosis) and two local measures based on co-occurrence matrices. Neither the local nor the global measures separated mammograms into Wolfe's four classes. Kimme-Smith et al. [12] applied a variety of statistics to sections of images from a small number of patients. They present only a subset, selected to distinguish prominant ducting.

Caldwell et al.[3] compute two parameters: the average fractal dimension of the image and the difference between this average and that of a computer selected region of interest near the nipple. Based on a limited data set, they conclude that a fractal parameter could distinguish "low risk" (N and P1) from "high risk" (P2 and DY) mammograms, but are less optimistic about separation into four classes. For this two-class separation (which seems pertinent to the fatty/dense distinction investigated here) they report good agreement (about 87%) between their classifier and the radiologists.

Miller and Astley [19] compare granulometry with texture energy for the task of segmentation of glandular tissue from fatty tissue. They conclude that one of Laws' texture energy measures [16] produces a correct pixel classification rate of 80% when tested against segmentations drawn by expert radiologists. Laws' methods are local property statistics: they compute a property (in this case the result of convolution with a mask) at each point, and then a macrostatistic (standard deviation) of that property within a larger window centred at each point.

From this review, it seems that the two most promising techniques are fractal dimension and Laws' texture energy. However, the proposed task is both different from, and simpler than, Wolfe grading or segmentation, and simpler statistical techniques may also be appropriate. As reported by Magnin, global grey-level statistics do not distinguish between the classes. However, grey-level statistics in smaller regions were not investigated. This is analogous to computing local property statistics, where the local properties are themselves gray-level statistics in a small area. For overall classification, as opposed to pixel segmentation, it is sufficient to divide the image into tiles (rather than have a small window centred at every point). In this paper this approach is applied over different tile sizes and resolutions, using the local statistics of standard deviation and skewness and the simplest possible macrostatistic: the mean. The results are compared with the two techniques identified above.

4. Images

Images were provided by the Fondation Bergonié, a regional cancer centre in Bordeaux, France. The images used were 'mediolateral oblique' views. This is the single view used in the UK screening programme; the images however were not all from women within the screening age group. The initial set of 20 image pairs (hereafter referred to as the 'training set') was selected by the radiologists as being illustrative of the fatty/dense distinction.

The second series of 103 (the 'test set') was unselected except that, given the high proportion of symptomatic women seen at the Fondation and the desire to simulate a screening programme, it was decided to use only those images that were considered to be free of lesions. The implications of this decision are discussed later.

All images were classified by two senior radiologists at the Fondation Bergonié. No specific instructions or definitions were given: the radiologists were free to classify the images according to their own usage of the terms 'fatty' and 'dense'. As described earlier, the level of agreement between the radiologists is high. In both sets of images the proportions of fatty and dense were approximately equal. Note that the screening population contains a much higher proportion of fatty images (see Section 6).

In the training set, two of the 20 were deemed borderline by the radiologists. In the test set they classified all images independently, disagreeing on the classification of only six. These are marked unclassified in the results tables.

The images were captured by a CCD camera using a Screen Machine board and software on an Apple Macintosh. The resulting digital images were 740 by 480 pixels, with 7 bits per pixel. They were transferred to a Sun SPARCstation IPC for display and processing.

5. Experiments

One strategy for comparing the performance of various measures is to test them first on sections of images selected from the breast area. This allows the substantial problem of segmenting the image, in order to separate the breast from the background and the pectoral muscle from the breast, to be set aside until after a reasonably powerful discriminant has been developed. This is the strategy followed here.

The work is presented in three sub-sections corresponding to three distinct experiments. In each we present results and summarise the conclusions. Discussion of all three is presented in Section 6.

Firstly (Section 5.1), a series of different measures were compared on patches manually selected from the breast images. In the second experiment (Section 5.2), two different strategies for incorporating the most successful measure into an automated procedure were compared: the first automating the selection of the patch, and the second applying the measure to the whole breast area. In Section 5.3 we describe refinements to the more successful strategy, resulting in an almost completely automated procedure for sorting mammograms, and test the performance of that procedure.

5.1. Choice of measure

The measures compared were:

a) Dividing a patch into tiles, measuring statistics within each tile and taking the mean over all tiles. The statistics of skewness and standard deviation were used, over a range of tile sizes and image resolutions.

b) Laws' normalised R5R5 texture energy measure (defined in the Appendix), which Miller and Astley [19] found most promising.

c) Fractal dimension, as described by Caldwell [3]. Caldwell used two parameters, but the method of selecting the region of interest required for the second parameter is not described. The plots of the results suggest that most of the discrimination of interest to this application is found in the first parameter, the overall average fractal dimension.

5.1.1. Experiment

A 128*128 pixel square was cut from one image from each pair. The squares were selected by the authors to provide a representative sample of the tissue from each breast, avoiding the pectoral muscle, the skin and the nipple.

a) For each 128*128 image patch, a Gaussian pyramid of images at different resolutions was created, yielding image sizes 128*128, 64*64, 32*32, 16*16 and 8*8. At each resolution the image was divided up into non-overlapping tiles, of various sizes up to the image size. Skewness (a measure of the asymmetry of the grey-level histogram, see for example [2]) and standard deviation were calculated for each tile and the mean taken.

b) Laws' normalised R5R5 texture energy measure (defined in the Appendix) was calculated on the full resolution patch.

c) Fractal dimension was calculated on the full resolution patch, as described in [3,17]. For this method it is convenient to use dimensions which allow the area to be broken on exact boundaries. The measure was therefore computed on a 121*121 pixel square centered in the patch (allowing edge sizes 1-6).

5.1.2. Results

Receiver operating characteristic (ROC) curves were plotted to compare the separation afforded by each of the measurements. Each measurement yields a single number for each image patch. The images can be divided into two classes using a value of this number as a threshold. The ROC curves plot the percentage of true dense (the proportion of the images classified by the radiologists as dense which are classified as dense by the threshold) against false dense (the proportion of images classified by the radiologists as fatty which are classified as dense by the threshold), for thresholds between the possible extremes. An optimum separation would be 100% true dense, 0% false dense, which corresponds to the top left-hand corner of the plot. Measures can be compared by seeing which curve passes closest to this point.

ROC curves were plotted for the training set in order to find the optimum tile size and resolution for the different measures. Figure 1a shows the results for skewness at full resolution. (The curves for 8*8 and 64*64 tiles gave intermediate results for skewness and are omitted for the sake of clarity.)

(a)

(b)

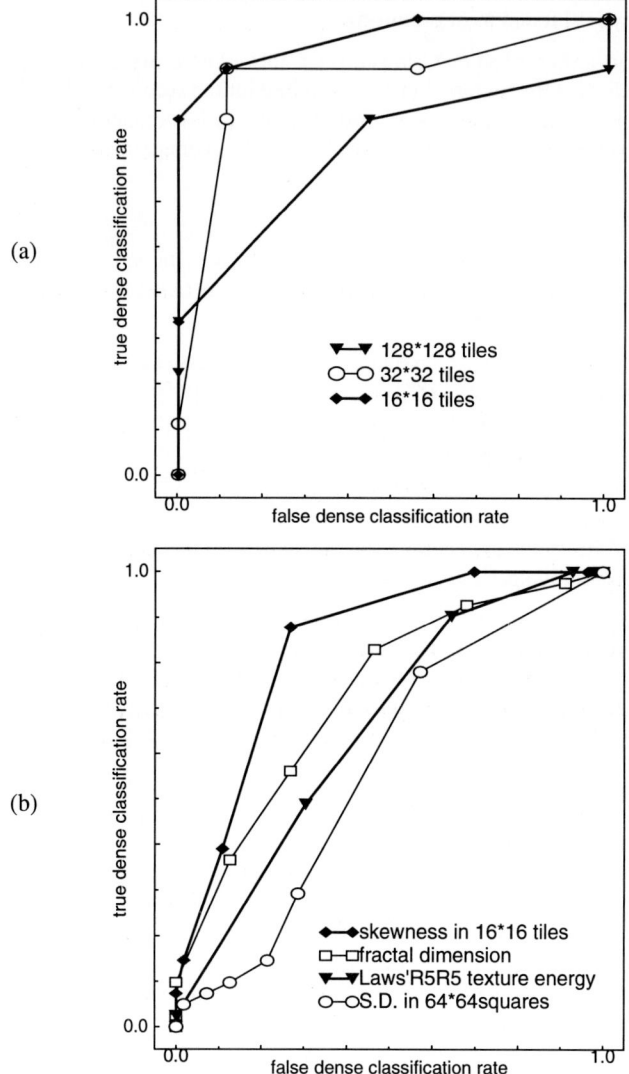

Figure 1: (a) Skewness measured in non-overlapping tiles of different sizes over the training set at full resolution. (b) Comparison of best skewness, standard deviation, fractal dimension and Laws' texture energy, for the test set.

The skewness measure which gave the best separation was for 16*16 tiles at full resolution. A similar comparison for standard deviation showed 64*64 tiles at full resolution to be the best measure.

Once the optimum parameters had been established for the skewness and standard deviation measures on the training set, they could then be compared, together with the fractal dimension and Laws' texture energy measures, on the test set. Figure 1b shows the ROC curves for this comparison.

5.1.3. Conclusions

Of the measures calculated the mean local skewness gives the best separation into the two classes as defined by the radiologists.

5.2. Strategy for automation

The procedure reported above used a manually selected patch taken from the image as the basis for classification. This step allowed the investigation to concentrate on the textural differences between tissue types without being complicated by issues of segmentation. However, a complete automation of the process requires either that the manual selection of the patch be automated or that the measure be applied to the whole breast. In this section we present a comparison of these approaches.

Both require an initial step in which the area of the image corresponding to the breast is identified. A reduced scale image, in which each pixel represented a 16*16 pixel square in the original image, was created by repeated cycles of Gaussian smoothing and resampling. A global threshold was used to segment the reduced image into foreground and background regions and the largest foreground region was taken to be the breast. The corresponding region on the original image was assumed to represent the breast area.

The segmentation produced was by no means perfect and in a few cases was grossly inaccurate, but adequate for the purpose. The segmentation was not fully automatic in that the threshold was chosen by the authors. However, studies using better digitisation equipment [19] indicate that it is possible to segment the image adequately on the basis of a threshold calculated from the grey-level histogram.

We compared measuring skewness over the whole of the breast area with measuring skewness in a 128*128 pixel square placed within the breast area by an automated procedure.

Almost all mammograms with a significant dense region have dense tissue in the area above the nipple and towards the front of the breast area. We used, therefore, the following algorithm to place the square within the breast area: in the case of a left breast, place the square so that its bottom right-hand corner is on the rightmost foreground pixel, adjust the position of the square by moving to the left until only foreground pixels are found within the square. This placement is illustrated in Figure 2.

The skewness measure used in both cases was that found in the earlier experiment to be the most powerful: the mean of the skewness of the grey-level histogram measured in 16*16 tiles across the image.

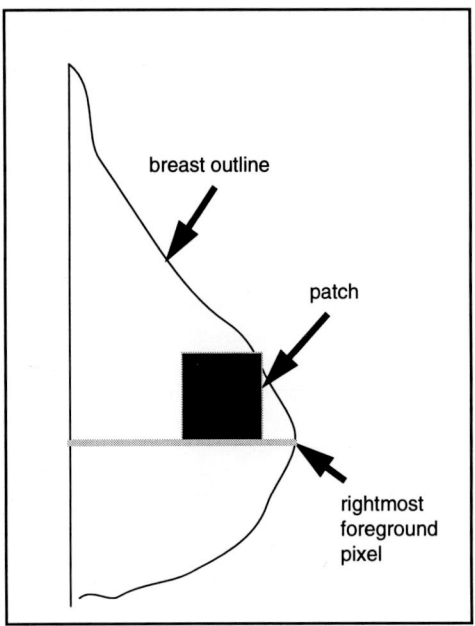

Figure 2: Automatic placement of the patch within the breast: initial procedure.

5.2.1. Results

The two methods were applied to the mammograms in both the training and the test sets and the results combined. The automatic placement routine was unable to fit a patch within the segmented region on 23 out of the 123 mammograms in the study. These 23 cases are excluded from the results of both sets of measurements. ROC curves plotted for the two sets of measurements (Figure 3) suggest that automatic placement is the more powerful. The whole-breast measure (lower curve) remains well below the top axis, this means that any threshold which falsely classifies only a few dense images as fatty will classify almost all images as dense.

5.2.2. Conclusion

The purpose of this comparison was to decide between two distinct strategies for incorporating the measure into a fully automated procedure. The examples of each strategy could be improved and both required manual interventions. The comparison was, however, sufficiently informative to guide the development of the procedure. From these results automatic patch placement is the most promising strategy. However the procedure used in this experiment is inadequate: in too many cases it is unable to fit the patch within the breast and it is less successful than the method using manually selected patches.

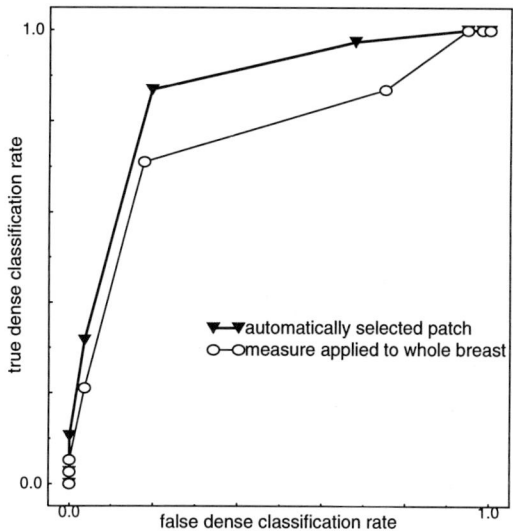

Figure 3: Skewness measured in tiles over the whole breast compared with skewness measured in an automatically selected patch.

5.3. Refinement of the procedure

In consultation with radiologists the method of patch placement was revised in the following ways: by varying the height of the patch, the width of the patch, the position of the patch relative of the breast outline and by making the size of the patch depend upon the width of the breast. Although many of these changes produced only marginal effects, increasing the size of the patch made the measure more accurate and varying the width allowed the patch to be placed in all cases. The best performance was discernibly better than the earlier automatic patch placement tested above, and merited comparison with the original manual patch placement.

The revised automatic patch placement measure was applied to all the left breast images in the study. The detail of the algorithm is as follows: a simple global threshold is used to segment the background from the foreground. A line 160 pixels long is then drawn vertically through the rightmost foreground pixel, positioned so that 80% of the line is above this pixel. This line is moved to the left until it lies entirely within the foreground. At this point the distance from the line to the back of the breast is measured and 80% of that distance taken as the width of the patch. The patch is therefore of variable width but constant height (160 pixels) and lies 80% above the rightmost foreground pixel. This procedure is illustrated in Figure 4.

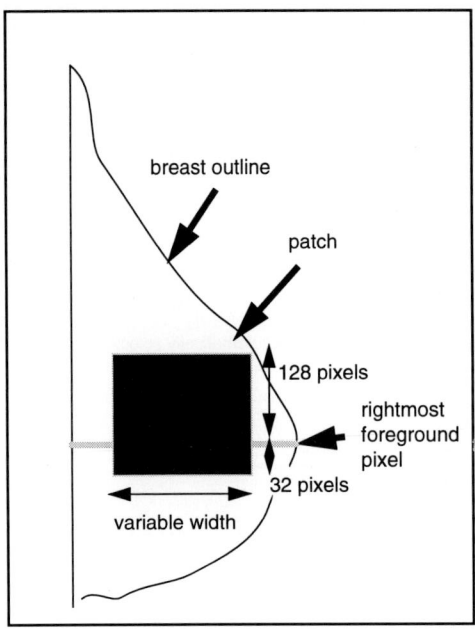

Figure 4: Automatic placement of the patch within the breast: revised procedure.

The skewness measure taken within this area was that used in the previous study. The skewness of the grey-level histograms of 16*16 pixel tiles was calculated and the mean of these values used as the measure.

5.3.1. Results

The results from this measure were compared with those from the manually selected patches and it is clear from the ROC curves (Figure 5) that there is no substantial difference between the two.

Figure 6 shows the distributions of the resulting measure for the two classes. The difference between the means is statistically significant (P<0.001).

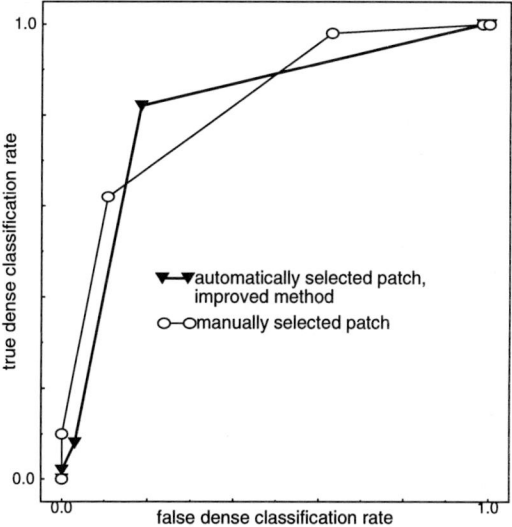

Figure 5: Skewness measured in an automatically selected patch compared with skewness measured in a manually selected patch.

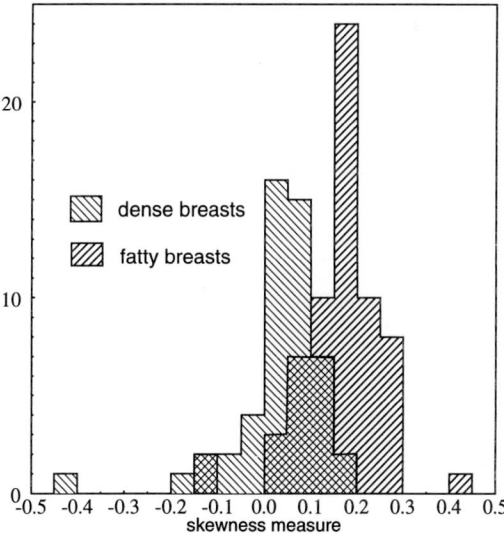

Figure 6: Histograms of the distribution of skewness values for fatty and dense breasts.

Setting an optimal threshold requires a consideration of both the expected relative sizes of the distributions in the screening population and the relative costs of the two types of errors. In the screening population there will be four times as many fatty as dense images but in the given data the proportions are roughly equal. For the intended application, the false classification of a dense image as fatty is a much more serious error than the reverse. We present, as an illustration, a classification based on a threshold which was set so as to generate five times as many false dense as opposed to false fatty classifications, assuming the proportions of fatty and dense in the sample to be equal.

If the two distributions are assumed to be Normal, statistical tables relating standard deviations to areas under the curve can be consulted to find an appropriate threshold [2]. For these data the threshold is 0.16, since this is 1.33 standard deviations away from the mean of the dense distribution and 0.06 away from that of the fatty, and thus the region of the fatty distribution on the wrong side of the threshold will be five times as large as the misclassified region of the dense distribution. If the data were representative samples from two Normal distributions, 48% of the fatty breasts and 9% of the dense would be wrongly classified by this threshold.

Applying the threshold to the data gives the classification summarised in Table 1. The errors generated are rather fewer than predicted by the tables for Normal distributions, suggesting that the data may not be Normal, and that to calculate the threshold they could be modelled as skewed distributions. This has not been attempted.

Table 1: Classification of all images by the automated procedure, threshold 0.16

	True Fatty	True Dense	Unclassified
Classed Fatty	40	1	0
Classed Dense	25	49	8

5.3.2. Conclusion

This study indicates that a fully automated procedure sorting images of fatty from dense breasts could be as reliable as a procedure based on manually selected image patches.

6. Discussion

Of the measures compared, the mean tile skewness gives the best separation into the two classes as defined by the radiologists.

Local standard deviation separates out some fatty and some dense patches, but gives a large overlapping region. It seems that skewness is better at distinguishing these cases. We assume that because fatty tissue appears as light structure on a dark background there will be a preponderance of dark pixels and (if brighter shades are represented by higher numbered grey-levels) histograms of fatty tissue will be skewed to the left. Dense tissue, being predominantly white, will lead to histograms being skewed the other way. Thus the two tissue types would have different skewness even though they might have identical variance. If this explanation of the measure's success is true, it would be difficult to distinguish pure fat from smooth dense tissue (cf. Miller and Astley's remark that 'The most significant error occurs ... where areas of the glandular disc appear to be relatively smooth and are falsely classified as fat' [19]). This was not a problem in these experiments. Removing tiles with very low variance from the calculations did not improve the results.

Laws uses a measure related to standard deviation as the macrostatistic in calculating the texture energy, but comments that to distinguish asymmetrical textures (where light or dark pixels predominate), a different statistic should be used (POSAVE instead of ABSAVE) [16]. This corresponds to the above explanation of the advantage of using skewness rather than standard deviation, although these results are on the raw grey-level distribution and not filtered images as in the texture energy measure. Miller and Astley's results on texture energy suggest that the measure should give distinguishable values for fat and dense areas in many cases. They (and Laws) were using the measure for segmentation on a pixel-by-pixel basis.The system of averaging the results used here is clearly different. Nonetheless, one would expect a measure which produced good segmentations to give separable average values as well. This does not appear to be the case with these data. Using skewness instead of standard deviation as the macrostatistic in the texture energy measure had little effect.

The range of values of fractal dimension found in the patches was 2.13 - 2.30 (cf. 2.20 - 2.50 reported by Caldwell for the whole breast [3]). Calculating the fractal dimension of an image can be understood if the image is viewed as a three-dimensional surface with intensity as the third dimension. The fractal dimension indicates how the surface area depends on the size of the ruler used to measure it. A fractal model is only appropriate if the relationship between log(surface area) and log(ruler size) is linear. Caldwell quotes very high correlation coefficients. In the experiment reported here, although the values vary somewhat more widely, they are all above 0.984. This suggests that fractal dimension is a reasonable property to measure for these images. For this application, the separation it provides is intermediate.

Comparing automatic patch placement with measures applied to the whole breast shows that automatic placement is the more promising strategy. This could be because applying the measure to the whole breast would require a more accurate segmentation and a special treatment of the pectoral muscle.

The procedure developed by refining the automatic patch placement, given a rough initial segmentation, produces similar results to that employing a manually selected patch.

The selection of a segmentation threshold is the last remaining manual step, and is made necessary by shortcomings of the digitisation equipment. We have not tried to overcome this, since other investigators report success using global thresholds for rough segmentations [3]. An evaluation of this work using slightly better digitisations is in progress, and it appears that a threshold calculated from the grey-level histogram does segment the images adequately. If this evaluation is successful, the proven procedure will be fully automatic.

The choice of a threshold between the means carries the usual trade-off between sensitivity and specificity. In this application, the cost of a false negative is higher than that of a false positive. By choosing a conservative threshold (few dense images wrongly classified), a proportion of fatty images fall below the threshold. Nonetheless, the results indicate that nearly two-thirds of the fatty images could be reliably separated off. Given a frequency of 80% fatty images in the screening population, the resulting category (about half the total number of images) represents a very large number of mammograms.

In considering these positive results the following points should be borne in mind:

- **The images were all classified by the same two radiologists.**

    We acknowledge that the classification of mammograms may be subjective. Different radiologists might define the terms 'fatty' and 'dense' in subtly different ways. The two radiologists involved in this work agree with each other to a very great extent, but this may be because they are colleagues working in the same hospital. Our concern is not with the definitions of the terms, but with the hypothesis that sorting may make it possible to improve screening by differentially allocating difficult images to more experienced readers. A justification for the criterion used in sorting should come from a clinical test of this hypothesis.

- **No abnormalities were present.**

    This study used only images of normal breast tissue. Clearly abnormalities are present in the screening population; indeed their discovery is the purpose of the screening programme. In the context of this research, 'errors' which falsely classified abnormalities as regions of dense tissue would be entirely acceptable, even desirable. We are not aware of any malignant abnormality which would cause a dense breast to be classified as fatty. However, future work will take into account the response to abnormalities of any techniques which are developed.

7. Conclusions

We have investigated whether mammograms can be sorted into fatty and dense categories by a computerised procedure.

An operator based on grey-level skewness, measured over tiles within an automatically placed patch of the image, separates fatty from dense images.

The distributions of the measure for the two classes show that although the peaks are close together the means are distinct.

Given a frequency of 80% fatty images in the screening population, treating misclassification of dense images as the more serious error still allows a threshold to be set that classifies nearly half the total number of mammograms as fatty. If this category could be reliably screened by less experienced readers, the time saved by the most experienced radiologists would be considerable.

Future work will evaluate the procedure further and will investigate the hypothesis that computer-aided detection of abnormalities is also more tractable for fatty mammograms. If this is confirmed, the efficiency and reliability of screening procedures may be further improved.

8. Acknowledgements

This research was supported by the Imperial Cancer Research Fund and the Caisse Régionale d'Assurance Maladie d'Aquitaine.

We wish to thank George Holt for digitising the images, and John Fox, Peter Sasieni, Mike Michell and Ralph Highnam for helpful discussions.

9. Appendix: Definition Of Laws' Texture Energy

Laws defines a set of filters, each of which can be used to provide a texture energy measure. This experiment used the R5R5 filter. The *raw texture energy* is calculated by first convolving the image with the 5*5 filter. On the convolved image, the local variance in a 31*31 moving window is calculated. Separately, a map of local contrast values is obtained by convolving the original image with a smoothing filter (Laws' L5L5) and measuring the local variance of the resulting image with a 31*31 moving window. The *normalised texture energy* is computed by dividing values in the raw texture energy image by those in the map of local contrast values. The two filters are defined as follows:

Laws' R5 filter   [1   -4   6   -4   1]
Laws' L5 filter   [1   4   6   4   1]

The two-dimensional R5R5 filter is made by convolving R5 with itself, and similarly for the L5L5 filter.

This is the procedure followed by Miller and Astley to segment images. Since this study aims to classify images, the measure used was the mean normalised texture energy over the whole image patch.

10. References

1. Astley, S., Hutt, I., Adamson, S., Miller, P., Rose, P., Boggis, C. Taylor, C. Valentine, T., Davies, J. and Armstrong, J. Automation in Mammography: Computer Vision and Human Perception. *SPIE Biomedical Image Processing IV* (San Jose, Jan. 1993).

2. Altman, D. G. *Practical Statistics for Medical Research* (Chapman and Hall,

1991).

3. Caldwell, C. B., Stapleton, S. J., Holdsworth, D. W., Jong, R., Weiser, W., Cooke, G., and Yaffe, M. J. Characterization of Mammographic Parenchymal Pattern by Fractal Dimension. *SPIE Vol. 1092 Medical Imaging III: Image Processing*, **1092** (1989) 10-16.

4. Caseldine, J., Blamey, R., Roebuck, E., and Elston, C. *Breast Disease for Radiographers* (Butterworth, Wright imprint, 1988).

5. Chan, H.-P., Doi, K., Vyborny, C. J., Lam, K.-L., and Schmidt, R. A. Computer-Aided Detection of Microcalcifications in Mammograms: Methodology and Preliminary Clinical Study. *Investigative Radiology*, **23(9)** (1988) 664-671.

6. Davies, D. H., Dance, D. R., and Jones, C. H. Automatic Detection of Microcalcifications in Digital Mammograms Using Local Area Thresholding Techniques. *SPIE Vol. 1092 Medical Imaging III: Image Processing*, **1092** (1989) 153-159.

7. Du Buf, J. M. H., Kardan, M. and Spann, M. Texture Feature Performance for Image Segmentation. *Pattern Recognition*, **23(3/4)** (1990) 291-309.

8. Fam, B. W. and Olson, S. L. The Detection of Calcification Clusters in Film-Screen Mammograms: A Detailed Algorithmic Approach. *SPIE Vol. 914 Medical Imaging II*, **914** (1988) 620-634.

9. Feig, S., Shaber, G., Patchefsky, A., Schwartz, G., Edeiken, J., Libshitz, H., Nerlinger, R., Curley, R., and Wallace, J. Analysis of Clinically Occult and Mammographically Occult Breast Tumours. *American Journal of Roentgenology*, **128** (1977) 403-408.

10. Forrest, P. *Breast Cancer: the Decision to Screen.* Fourth H. M. Queen Elizabeth the Queen Mother Fellowship (Nuffield Provincial Hospitals Trust, 1990).

11. Haralick, R. M. Statistical Image Texture Analysis. In *Handbook of Pattern Recognition and Image Processing,* ed. T. Y. Young and K.-S. Fu (Academic Press, 1986).

12. Kimme-Smith, C., Frankl, G., Wassel, G., and Sklansky, J. Toward Reliable Measurements of Breast Parenchymal Patterns. *IEEE Computer Applications in Radiology and Analysis of Radiological Images*, **VI** (1979) 118-121.

13. Kimme-Smith, C., Dardashti, S. and Bassett, L.W. Glandular Tissue Contrast in CCD Digitized Mammograms. *SPIE Biomedical Image Processing IV* (San Jose, Jan. 1993).

14. Lau, T. K. and Bischof, W. T. Automated Detection of Breast Tumours using the Asymmetry Approach. *Computers and Biomedical Research*, **24** (1991) 273-295.

15. Law, J. Improved Image Quality for Dense Breasts in Mammography. *British Journal of Radiology*, **65(769)** (1992) 50-55.

16. Laws, K. I. Textured Image Segmentation. *Report 940* (University of Southern California Image Processing Institute, 1980).
17. Lundahl, T., Ohley, W. J., Kuklinski, W. S., Williams, D. O., Gewirtz, H., and Most, A. S. Analysis and Interpolation of Angiographic Images by Use of Fractals. *Conference on Computers in Cardiology* (1985) 355-358.
18. Magnin, I. E., Cluzeau, F., and Odet, C. L. Mammographic Texture Analysis: An Evaluation of Risk for Developing Breast Cancer. *Optical Engineering*, **25(6)** (1986) 780-784.
19. Miller, P. and Astley, S. Classification of Breast Tissue by Texture Analysis. *Image and Vision Computing*, **10(5)** (1992) 277-282.
20. *NHS Breast Screening Programme Review 1993* (NHS BSP Publications, Sheffield, UK, 1993).
21. Reed, T. R. and Du Buf, J. M. A Review of Recent Texture Segmentation and Feature Extraction Techniques. *CVGIP: Image Understanding*, **57(3)** (1993) 359-372.
22. Shadagopan, A., Alcorn, F. S., Semmlow, J. L., and Ackerman, L. V. Computerized Quantification of Breast Duct Patterns. *Radiology*, **143** (1982) 675-678.
23. Tabar, L. and Dean, P. B. Mammographic Parenchymal Patterns. Risk Indicator for Breast Cancer? *Journal of the American Medical Association*, **247(2)** (1982) 185-189.
24. Taylor P. A Study of Radiologists' Consistency in Judgements of Density *Internal Technical Report 163* (Advanced Computation Laboratory, Imperial Cancer Research Fund, London, UK, 1992).
25. Warner, E., Lockwood, G., Math, M., Tritchler, D., and Boyd, N. The Risk of Breast Cancer Associated with Mammographic Parenchymal Patterns: A Meta-Analysis of the Published Literature to Examine the effect of Method of Classification. *Cancer Detection and Prevention*, **16(1)** (1992) 67-72.
26. Warren, R. and Skrabanek, P. The Debate Over Mass Mammography in Britain. *British Medical Journal*, **297** (1988) 969-972.
27. Winsburg, F., Elkin, M., Macy, J., Bordaz, V., and Weymouth, W. Detection of Radiographic Abnormalities in Mammograms by Means of Optical Scanning and Computer Analysis. *Radiology*, **89** (1967) 211-215.
28. Wolfe, J. N. Breast Patterns as an Index of Risk for Developing Breast Cancer. *American Journal of Roentgenology*, **126** (1976) 1130-1139.
29. Wolfe, J. N. Breast Parenchymal Patterns and Their Changes With Age. *Radiology*, **121** (1976) 545-552.

COMPUTER-AIDED DETECTION AND DIAGNOSIS OF MASSES AND CLUSTERED MICROCALCIFICATIONS FROM DIGITAL MAMMOGRAMS

Robert M. Nishikawa, Maryellen L. Giger, Kunio Doi,
Carl J. Vyborny, Robert A. Schmidt

Kurt Rossmann Laboratories for Radiologic Image Research,
Department of Radiology, The University of Chicago, Chicago IL 60637

1. Introduction

We are developing an extensive package of computer-aided techniques to assist radiologists in diagnosing breast cancer from mammograms. This package includes computerized schemes for the automated detection and classification (benign versus malignant) of both clustered microcalcifications and breast masses, and techniques for identifying secondary indicators of breast cancer, such as skin thickening. Our ultimate goal is to develop an "intelligent" mammography workstation that would provide a "second opinion" to mammographers on a routine clinical basis. With such a workstation, computer-aided diagnosis (CAD) could become a clinical reality. We define CAD as a diagnosis made by a radiologist who uses the results of a computer analysis of the radiographic image in making a diagnosis. In all cases, the final diagnostic decision and recommendations for appropriate patient management are made by the radiologist. We believe that CAD can improve radiologists' accuracy by reducing the number of false negatives (i.e., missed diagnoses) and by improving the overall reproducibility of image interpretation.

This chapter reports on the research carried out at the University of Chicago for the development of computer-aided diagnosis in mammography, which we have reported on extensively in the literature.[1-25] The purpose of this chapter is to provide an overview of the different computerized schemes and how they will form a cohesive package. Figure 1 shows a flowchart showing the planned and existing connections among the various CAD schemes.

This chapter is based on a paper presented at the 1993 IS&T/SPIE Symposium on Electronic Imaging, held in San Jose in February, and the subsequent publication in the conference proceeding.[18] We have updated the contents of the proceedings paper and have added a discussion on three factors (other than the actual computer-vision techniques used) that affect the measured performance of CAD schemes -- namely, the method used to evaluate performance, the method used to score true and false detections, and the difficulty

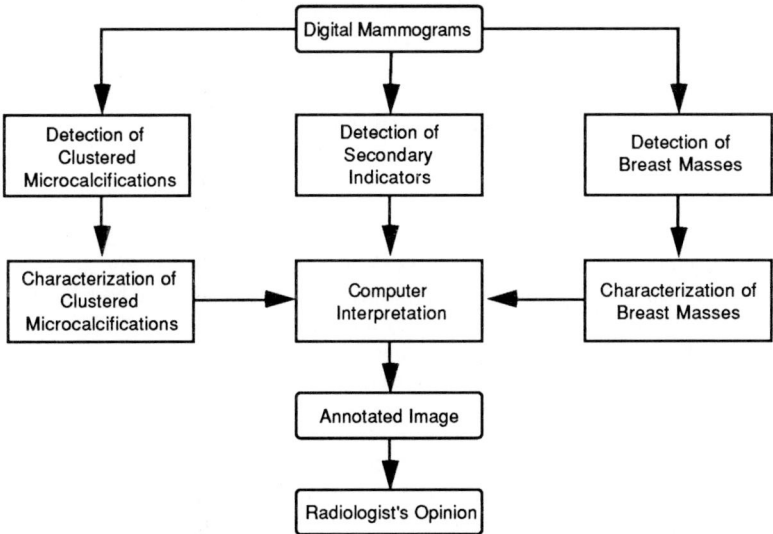

Figure 1. Overview of the computer-aided diagnostic schemes for detecting and classifying breast lesions.

of cases used in the evaluation. We begin with a description of our different CAD schemes.

2. Image Digitization and Breast Segmentation

Currently four films are digitized per case -- the cranio-caudal and the mediolateral-oblique views of the left and the right breasts. In the future, special view mammograms, such as spot compression films, will also be digitized. Currently, the images are digitized to a 0.1 mm pixel size with 10 bit resolution, so that an 8"x10" film contains 2048x2580 pixels.[26,27] For the mass detection scheme, the image is subsampled to a 512x512 matrix with effective pixel size of 0.4 mm. In the future, 0.05 mm pixel size will be used, particularly when determining the characteristics of microcalcifications.

The first step in the overall CAD scheme is the identification of the skinline,[8,22,24] which is used to segment the breast. A global thresholding is applied, followed by a morphological close operation. A tracking scheme is then used to trace the skinline. Once the skinline is known, the breast can be segmented. The two detection programs, which are described in the following two sections, analyze only the regions of the image that contain imaged breast tissue. We are currently investigating more efficient methods for outlining the border of the breast. Also, once the skinline has been identified, distortions in or thickening of the skin can be detected. Techniques to detect such possible secondary indicators of breast cancer are under development.[24]

3. Detection of Clustered Microcalcifications

3.1. Method

For the automated detection of clustered microcalcifications, we are developing a technique that consists of three basic steps, as shown in the flowchart in Fig. 2. First, the signal-to-noise ratio of microcalcifications is increased by suppressing the background structure of the breast. This is accomplished by matched filtering the image (3x3 pixel kernel) to enhance small signals, and subtracting from this enhanced image an image in which the signals have been suppressed by means of a box-rim filter (outer width 9 pixels, inner width 5 pixels).[1]

The second step, signal extraction, is accomplished in a series of three procedures. An initial global thresholding is used to set all but the 2% of the pixels with the highest pixel values to a background value of 512 (the average pixel value in the difference image).[1] Then a morphological erosion is performed using the structuring elements shown in Fig. 3.[5] This eliminates very small signals, 1 or 2 pixels in area, that are caused by image noise and not by actual microcalcifications. Finally, a local adaptive grey-level thresholding is applied to the processed image. The threshold value is chosen to be the mean pixel value (grey level) plus 3.4 times the standard deviation in the mean of a 5.1x5.1 mm region.[1] For evaluating the performance of the scheme, a range of multipliers from 3.0 to 4.0 is used in place of the value of 3.4. In this way, pairs of true-positive and false-positive rates are generated with which free-response receiver operating characteristic (FROC) curves[28-30] are created.

The third step is feature analysis, which is used to reduce the number of falsely identified signals. Three different techniques are used: texture analysis,[3] area-contrast analysis,[10,17] and a nonlinear clustering technique.[14] The texture analysis technique takes advantage of the change in the shape of the power spectrum of a local region when a microcalcification is present. In the texture analysis, the region around the signal of interest (6.4x6.4 mm) is first corrected to remove any low frequency trends in the background. This is done by fitting a polynomial of degree three to the ROI and then subtracting this fitted data from the original data in the ROI. As illustrated in Fig. 4, the presence of a microcalcification causes the first moment of the power spectrum to shift to a lower spatial frequency. Note that the spectrum for background contains more high frequency power than that for microcalcifications because of the presence of film granularity, which is the dominant source of high frequency noise in a mammogram.[31-33] We have found that the first moment of the power spectrum of a true microcalcification is generally less than 3.0 cycles/mm. Figure. 5 shows the distribution of the first moment of the power spectrum for true and false signals detected by the CAD scheme. A threshold value of 3.0 cycles/mm for

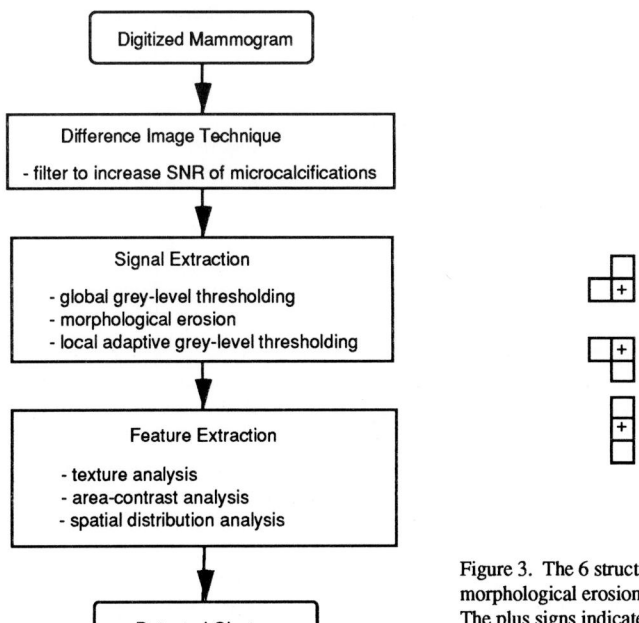

Figure 3. The 6 structuring elements used by the morphological erosion operator in the area filter. The plus signs indicate the operating point of the elements.

Figure 2. Flowchart of the automated scheme for detection of clustered microcalcification.

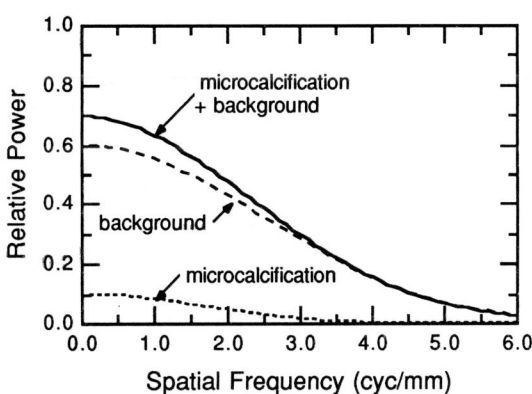

Figure 4. An illustration of how the presence of a microcalcification in an ROI shifts the first moment of the power spectrum to a lower value. The curve labeled background is the power spectrum of an ROI without a microcalcification present.

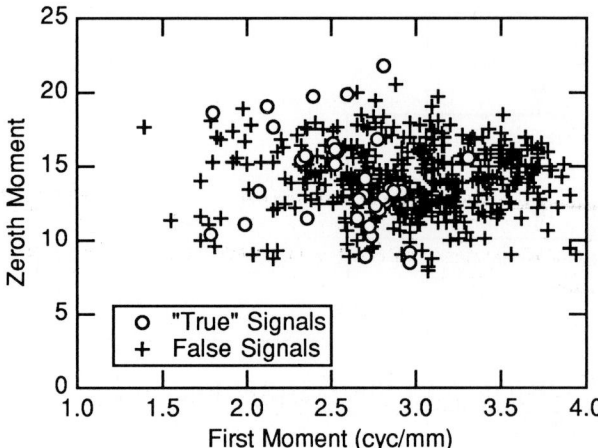

Figure 5. Distribution of the zeroth and the first moments of the power spectra of "true" and false signals. Above a first moment of 3.0 cycles/mm, there is only one true signal and approximately 200 false signals.

the first moment can eliminate approximately half of the false signals while keeping all but one true signal.

The second feature extraction technique compares the size (projected area) of a microcalcification with its radiation contrast. Region growing using a grey-level threshold value of 50% of the maximum pixel value in the signal is used to identify the size of the signal, as measured in pixels. The radiation contrast is calculated by correcting the measured radiographic contrast (measured by the difference in pixel value between the average signal pixel intensity and the average background pixel value in the area surrounding the signal) using the characteristic (H&D) curve of the screen-film system. Two types of false positives, i.e., film artifacts and image noise, can be removed using this technique. Film artifacts such as scratches on the original mammogram can lead to computer-detected false signals. These false signals, however, have a very high contrast for their small size compared to true microcalcifications.

The second types of false positives are those that have very low contrast and are caused by random fluctuations (noise) in the image. The reason noise in the image can lead to false detections can be understood by examining Fig. 6. Figure 6 shows a hypothetical example of two microcalcifications, one in a part of the breast with average thickness, and the other in a thick region of the breast. In terms of logarithmic x-ray intensity, both signals are easily identified above the background intensity level (left profile in Fig. 6). X-ray intensity, however, is converted in a nonlinear manner to film optical density, as characterized by the screen-film system's H&D curve (shown in the middle of Fig. 6). The

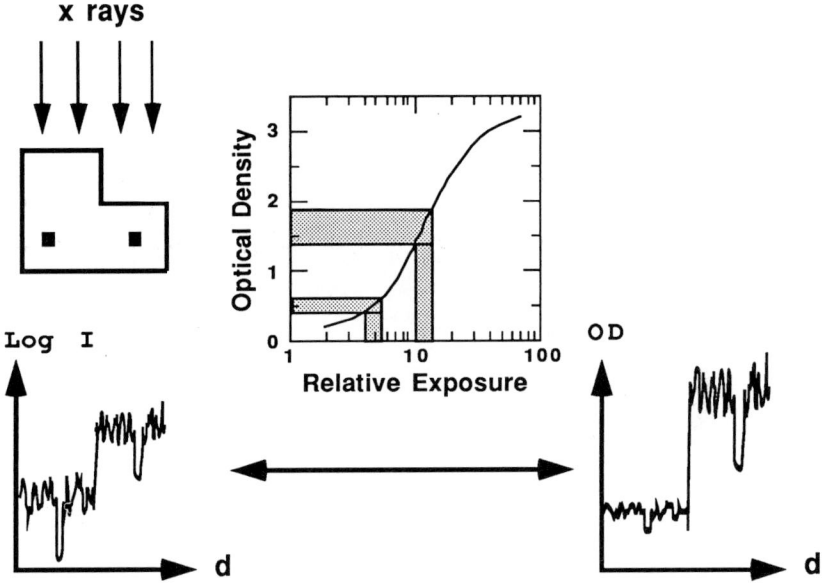

Figure 6. An illustration of the nonlinear conversion of x-ray exposure to film optical density. The noise fluctuations in the properly exposed region of the film can be as large as the difference in film density for the signal in the under exposed region of the film.

resulting distribution in optical density of the two microcalcifications is dependent on the background x-ray intensity. The signal in the low intensity region has a much lower contrast than the other signal. As a result, to set a global threshold to keep both signals, some noise fluctuations in the higher intensity region will also be included leading to possible false detections. By correcting for the H&D curve, both true signals will have appreciably higher contrast than the falsely detected noise signals. Therefore, by using both an upper and lower threshold, the number of false signals detected can be reduced. Correcting for the H&D curve is also used in a technique developed by Karssemeijer,[34] but he applies the correction as a preprocessing step and also takes into account image noise in the correction. We apply the correction only to detected signals, which is less time consuming computationally.

The third feature used to reduce the false-positive rate is the spatial distribution of signals within the cluster.[14] As shown in Fig. 7, the minimum distance between any two signals in a cluster tends to be smaller for true clusters than for false clusters. False signals are often caused by random noise in the image and therefore tend to be somewhat randomly

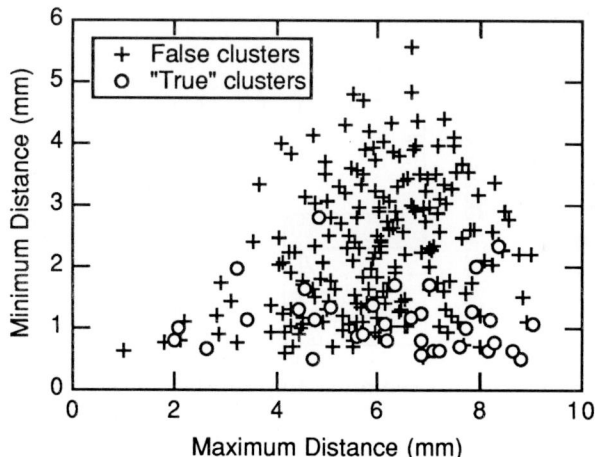

Figure 7. Distribution of the minimum and maximum distances between any two signals within a "true" or a false cluster. "True" clusters tend to be more closely packed than are computer-detected false clusters.

distributed. True clusters, however, are caused by some physiological process and thus tend to be quite localized (at least for clinically relevant clustered microcalcifications; scattered calcifications are not clinically relevant). To take advantage of this difference, we group the detected signals by passing a 3.2x3.2-mm square box over the processed image. Only if there are three or more signals within the box are these signals passed to the output image. Every point in the image is examined in this way. The resulting output image contains the detected clustered signals; scattered signals are rejected. The detected location of the clustered signals is indicated on the image with an arrow.

3.2. Performance

For this study, our database consisted of 78 screen-film mammograms -- half containing at least 1 cluster of microcalcifications (2 films had 2 clusters each) and the other half containing no clusters. All 39 films that contained clusters were sent to biopsy, except for 2 films that the radiologist felt were obviously benign. The x-y locations of the microcalcifications in all 78 images were determined by an experienced mammographer.

The 78 mammograms were chosen over a period of three years by two experienced mammographers as being representative of subtle cases. The 41 clusters had an average of 14.3 microcalcifications per cluster with a standard deviation of 12.0. The average area (size) of the microcalcifications was 8.8 pixels (equivalent to approximately a 0.3x0.3 mm

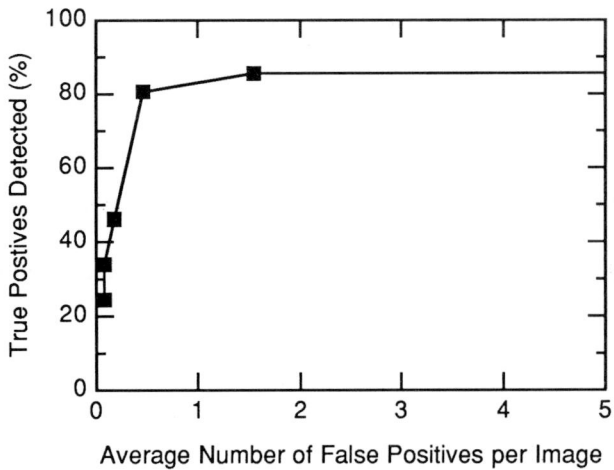

Figure 8. FROC curve for the clustered microcalcification scheme.

microcalcification) with a standard deviation of 7.8. The average contrast of the microcalcifications (measured as the difference in film optical density between the microcalcification and its background) was 0.11 with a standard deviation of 0.04.

These films were digitized to 0.1-mm square pixels and 10 bits using a Fuji drum scanner.[26] Both the scanning aperture and the scanning distance were 0.1 mm for this digitizer. Because of computer memory limitations, an 8x10 cm central region of the mammogram was analyzed. With an upgrade to a new computer, the full image can be analyzed.

For the 78 films in the database, the performance of our detection scheme is given by the FROC curve shown in Fig. 8. The scheme was able to identify 85% of the "true" clusters with about 1.5 false detections per image. It should be noted that the mean size and contrast of the microcalcifications in our database are smaller than those reported by other investigators. This is discussed in Section 7.1.

3.3. Application of Artificial Neural Networks to the Detection of Clusters

Recently, we have used an artificial neural network (ANN) to examine the computer-detected clusters in an effort to reduce further the false-positive rate.[12] The ANN used was a three-layer feed-forward network with 32x16 input units, 15 hidden units and 1 output unit. The input to the ANN were the power spectral values of the cluster (only half the power spectrum is used since it is symmetric). The power spectrum was calculated by taking the magnitude of the 2-dimensional Fourier transform of a 32x32 pixel region centered on the computer-detected cluster, which is either a true cluster or a false one. Before taking the Fourier transform of the region of interest (ROI), a polynomial of degree three is fitted to the ROI and these fitted data are subtracted from the original ROI.[35] This reduces low spatial frequency variations in the ROI.

In a preliminary study, a "jack-knife" method was used for training and testing using 56 ROIs containing "true" clusters and 56 ROIs containing computer-detected false clusters. The ANN was able to distinguish actual clustered microcalcifications from false-positive regions. Approximately 50% of the false clusters were removed, while preserving 95% of the true clusters.

Even more recently, we have tested a novel shift-invariant neural network as means for reducing the number of false positives detected.[25,36,37] The advantage of the shift-invariant neural network is that it can use the image data directly as input. The conventional neural network that we tested is not shift invariant and therefore power spectra were used as input to effectively "center" the cluster in the region of interest. Initial studies indicate that the shift-invariant neural network can eliminate 70% of the computer-detected false positive clusters without the loss of any true-detected clusters.[25]

4. Detection of Breast Masses

4.1. Method

For the automated detection of breast masses, we are developing a technique that identifies asymmetric densities between the right and left breasts,[4,8,13,22,23] since asymmetries indicate potential masses. An outline of the scheme used is shown in Fig. 9. The input to the computerized scheme, for a given patient, is a pair of mammograms -- left and right views of either the cranio-caudal or the medio-lateral-oblique view. After automatic registration of the left and right breast images,[8,22] a nonlinear subtraction technique is employed in which grey-level thresholding is performed on the individual mammograms prior to the subtraction. Ten thresholded images of both the left and right breasts are created using one of 10 different cutoff grey levels. The thresholds range from 5% to 50%, in increments of 5%, of the total area under the grey-level histogram of the particular mammogram. As an example, Fig. 10 shows the pixel value (average over a 10x10-pixel region) at the 10 different cutoff grey levels, for four different regions in a pair of mammograms. Next, the corresponding right and left breast images are subtracted to generate 10 bilateral-subtraction images. Runlength analysis is then used to combine the 10 pairs of images into a single pair of processed images, which contain locations of suspected masses for the left and right breasts.[8]

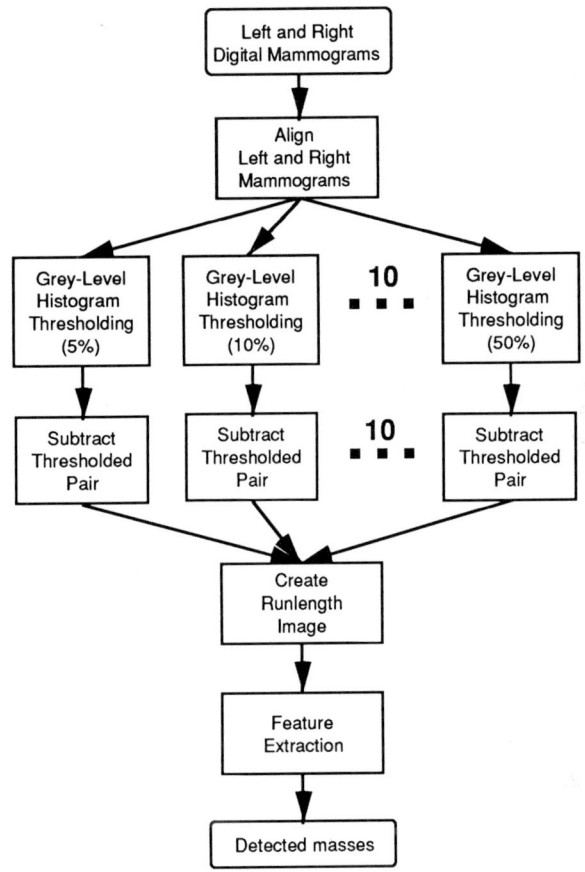

Figure 9. Overview of the automated scheme for the detection of breast masses.

    Runlength analysis is a linking process that accumulates the information from the set of 10 subtraction images into two images. Grey-level thresholding is applied to each of the ten subtraction images. Two thresholds, an upper and lower threshold, are applied simultaneously, since masses in the right breast will appear as black on grey and masses in the left breast will appear as white on grey. The two threshold levels are chosen so that 50% of the pixels above a grey level of 255 (the mean pixel value of the subtracted image) and 50% of the pixels below 255 will be eliminated. These 10 thresholded images are then linked through runlength analysis. For each pixel in the image, the number of non-zero

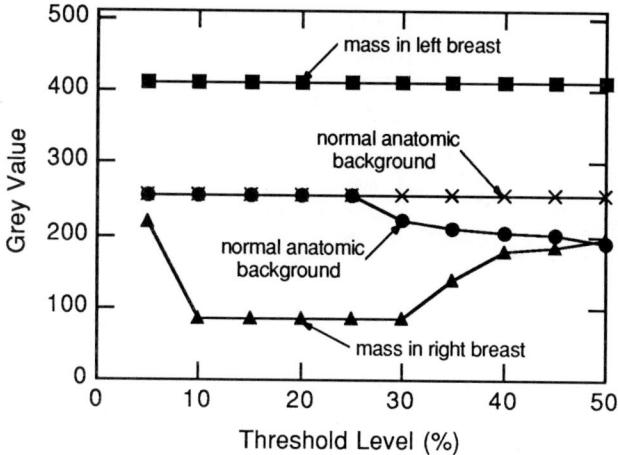

Figure 10. The grey-level variation in normal and abnormal regions of the subtracted breast images at different grey-level threshold values.

values in the 10 thresholded subtraction images are counted and stored in the runlength image. The two images, one for the right breast and one for the left, contain locations of potential masses. Finally a third threshold is applied, this time to the runlength image, and a threshold value of 5 is used. That is, if a pixel in the initial subtracted image appeared in at least 5 of the threshold images, then that pixel is retained in the final binary image. A final morphological operation (closing followed by opening using a square of 3x3 pixel structuring element) is performed to eliminate isolated pixels. The final images contain locations of possible breast masses.

Feature-analysis techniques are applied next to reduce the number of false detections.[23] Features of the potential masses include: size (area), circularity, contrast, and distance from border. The border test is used to eliminate detections of artifacts caused by slight misalignments of the right and left breasts. Minimum and maximum size criteria are imposed on both the processed image and the original digital mammogram. Circularity and contrast were derived from measurements using the original image. Using the location of potential masses in the runlength image as a template, region growing is used to segment the potential mass in the original image. Pairs of true and false positive rates were calculated by using 10 different cutoffs for the size criteria, from which an FROC curve was plotted. After the feature-analysis techniques, the results are used to annotate a copy of the original image with arrows indicating computer detected masses.

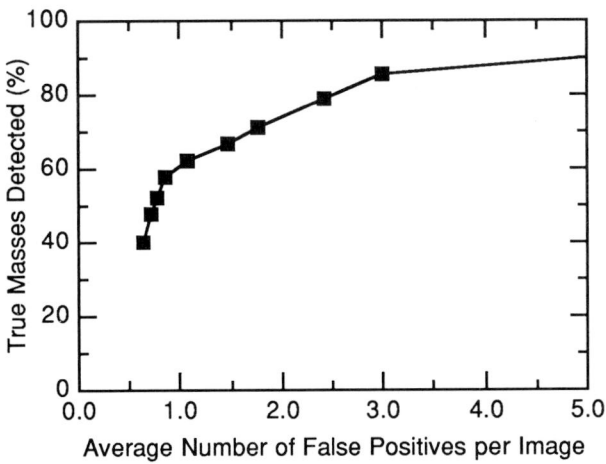

Figure 11. FROC curve for the mass detection scheme.

4.2. Performance

For this analysis, 154 pairs of clinical mammograms were used. Ninety pairs contained a single mass while the other 64 had no masses. The presence of a mass was verified from biopsy reports or clinical follow-up studies. The mean area of the masses was 19.5 pixels (which corresponds to a tumor slightly less than a 2 cm in diameter) with a standard deviation of 9.4. The mean contrast (measured as the difference in film optical density between the mass and its background) was 0.49 with a standard deviation of 0.25. Using this database, the FROC curve shown in Fig. 11 was generated. The mass detection scheme achieved a true-positive rate of approximately 85% with an average of 3.0 false-positive detections per image.

5. Classification of Breast Lesions

We are also applying an ANN to the decision-making task in mammography.[16] A three-layer, feed-forward neural network with a back-propagation algorithm was trained for the interpretation of mammograms on the basis of features extracted from mammograms by experienced radiologists. There were 14 input units, 5 hidden units and a single output unit. The 14 input features are listed in Table 1.

The ANN was trained and tested on 14 features extracted by experienced mammographers from 133 textbook cases and 60 clinical cases (obtained from our radiology department) for which biopsy proof was known. A modified round robin (or "leave-one-out") technique was used. That is, one of the clinical cases was removed and the 133 textbook cases and the remaining 59 clinical cases were used to train the network. Then the clinical case that was not in the training set was used for testing. This was repeated 60 times until the ANN was tested with all 60 clinical cases. The 14 features used in the analysis were selected from an initial number of 43. It remains to be seen whether these 14 features are the optimum choice.

Receiver operating characteristic (ROC) analysis was used to evaluate the performance of the ANN against the performance of radiologists.[38] Using the data shown in Fig. 12, the area under the ROC curve (A_z) was used as a measure of performance. The ANN had higher accuracy ($A_z = 0.89$) than either radiology residents ($A_z = 0.80$) or attending radiologists ($A_z = 0.84$). These differences were significant at the $P < 0.01$ level, for the 60 cases used in the test. From the ROC study measures of performance were obtained. The ANN was able to classify all malignant cases correctly (100% sensitivity) with a false-positive classification rate of 41%. This compares favorably to the average performance of radiologists who had a sensitivity of 89% at a false-positive classification rate of 60%.

At present the results of the ANN are very promising. However, the features of the mammograms that were used as input to the ANN were based on radiologists' subjective

Table 1. The 14 radiographic features used as input to the artificial neural network for classifying breast lesions.

Density-Related Features	Microcalcification-Related Features	Secondary Features
- number of spiculations	- rounded to irregular	- subtlety of distortion
- length of spiculations	- presence of linear microcalcifications	- distortion definable on two views
- difference between spicules and local linear features	- microcalcifications elsewhere in breast	- presence of similar pattern elsewhere in breast
- presence of well-defined lucencies	- presence of branched calcifications	
- opacity relative to size	- shape of cluster (geometric to irregular) - radiation of microcalcifications along duct	

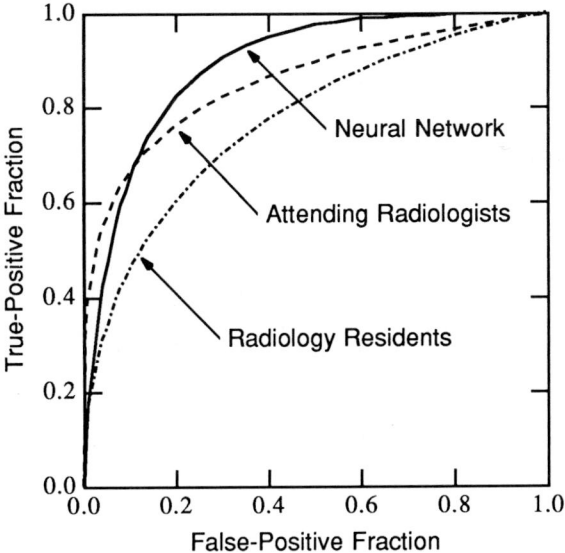

Figure 12. Comparison of the performance of attending radiologists, radiology residents, and of a neural network for distinguishing between benign and malignant cases.

ratings of 14 different radiographic features, which reduces the ANN's clinical utility. Therefore, we are developing computer-vision techniques to extract the relevant features.[4,17] Initial work on characterizing the degree of spiculation of masses and the variation of size and contrast of microcalcifications within a cluster have shown promise as measures capable of distinguishing benign from malignant lesions.

6. "Intelligent" Mammography Workstation

We are developing an "intelligent" workstation[6,19,20] that will consist of a high-speed computer, four 2kx2k CRT monitors, a film digitizer and a high-volume local storage device. The workstation will be placed in the mammography reading area of our radiology department. It will offer radiologists a "second opinion" on mammograms that they are reading.

At present, and at least for the near future, radiologists will still do their primary interpretation from film on a view box, but will have the results of the computer analysis available either on a CRT monitor or on hardcopy (film). The computer output will contain arrows indicating suspicious areas identified by the computer. Each arrow will have associated with it a number indicating the computer's estimate of the probability that the lesion is malignant. Initially, only arrows indicating suspicious regions will be available to the radiologists, as the computer schemes for classification are still at an early stage of development. We expect that, after a few months of use, we will have enough preliminary results to design and to conduct a controlled clinical study to measure the efficacy of CAD in mammography.

7. Discussions

There are many factors that can influence the measured performance of automated detections scheme. Perhaps the three most important are: (1) the cases used for testing, (2) the method used for scoring, and (3) the method used for evaluating performance.

7.1. Case Selection

Intuitively, the accuracy of a CAD scheme is inversely related to the percentage of difficult or subtle cases in the database. In principle, therefore, any accuracy from 0 to 100% is possible depending on the nature of the database. However, investigators, who are developing CAD schemes, each have their own database, which is not only different from other databases, but may contain different proportions of subtle cases and obvious cases. As a result, comparison of performance of different techniques may not be valid if different cases were used in the evaluation.[21] As an example of the effect that case selection can have on measured performance, Fig 13 shows FROC curves for our mass detection scheme for three different testing databases. The scheme is identical for each curve, only the testing cases varied -- from cases containing only small size masses to cases containing only large masses. Clearly, when testing the scheme with cases containing large (somewhat obvious) masses a superior performance can be measured compared to testing with cases containing (subtle) small masses.

Meaningful comparisons of different schemes require that the testing databases either be the same or be matched in difficulty by some objective method. Currently, neither option is available or practiced. A minimum solution to this problem would be for investigators to report physical measures of lesion characteristics such as mean and standard deviation of size and contrast. This would allow a qualitative estimate of the degree of difficulty of the testing cases to be made.

For example, two other investigators have reported extremely good performance (95-100% sensitivity with 0.1 false positive clusters per image) for their computerized schemes for the detection of clustered microcalcifications. While this is better than our scheme's measured performance, different cases were used in testing the three different schemes. The average size of the microcalcifications in our testing database was 0.3 mm with an average contrast (in terms of difference in optical density) of 0.12. Fam *et al.*[39]

stated that the microcalcifications in their database had an average contrast of 0.4, and although they did not give the size of microcalcifications, the pixel size in their images was 0.2 mm suggesting that the microcalcifications must have been significantly larger than 0.2 mm. Based on values of different parameters used by Davies and Dance,[40] the microcalcifications in their database ranged from 0.2 mm to 1.6 mm in size with a contrast ranging from 0.2 to over 1.0. Therefore, we believe that the differences in performance between our computer scheme and others' are due to the much more subtle nature of the cases used in testing our scheme.

7.2. Scoring Method

There is no universal scoring method currently in use. The criterion used for determining a true detection from a false one varies between investigators. We used different criteria for our two different detection schemes. For the clustered microcalcification scheme, a computer detection was scored as a true detection if the center of mass of the true cluster and the computer detected cluster were within 6 mm and that the computer detected at least one true microcalcification. For the scheme to detect masses, initially the computer detection was considered correct if there was at least one pixel in common between the true and computer-detected mass. These are arbitrary rules with the former being perhaps too strict and the latter somewhat lenient.

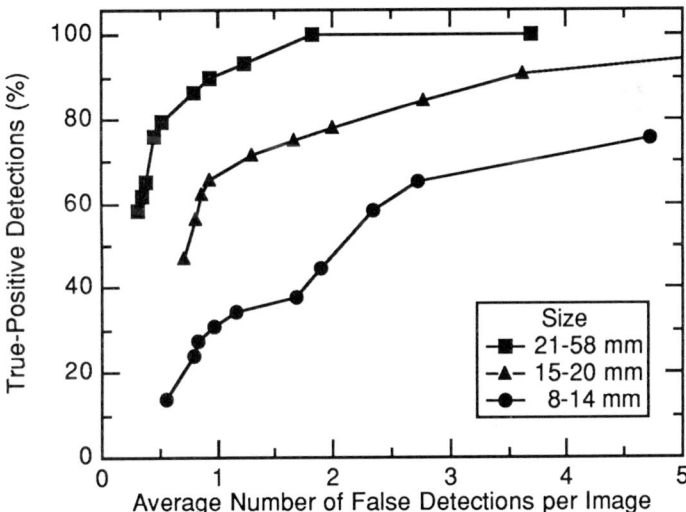

Figure 13. FROC curves for the mass detection scheme for three different testing databases based on the size of the mass.

The scoring method should take into consideration the objective of the detection scheme. For our schemes, the goal is to alert radiologists to suspicious areas on the mammogram. Therefore, the computer-detected lesion need only be "close" to the actual lesion such that when the radiologist scrutinizes the area containing the computer-detected lesion, the true lesion can be seen (i.e., it is within the radiologist's concentrated field of view). Requiring that the computer detect at least one true microcalcification to be correct is not necessarily necessary, since as long as the computer detected cluster is close enough to the true cluster (they could in fact overlap), the radiologist will "see" the true cluster and the scheme will have fulfilled its purpose. Also, clustered microcalcifications are clinically important, while isolated calcifications are not. Therefore, scoring the scheme by its ability to accurately detect individual microcalcifications is not addressing the clinical situation.

Because there is no accepted method for scoring, investigators should explicitly state how they scored true and false detections.

7.3. Performance Evaluation Method

There are several different methods currently employed to evaluate the performance of a detection scheme. In our laboratory, we use receiver operating characteristic (ROC) analysis[38] and other associated measures such as FROC analysis.[28-30] We believe that these are appropriate measures, because generally for all schemes there will be a tradeoff between sensitivity and false-positive rate. A scheme with a high sensitivity and a high false positive rate may have the same accuracy as a scheme with moderate sensitivity and moderate false-positive rate. That is, the two schemes could have the same FROC curves, but different points on the curve may be used to report sensitivity and false-positive rate. Therefore, reports of just sensitivity and false-positive rate makes comparison of different schemes difficult.

8. Summary

We are developing an "intelligent" workstation to assist radiologists' interpretation of mammograms. The "intelligence" of the workstation is derived from a group of interconnected computer detection and classification schemes. Currently, our detection schemes have a sensitivity of 85% for the detection of masses and microcalcifications, with false-positive detection rates of 3.0 false masses per image and 1.5 false clusters per image. Running on an IBM Powerstation 560, the mass detection program requires approximately 17 s to analyze a pair of mammograms, while the cluster detection program takes approximately 30 s for a single film. We have also developed an ANN for the classification of breast lesions that in initial testing had a sensitivity of 100% with a specificity of 60%. Currently we are developing techniques to extract, from the lesions identified by our detection schemes, the 14 radiographic characteristics that are used by the ANN. The classification schemes are still at an early stage of development. However, the two detection schemes, particularly the microcalcification detection scheme, are at a sufficiently high level of performance to undergo preliminary clinical testing, which will be conducted in the near future.

9. Acknowledgments

Over the past seven years, many individuals have contributed to the work reported here. We acknowledge the contributions of H-P. Chan, K. Lam, H. MacMahon, S. Galhotra, Y. Ogura, and P.M. Jokich during the initial phases of the projects; the more recent contributions of F-F. Yin, Y. Wu, Y. Jiang, U. Bick, W. Zhang, T. Ema, Z. Huo, R.H. Nagel, P. Lu, J. Papaioannou, and S. Cox; and the continuing contributions of C.E. Metz. This work was supported by the Whitaker Foundation, the American Cancer Society (FRA 390), and USPHS grants CA 48985, CA 09649, and CA 24806.

10. References

1. H.-P. Chan, K. Doi, S. Galhotra, C. J. Vyborny, H. MacMahon and P. M. Jokich, "Image feature analysis and computer-aided diagnosis in digital radiography. 1. Automated detection of microcalcifications in mammography," Med. Phys. 14, 538-548 (1987).
2. H.-P. Chan, K. Doi, C. J. Vyborny, K. L. Lam and R. A. Schmidt, "Computer-aided detection of microcalcifications in mammograms: Methodology and preliminary clinical study," Invest. Radiol. 23, 664-671 (1988).
3. H.-P. Chan, K. Doi, C. J. Vyborny, R. A. Schmidt, C. Metz, K. Lam, T. Ogura, Y. Wu and H. MacMahon, "Improvement in radiologists' detection of clustered microcalcifications on mammograms: The potential of computer-aided diagnosis.," Invest. Radiol. 25, 1102-1110 (1990).
4. M. L. Giger, F.-F. Yin, K. Doi, C. E. Metz, R. A. Schmidt and C. J. Vyborny, "Investigation of methods for the computerized detection and analysis of mammographic masses," Proc. SPIE 1233, 183-184 (1990).
5. R. M. Nishikawa, K. Doi, M. L. Giger, H. Yoshimura, Y. Wu, C. J. Vyborny and R. A. Schmidt, "Use of morphological filters in the computerized detection of microcalcifications in digitized mammograms," Med. Phys. 17, 524 (1990).
6. M. L. Giger, R. M. Nishikawa, K. Doi, F.-F. Yin, C. J. Vyborny, R. A. Schmidt, C. E. Metz, Y. Wu, H. MacMahon and H. Yoshimura, "Development of a "smart" workstation for use in mammography," Proc. SPIE 1445, 101-103 (1991).
7. R. M. Nishikawa, M. L. Giger, K. Doi, C. J. Vyborny and R. A. Schmidt, "Computer-aided detection of microcalcifications in digital mammograms," Image Technology and Information Display 23, 1092-1096 (1991).
8. F.-F. Yin, M. L. Giger, K. Doi, C. E. Metz, C. J. Vyborny and R. A. Schmidt, "Computerized detection of masses in digital mammograms: Analysis of bilateral-subtraction images," Med. Phys. 18, 955-963 (1991).

9. M. L. Giger, Future of breast imaging. Computer-aided diagnosis, in Syllabus: Categorical Course in Physics. Technical Aspects of Breast Imaging, A. Haus and M. J. Yaffe, ed. (Radiological Society of North America, Oak Brook, IL, 1992) pp 257-270.
10. Y. Jiang, R. M. Nishikawa, M. L. Giger, K. Doi, C. J. Vyborny and R. A. Schmidt, "Method of extracting microcalcifications' signal area and signal thickness from digital mammograms," Proc. SPIE 1778, 28-36 (1992).
11. R. M. Nishikawa, Y. Jiang, M. L. Giger, K. Doi, C. J. Vyborny and R. A. Schmidt, "Computer-aided detection of clustered microcalcifications," Proceedings of IEEE International Conference on Systems, Man, and Cybernetics 2, 1375-1378 (1992).
12. Y. Wu, K. Doi, M. L. Giger and R. M. Nishikawa, "Computerized detection of clustered microcalcifications in digital mammograms: Applications of artificial neural networks," Med. Phys. 19, 555-560 (1992).
13. F.-F. Yin, M. L. Giger, C. J. Vyborny, K. Doi and R. A. Schmidt, "Comparison of bilateral-subtraction and single-image processing techniques in the computerized detection of mammographic masses," Invest. Radiol. 28, 473-481 (1993).
14. R. M. Nishikawa, M. L. Giger, K. Doi, C. J. Vyborny and R. A. Schmidt, "Computer-aided detection of clustered microcalcifications: An improved method for grouping detected signals," Med. Phys. (accepted for publication, 1993).
15. R. M. Nishikawa, M. L. Giger, K. Doi, C. J. Vyborny and R. A. Schmidt, "Computer-aided detection of microcalcifications on digital mammograms," Medical and Biological Engineering and Computing (accepted for publication, 1993).
16. Y. Wu, M. L. Giger, K. Doi, C. J. Vyborny, R. A. Schmidt and C. E. Metz, "Artificial neural networks in mammography: Application to decision making in the diagnosis of breast cancer," Radiology 187, 81-87 (1993).
17. R. M. Nishikawa, Y. Jiang, M. L. Giger, C. J. Vyborny, R. A. Schmidt and U. Bick, "Characterization of the Mammographic Appearance of Microcalcifications: Applications in Computer-Aided Diagnosis," Proc. SPIE 1898, (in press, 1993).
18. R. M. Nishikawa, M. L. Giger, K. Doi, C. J. Vyborny, R. A. Schmidt, C. E. Metz, Y. Wu, F.-F. Yin, Y. Jiang, Z. Huo, P. Lu, W. Zhang, T. Ema, U. Bick, J. Papaioannou and R. H. Nagel, "Computer-aided detection and diagnosis of masses and clustered microcalcifications from digital mammograms," Proc. SPIE 1905, (in press, 1993).
19. M. L. Giger, K. Doi, H. MacMahon, R. M. Nishikawa, K. R. Hoffmann, C. J. Vyborny, R. A. Schmidt, H. Jia, K. Abe, X. Chen, A. Kano, S. Katsuragawa, F.-F. Yin, N. Alperin, C. E. Metz, F. M. Behlen and D. Sluis, "An "intelligent" workstation for computer-aided diagnosis," RadioGraphics 13, 647-656 (1993).
20. M. L. Giger, R. M. Nishikawa, R. A. Schmidt, C. J. Vyborny, P. Lu, Y. Jiang, Z. Huo, J. Papaioannou, Y. Wu, S. Cox and K. Rosculet, "Preliminary evaluation of an intelligent mammography workstation," Proc. SPIE 1898, (in press, 1993).
21. R. M. Nishikawa, M. L. Giger, K. Doi, F.-F. Yin, C. J. Vyborny and R. A. Schmidt, "Effect of case selection on the performance of computer-aided detection schemes," Med. Phys. (submitted, 1992).

22. F.-F. Yin, M. L. Giger, K. Doi, C. J. Vyborny and R. A. Schmidt, "Computerized detection of masses in digital mammograms: Automated alignment of breast images and its effect on bilateral-subtraction technique," Med. Phys. (submitted, 1992).
23. F.-F. Yin, M. Giger, C. Metz, K. Doi, C. Vyborny and R. Schmidt, "Computerized detection of masses in digital mammograms: Investigation of feature-extraction techniques," Journal of Digital Imaging (in press, 1993).
24. U. Bick, M. L. Giger, Z. Huo, R. A. Schmidt, K. Doi, R. M. Nishikawa and C. J. Vyborny, Automated Detection of Skin Thickening in Mammograms, in CAR'93 Computer Assisted Radiology, H. U. Lemke, K. Inamura, C. C. Jaffe and R. Felix, ed. (Springer-Verlag, Berlin, 1993) pp 461-465.
25. W. Zhang, K. Doi, M. L. Giger, R. M. Nishikawa and Y. Wu, "Computerized detection of clustered microcalcifications in digital mammograms using a shift-invariant artificial neural network," Med. Phys. (submitted, 1993).
26. M. Ishida, H. Kato, K. Doi and P. H. Frank, "Development of a new digital radiographic image processing system," Proc. SPIE 347, 42-48 (1982).
27. F.-F. Yin, M. L. Giger, K. Doi, H. Yoshimura, X.-W. Xu and R. M. Nishikawa, "Evaluation of imaging characteristics of a laser film digitizer," Physics and Medicine in Biology 37, 273-280 (1992).
28. P. C. Bunch, J. F. Hamilton, G. K. Sanderson and A. H. Simmons, "A free response approach to the measurement and characterization of radiographic observer performance," Proc. SPIE 127, 124-135 (1977).
29. D. Chakraborty, "Maximum likelihood analysis of free-response receiver operating characteristic (FROC) data," Med. Phys. 16, 561-568 (1989).
30. D. Chakraborty, "Free-response methodology: Alternate analysis and a new observer-performance experiment," Radiology 174, 873-881 (1990).
31. G. T. Barnes and D. P. Chakraborty, "Radiographic mottle and patient exposure in mammography," Radiology 145, 815-821 (1982).
32. R. M. Nishikawa and M. J. Yaffe, "Signal-to-noise properties of mammographic film-screen systems," Med. Phys. 12, 32-39 (1985).
33. P. C. Bunch, K. E. Huff and R. Van Metter, "Analysis of the detective quantum efficiency of a radiographic film-screen combination," J. Opt. Soc. Am. A 4, 902-909 (1987).
34. N. Karssemeijer and L. van Earning, "Iso-precision scaling of digitized mammograms to facilitate image analysis," Proc. SPIE 1444, 166-177 (1991).
35. S. Katsuragawa, K. Doi and H. MacMahon, "Image feature analysis and computer-aided diagnosis in digital radiography: Detection and characterization of interstitial lung disease in digital chest radiographs," Med. Phys. 15, 311-319 (1988).
36. W. Zhang, K. Itoh, J. Tanida and Y. Ichioka, "Parallel distributed processing model with local space-invariant interconnections and its optical architecture," Applied Optics 29, 4790-4797 (1990).
37. W. Zhang, A. Hasegawa, K. Itoh and Y. Ichioka, "Image processing of human corneal endothelium based on a learning network," Applied Optics 30, 4211-4217 (1991).

38. C. E. Metz, "ROC methodology in radiologic imaging," Invest. Radiol. 21, 720-733 (1986).
39. B. W. Fam, S. L. Olson, P. F. Winter and F. J. Scholz, "Algorithm for the detection of fine clustered calcifications on film mammograms," Radiology 169, 333-337 (1988).
40. D. H. Davies and D. R. Dance, "Automatic computer detection of clustered calcifications in digital mammograms," Phys. Med. Biol. 35, 1111-1118 (1990).

MAMMOGRAM SCREENING USING MULTIRESOLUTION-BASED IMAGE SEGMENTATION

D. Brzakovic and M. Neskovic
Department of Electrical Engineering and Computer Science
Lehigh University
Bethlehem, Pa 18015

Abstract

This paper describes the design, implementation, and testing of an adaptive digital image segmentation method that detects cancerous changes in mammograms and can potentially aid medical experts in establishing the diagnosis. The essence of the method is hierarchical region growing that uses pyramidal multiresolution image representation. The relationships between pixels at different resolution levels are established using a fuzzy membership function, thus enabling detection of very small and/or low contrast objects in a highly textured background. The selection of the parameters of the fuzzy membership function allows for fine-tuning the method to specific segmentation objectives. This paper discusses two versions of the method: the first is aimed at the detection of microcalcifications and the second at the detection of benign and malignant nodules. The two versions are fully automated and differ in the procedure applied to automatically select the appropriate parameters of the fuzzy membership function. Both versions were evaluated in two ways: (i) using synthetically generated objects superimposed on normal mammograms and (ii) using mammogram images for which the corresponding truth images were generated by human experts. The objective of the first evaluation was to precisely determine the method's capabilities and its sensitivity to object size, shape, and contrast. The objective of the second evaluation was to establish the method's usefulness in helping medical experts to establish the diagnosis.

1. Introduction

Breast cancer is currently the second cause (next to lung cancer) of cancer-related mortality in the female population [4],[12]. It is estimated that 150,000 new cases of breast cancer were detected in 1990 and 44,000 deaths were caused by it in the same year in the USA [4]. It is also predicted that these numbers will increase in the future [17]. Early detection of breast cancer is the key to successful treatment and reduction of mortality. Consequently, routine mammograms are recommended for a large percentage of the female population as the most reliable detection method. On average, a mammogram can detect breast cancer two years before it is palpable. Studies have shown that properly administered mammograms can reduce the overall mortality from breast cancer in specific groups of the population by 30%. Consequently, NCI has chosen breast cancer screening as one of its high priorities for the year 2000. One of the major obstacles towards achieving this goal is the high cost of the procedure. Part of this cost is associated with mammogram readings, which are performed by highly skilled experts. Considering that typically there are four mammograms associated with an individual, a viable means of reducing this cost is to replace part of the manual readings by automated, computer-based mammogram analysis. In addition, automation offers consistency in performance since it is not subject to fatigue.

Automated mammogram analysis has attracted considerable attention in recent years. Due to the complexity of the problem, researchers have considered specific subproblems, emphasizing mammogram enhancement [11],[18],[20],[22], [25], [26], detection of microcalcifications [9],[10],[16] , and detection of particular classes of tumors [14],[21]. Rudimental studies have been done in designing and implementing complete expert systems for mammogram analysis, e.g., [2],[6]. These studies have shown that automated mammogram screenings are feasible in the near future.

This paper details an image segmentation method that pre-screens mammograms and separates them into two groups: those containing potential cancerous signs and those containing no suspicious signs. The mammograms in the first group are segmented into "suspicious regions" and normal tissue, thus drawing the attention of the human expert to specific regions in the mammogram. In the present form, the method detects microcalcifications and nodules (benign and malignant).

The heart of the method is multiresolution image segmentation, which allows, similarly to human perception, comprehension of the global structure of a mammogram (normal tissue) followed by search for fine detail (abnormality). The relationships between pixels at different resolution levels are established using the notion of "fuzzy links". The selection of the function modeling fuzzy links and the selection of specific parameters of this function determine the size and contrast of the objects that the method detects. The paper details two versions of the method: the first version searches for the presence of microcalcifications and the second for the presence of nodules (benign or malignant). Both of the versions are fully automated, and the difference between the two is in the automated selection of segmentation parameters.

The performance of the method in both cases was evaluated in two ways. First, the performance was evaluated using synthetically generated objects superimposed on normal mammograms. This allowed us to measure objectively the capabilities of the method to detect objects of low contrast and small size. Next, the performance was evaluated on mammograms for which the truth images were generated by human experts. In both cases the primary concern was that the method always detects potential cancerous signs considered (assuming that these cancerous signs are visible). The secondary concern was that the method minimizes false alarms.

The paper is organized as follows. Section 2 describes the proposed multiresolution segmentation method. Section 3 describes the two versions of the method which detect microcalcifications and nodules, respectively. Section 4 describes the performance evaluation, starting with synthetic object generation, followed by a summary of the results.

2. Texture Image Segmentation

Ideally the segmentation of mammograms should yield two regions: potentially cancerous changes and normal tissue. Variations within the limits of normality of highly textured breast tissue pose the basic obstacle in achieving this objective. Cancerous changes may be very subtle, be of low contrast, and have hazy borders. Consequently, the cancerous changes are frequently less visible than the variations in the normal tissue.

Highly textured backgrounds in mammograms dictate the selection of image segmentation methods that are successful in dealing with texture regions and precludes the selection of simpler methods, such as edge detection. Guided by our previous experience with texture segmentation, we have chosen multiresolution pyramid-based image segmentation as the basis of our present work. Specifically, the work described in this paper is based on *the fuzzy pyramid linking method* that we proposed earlier for detection of fine detail in complex texture background [5]. This method has shown promise in segmenting low resolution mammograms containing large tumors, as described in [6]. In the present paper we have modified fuzzy pyramid linking to detect subtle intensity changes and small detail (microcalcification).

This section describes the fuzzy pyramid linking method. First, the notion of pyramids and pyramid linking is briefly described in Sections 2.1.1 and 2.1.2, respectively. Next, the details of fuzzy pyramid linking and the role of specific parameters are discussed in Section 2.2. Section 3 details the modifications and utilization of the method for the segmentation of mammograms.

2.1 Pyramid-based Image Segmentation

The segmentation methods employing pyramids are in essence hierarchical region growing methods that use efficient multiresolution image representation. In the following section we review common characteristics of many methods that fall into this category.

2.1.1 Image Pyramids

An image pyramid is a convenient and efficient representation of an image at multiple resolutions. It is created by using the original image I_0 of dimensions $2^n \times 2^n$ as the base of the pyramid. Each subsequent level of the pyramid, $I_1 \ldots I_n$, is a square array which is half the dimension of its predecessor. These arrays are lower resolution representations of the original image. The top level I_n of the pyramid is a 1×1 array. An element (node) of the array I_l ($l > 0$) is obtained by a weighted averaging of the I_{l-1} nodes within a $k \times k$ neighborhood. A pyramid is created using a specific weighting scheme. Subsequently, a pyramid may be redefined using an algorithm. This section discusses pyramid creation, and Section 2.1.2 reviews algorithms for redefining pyramid structures.

The selection of different weighting schemes for pyramid creation yields different types of pyramids. A convenient approach to choosing weights is to use a Gaussian weighted averaging technique. The image pyramid thus created is known as a Gaussian pyramid [7]. We have utilized the Gaussian pyramid in this work and the following discussion is limited to this pyramid; more general discussion on pyramids can be found in [1].

The creation of each level, I_l, $l = 1, 2, ..., n$, in the Gaussian pyramid is obtained by convolving the image one level below, I_{l-1}, with a 4×4 Gaussian mask $w(p,q)$; therefore, an element at location (i,j) at level l is created from elements at level $l-1$ using

$$I_l(i,j) = \sum_{p=-2}^{2} \sum_{q=-2}^{2} w(p,q) I_{l-1}(2i + p - \frac{p}{2|p|} + \frac{1}{2}, 2j + q + \frac{1}{2} - \frac{q}{2|q|}) \text{ for } p,q \neq 0. \quad (1)$$

Our implementation is based on the idea of the Hierarchical Discrete Correlation (HDC) [8]. Among various implementations of HDC involving odd or even neigbourhoods we have chosen the even neighbourhood size. The selection was made based on the fact that the even neighbourhood: (i) requires fewer calculations (computations are carried out over neighbourhood 4×4, rather than 5×5), and (ii) offers advantages in linking procedures. The reduced size pyramid is generated by retaining every second pixel at each of the levels. The relationships between pixels at different levels of the pyramid for 1-D case are shown in Figure 1. The extension to a 2-D case is straightforward. It should be noted that the Gaussian mask must be separable, normalized, and symmetric [7].

2.1.2 Pyramid Linking

Linking is the process by which nodes belonging to a given level of the pyramid are connected with nodes at adjacent levels, i.e., links establish relationships between pixels at different resolutions. Links are first used to redefine the pyramid iteratively and then to segment the image by replacing the nodes at level $l-1$ by the nodes at level l.

Since each Gaussian pyramid level is created by convolving the 4×4 weight mask with the preceding level of the pyramid, there exists a predetermined spatial relationship between nodes at two adjacent levels. From Equation (1) it follows that each node at level l, $l > 0$, has a 4×4 array of candidate child nodes at level $l-1$. Conversely, for each node at level l, $l < n-1$, there exists a 2×2 array of candidate parent nodes at level $l+1$. The links are established for all child nodes in the pyramid starting with the base of the pyramid and using a chosen link algorithm.

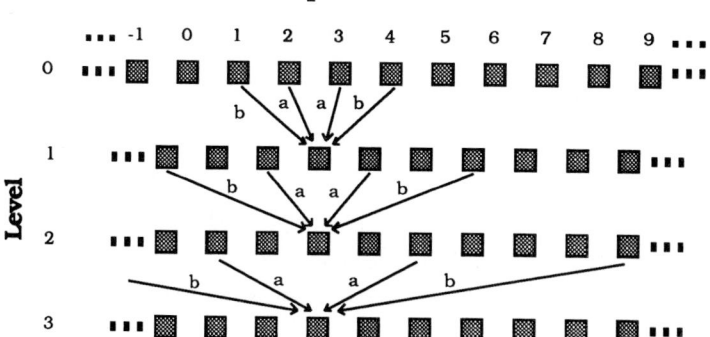

Figure 1: Even Hierarchical Discrete Correlation in a 1-D case. Relationships between successive levels of pyramid. Values a and b denote weights of the Gaussian mask.

The pyramid is redefined iteratively and new links are determined. The pyramid structure converges once the links within the pyramid stabilize.

Image segmentation can be achieved upon convergence by mapping the lower resolution image at the apex of the pyramid onto the original image at the base of the pyramid by following the linking paths through the intermediate levels. This form of segmentation by hierarchical region growing results in a number of regions equal to or less than the number of nodes at the apex of the pyramid, provided that there are no constraints limiting the propagation of the apex nodes to the base of the pyramid.

Various algorithms have been proposed for linking nodes at adjacent levels of the pyramid. Some of the proposed algorithms link a child node to the parent node that is the most similar based on a chosen property, e.g., intensity. These algorithms are frequently referred to as hard linking. In this paper, we propose a different algorithm where a child node is linked to all four candidate parent nodes. This algorithm differs from hard linking in that it allows connections between intensities that differ significantly, and the strength of the link is a function of the absolute difference between the value of a child node and its candidate parent node. By choosing different functions determining the strength of the link, various levels of detail can be extracted from texture images. It should be noted that this approach allows obtaining results identical to hard pyramid linking when choosing a particular type of linking function and/or its parameters.

2.2 Fuzzy Pyramid Linking

The linking algorithm used in this work is detailed in Section 2.2.1, followed by a discussion on the selection of the linking function (Section 2.2.2) and its parameters (Section 2.2.3).

2.2.1 Algorithm for Redefining Pyramid and Segmentation

In the proposed algorithm, the following variables are defined for the linking and ensuing iterative pyramid redefining process:

- $t_l(i,j)$: the *local image property* (in this paper intensity);
- $p_l(i,j)$: the *pointer* to the node's parent one level above having the maximum link strength, hereafter referred to as *the maximum link*;
- $s_l(i,j)$: the *strength value of the link* between the parent and the child nodes.

The iterations proceed in the following manner:

1. For level $l = 0$ set
$$s_0(i,j) = 1 \quad \text{and} \quad t_0(i,j) = I_0(i,j).$$

2. For each level l from 1 to $n-1$ set
$$s_l(i,j) = \sum_{i'j'} s_{l-1}(i',j') \phi_{i,j,i',j'},$$
where $\phi_{i,j,i',j'}$ denotes the strength of the link between the node (i,j) at level l and its child (i',j') at level $l-1$,
and
$$t_l(i,j) = \sum_{i'j'} t_{l-1}(i',j') \phi_{i,j,i',j'},$$
with summations performed over all children of the node.

3. For each node at level l, for $0 \leq l < n-2$, the pointer $p_l(i,j)$ points to the parent node at level $l+1$ that has the maximum link strength among the four candidate parent nodes. If two or more parents have the same link strength, a link is chosen randomly; however, if either link existed in the previous iteration, the link remains unchanged.

4. Once the links have propagated to the top of the pyramid the value of every node, except those at level 0, is recomputed in the following manner:
$$I_l(i,j) = t_l(i,j)/s_l(i,j) \quad for \ s_l(i,j) > 0.$$

5. If no link is reassigned during the current iteration, it is assumed that a steady state has been reached. If any number of links have been reassigned during the current iteration, the procedure is repeated starting from Step 2.

Upon reaching steady state, image segmentation is achieved in one top-down pass beginning from level $n-1$. In this pass, a child node at level l is replaced by the parent node pointed to by $p_l(i,j)$. The proposed algorithm limits the propagation of the links for specific nodes by requiring that the links between the child and parent nodes (pointed by $p_l(i,j)$) exceed a specified threshold τ.

2.2.2 Modeling Strength of the Link

The choice of the function ϕ, representing the strength of the link, determines the flexibility of the pyramid segmentation. We have considered various monotonically decreasing functions for modeling the strength of the link, including the linear-like, sigmoid-like, and fuzzy membership functions. Characteristics of the class of images to be segmented combined with the objectives of segmentation determine the best type of function. Considering Fisher ratios and false detections, the fuzzy membership function was found to be the most flexible of the three [24]. The linking algorithm employing this function is appropriately called *fuzzy pyramid linking*.

The fuzzy membership function is widely used in various applications based on the fuzzy set theory [27]. In these applications the objective is to establish imprecise relationships between objects and concepts, as is the case in this work. Therefore, the strength of the link between nodes (i,j) and (i',j') is modeled by

$$\phi_{i,j,i',j'}(u;\alpha,\beta,\gamma) = 1 - S(u;\alpha,\beta,\gamma), \tag{2}$$

where

$$S(u;\alpha,\beta,\gamma) = \begin{cases} 0 & \text{for } u \leq \alpha \\ 2\left(\frac{u-\alpha}{\gamma-\alpha}\right)^2 & \text{for } \alpha \leq u \leq \beta \\ 1 - 2\left(\frac{u-\gamma}{\gamma-\alpha}\right)^2 & \text{for } \beta \leq u \leq \gamma \\ 1 & \text{for } u \geq \gamma \end{cases} \tag{3}$$

and $u = |I_l(i,j) - I_{l-1}(i',j')|$. The parameters α and γ determine the shape of the function, and $\beta = \frac{\alpha+\gamma}{2}$. Values of $\phi_{i,j,i',j'}$ range between 0 and 1, and the assignment of specific values is determined by the selection of α and γ. The roles of these two parameters are discussed in the next section.

The function $\phi_{i,j,i',j'}$, described by Equations (2) and (3), makes the proposed pyramid linking method a special case of fuzzy isodata clustering [24]. Consequently, based on the convergence of fuzzy isodata clustering [3], the proposed pyramid linking is convergent [24]. (The relationship between pyramid linking and isodata clustering is discussed by Kasif and Rosenfeld [13].)

2.2.3 Parameter Selection: General Concerns

The discussion in this section is divided into two parts. First, we discuss the selection of the parameters for the fuzzy membership function. These parameters include α

and γ, both of which determine how the pyramid is redefined in the iterative process. Next, we discuss parameter selection for segmentation (that follows the iterative process). The segmentation parameters include the threshold value τ and the level of pyramid from which segmentation starts. The following discussion concentrates on general considerations, while the specific selection of parameters for segmenting mammograms is described in Sections 3.1-3.3.

Parameters for defining the pyramid

Parameters α and γ determine how intensities are weighted when generating the next level of the pyramid. Specifically, parameter α determines the difference between pixel values at adjacent levels below which the link strength is 1; while γ is the difference above which the link strength is 0. Combined they determine how much child nodes that differ from the parent node in the previous iteration contribute to the value of that parent node in the next iteration. Physically it makes sense to assign relatively small integer values to α, e.g., $\alpha = 0, 1, 2, ...5$, and considerably larger integer values to γ. The general considerations in choosing the values for these parameters are as follows.

Parameter α. Since parameter α allows two pixel values I_l and I_{l-1} (at levels l and $l-1$, respectively) to be considered as having the same value if $|I_l - I_{l-1}| \leq \alpha$, the selection of this parameter is dictated by (i) expected noise level and (ii) minimum contrast, μ_c, to be detected. Generally, parameter α should satisfy $\alpha << \mu_c$ and it should be larger than the expected variations due to noise. The two considerations may be conflicting. However, noise effects are of lesser importance due to the fact that through multiresolution processing the noise effects are reduced. Therefore, minimum contrast is the dominating criterion for selecting α. It should be noted that the selection of α in general does not impact the results significantly. We have obtained consistent results by employing $0 \leq \alpha \leq 15$ for different classes of images, including mammograms [5],[6].

Parameter γ. The impact of this parameter is significant as it has two effects: (i) it determines the intensity difference $|I_l - I_{l-1}|$ beyond which two pixels are unrelated, and (ii) it determines the weight values for parent (I_l) and child (I_{l-1}) nodes satisfying $\alpha < |I_l - I_{l-1}| < \gamma$. If γ is chosen close to α, function ϕ [Equation (2)] approaches a step function and the proposed algorithm approaches hard pyramid linking. This selection is appropriate when sharp edges are present and accurate segmentation is the objective. On the other hand, when objects are of low contrast, it is necessary to choose larger values for γ. It should be noted that γ can be chosen larger than the number of intensities in an image, thus implying that all intensities are related and allowing all child nodes to contribute on an almost equal basis to the parent node. The specific value for γ should be chosen based on the distribution of intensities in an image (image histogram) and the objective of segmentation, i.e., expected variations within statistically homogeneous regions.

Segmentation parameters

The segmentation results using the fuzzy pyramid structure are strongly influenced by the level from which segmentation starts and the threshold value τ. The impact of the two is as follows.

Pyramid Level. The level of the pyramid from which the segmentation starts determines the maximum number of regions that can be detected in an image when replacing child nodes with the parent nodes, starting from the top of the pyramid and going to the bottom and assuming that the maximum links exceed the threshold value. Fuzzy pyramid linking allows for the creation of a potentially larger number of regions since some pixels may retain their original values (and are not replaced) due to thresholding.

Threshold value τ. This parameter is the most critical and decides whether a child node can be replaced by a parent node in the segmentation procedure. Therefore, it determines the final number of regions in the segmented image since the maximum links whose values are below the threshold value do not propagate down to the base of the pyramid. Generally, $0 \leq \tau \leq 1$, and high values of the maximum links are associated with homogeneous regions, while low values appear around edges. Choosing a small τ will allow practically all links to propagate, thus generating few regions in a segmented image. On the other hand, large values of τ do not allow most of the maximum links to propagate, and the segmented image resembles the low-pass filtered original image. The range of the maximum links in an image is determined by the image intensities and the selection of γ. Therefore, it is appropriate to choose threshold value adaptively after studying the histogram of the maximum links for a specific image and taking into consideration the objectives of image segmentation.

Using the guidelines described in this section, we have adapted the fuzzy pyramid linking algorithm to mammogram segmentation. The selection of specific parameters and utilization of the algorithm is described in the next section.

3. Mammogram Segmentation

This section is divided into three parts. First, Section 3.1 discusses the characteristics of mammogram images and the appropriate selection of parameters α and γ. Sections 3.2 and 3.3 detail the utilization of fuzzy pyramid linking for detecting microcalcifications and nodules, respectively. These sections discuss the strategies employed, the appropriate pyramid level to start segmentation, and the selection of parameter τ. The segmentation procedures used for extracting microcalcifications and nodules are summarized in Table 1.

3.1 Selection of Fuzzy Membership Function Parameters

Generally, useful parts of mammogram images (breast region) are highly textured and contain a narrow range of gray levels; e.g., when digitized to 256 gray levels their histograms contain about 100 different intensities and typically the histograms are unimodal. The presence of cancerous changes is statistically insignificant except in cases of advanced cancer, which are not of interest in massive screening of mammograms. Noise arising from digitization is relatively low and of less concern than highly textured and varying characteristics of the normal breast tissue.

The objective of segmentation is to detect objects of low contrast (nodules) that vary in shape and size, and very small objects of somewhat higher contrast (microcalcifications). Taking into account these objectives, the characteristics of mammograms, and the general discussion in Section 2.2.3, we choose $\alpha = 1$. This selection is primarily motivated by our desire to detect objects of low contrast. As already mentioned, the results are stable for a range of values of α, and we have experimented with $0 \leq \alpha \leq 15$ without noticing any difference in the results. The selection of low values of α has little impact on digitization noise, which is taken care of by the very nature of multiresolution processing.

Table 1: Selection of parameters for extracting microcalcifications and nodules

objective	# of images used	links[1]	α	γ	τ	level[2]
microcalcifications	2	NP	1.	100.	ϕ^{min} [3]	4×4
		NP	1.	100.	$\phi^{min} + \delta$ [4]	4×4
small nodules	2	NP	1.	100.	$\phi_1^{(5)}$	4×4
		NP	1.	100.	$\phi_2^{(6)}$	4×4
large nodules	1	P	1.	100.	0.	$2^n/\sqrt{A}$ [7]

[1] NP-utilize only nodes whose maximum links do not propagate from the top of the pyramid; P-utilize only nodes whose maximum links propagate from the top of the pyramid.
[2] Level is chosen based on corresponding image size (actual level depends on the initial size of the image).
[3] Choose ϕ^{min} such that at $K = 40$ nodes have links smaller than ϕ^{min}.
[4] Choose δ such that $2K$ nodes have links smaller than $\phi^{min} + \delta$.
[5] Choose ϕ_1 such that $K = 2A$ nodes have links smaller than ϕ_1 (A is the expected maximum area of the objects of interest).
[6] Choose ϕ_2 such that $2K = 4A$ nodes have links smaller than ϕ_1 (A is the expected maximum area of the objects of interest).
[7] the chosen level is of size $2^n/\sqrt{A} \times 2^n/\sqrt{A}$; $2^n \times 2^n$ is the image size.

Considering that the range of gray levels is relatively low and that relationships between all intensities exist, we have chosen $\gamma = 100$, thus allowing all intensities to be weighted similarly and creating a truly fuzzy relationship between pixels at different pyramid levels. All images discussed in this paper were processed using the same values of parameters α and γ. Therefore, it is implicitly assumed that each of the images is subject to low noise level, the objects of interest are of low contrast and practically all intensities in an image are related. If either of these assumptions are violated it is necessary to choose different parameters using guidelines in Section 2.2.3.

Since there are only a few sharp intensity transitions in mammograms, our selection of values for parameters α and γ results in the maximum links close to 1 for most of the pixels. The only exceptions are very small objects, such as microcalcifications, which have somewhat smaller maximum links. It should be noted that all of the processed mammograms that contain no microcalcifications have high maximum links. Two typical histograms of the maximum links are shown, together with corresponding images, in Figure 2. The difference between the two images is that the image in Figure 2(a) contains more texture variation, in comparison to image in Figure 2(b).

3.2 Utilization of Fuzzy Pyramid Linking for Detection of Microcalcification

Individual microcalcifications are typically small, sometimes only one pixel in size, and vary slightly in intensity from the surrounding area. Therefore, the microcalcifications are associated with pyramid nodes that have relatively small maximum links close to the base of the pyramid. When choosing low values for threshold τ, with selection of parameters α and γ described in Section 3.1, most of the child nodes will be replaced by the parent nodes, thus generating large uniform regions in the segmented images. Only pixels corresponding to edges and small objects, such as individual microcalcifications, retain their original intensities in the segmented image. The two groups of pixels can be easily differentiated since the groups corresponding to edge pixels increase in size when τ is increased, while small objects retain their shape and size. Consequently, microcalcifications are detected in the following three steps.

1. Upon pyramid convergence, generate histogram of the maximum links $\phi_{max}(i,j,i',j')$, and determine the minimum value of the maximum links ϕ^{min}. It should be noted that it is necessary to quantize values of ϕ_{max}. A slightly larger value is chosen for ϕ^{min} if the number of nodes associated with the true minimum is very small. We have chosen value ϕ^{min} such that at least $K = 40$ nodes have $\phi_{max} \leq \phi^{min}$.

2. Generate segmented image, I_{s0}, using $\tau_0 = \phi^{min}$. Next, generate segmented image, I_{s1}, using $\tau_1 = \phi^{min} + \delta$, where δ is chosen such that at least $2K$ nodes have $\phi_{max} \leq \tau_1$.

3. Compare I_{s0} and I_{s1} and determine if there are pixel groupings in two images that have not changed shape and size. Extract these pixels and generate segmented image containing potential microcalcifications. Retain in segmented

image only the pixels whose maximum links did not allow them to be replaced by pixels at the very top of the pyramid.

Considering that a mammogram may contain nodules or other bright regions, we start segmentation at the pyramid level that has size 4×4, thus allowing the existence of 16 homogeneous regions. The choice of parameter K in Step 1 is determined by the expected number of pixels corresponding to microcalcifications, and K should be larger than that number. The selection of δ in Step 2 should be such that I_{s1} contains observable differences relative to I_{s0}. If $\tau_0 = \tau_1$, i.e., more than $2K$ pixels are associated with ϕ^{min}, the next value of ϕ_{max} is chosen for τ_1. Neither of the values K or δ is critical for the success of the method; however, the above guidelines keep the algorithm in Step 3 simple. The evaluation of the performance of this method on mammograms containing microcalcifications as well as normal mammograms containing synthetically superimposed microcalcifications is described and quantitatively summarized in Section 4. The evaluation incorporates both the ability to detect microcalcifications as well as false alarms.

3.3 Utilization of Fuzzy Pyramid Linking for Detection of Nodules

Nodules, benign and malignant, are generally characterized by higher intensities (relatively to the surrounding tissue) and are relatively homogeneous, at least in the center. However, they may have ill-defined boundaries. In contrast to microcalcifications, the nodules are relatively large. Depending on the size of the nodules we propose two approaches. The first is used for the detection of small nodules and uses the procedure described in Section 3.2. The only difference is that in Steps 1 and 2 the threshold values τ_0 and τ_1 are chosen differently, based on the expected maximum size of the object, A. Value τ_0 is chosen such that $K = 2A$ nodes have the maximum links smaller than this value. The threshold value τ_1 is chosen such that $2K$ nodes have the maximum links smaller than τ_1.

A different version of fuzzy pyramid linking is used for the detection of larger objects. There are two basic differences, the level from which the segmentation starts and the selection of parameter τ. The first is dictated by the size of the objects to be detected. The smaller the objects, the lower the level of pyramid is chosen; practically, this means that it is appropriate to choose the level of pyramid which allows the object "to be seen". Since our objective is to detect homogeneous regions, it is necessary that all links propagate through the pyramid. The image of interest, in contrast to microcalcification detection where we are interested only in pixels whose links did not propagate from the top of the pyramid, is the image where all pixels were replaced by the pixels at the top of the pyramid (i.e., the level from which the segmentation has started). The nodules are extracted in the following three steps.

1. Choose $\tau < \phi^{min}$ and perform segmentation as described in Section 2.2.

2. Linearly scale and threshold the result. (In this work we have used the thresh-

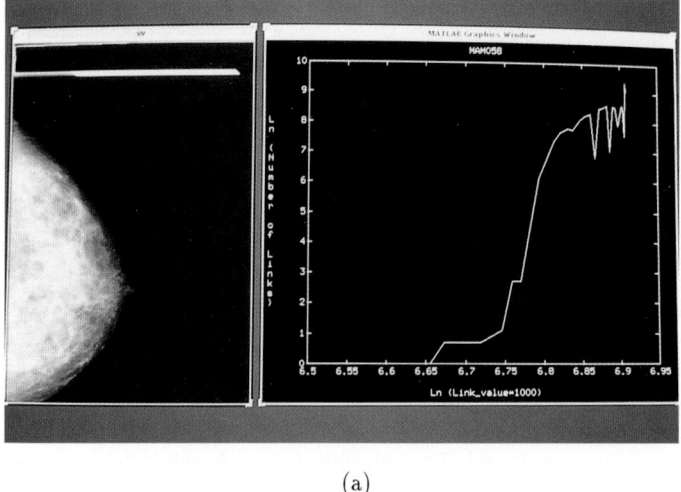

(a)

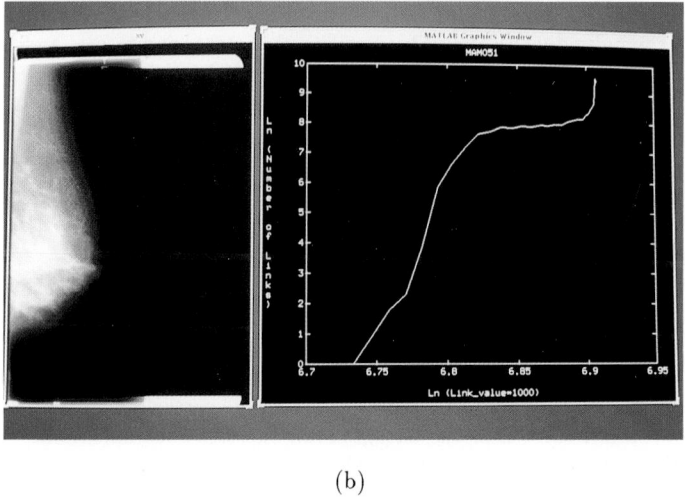

(b)

Figure 2: Examples of typical histograms of maximum links (shown on logarithmic scale): (a) textured mammogram and its maximum link histogram, and (b) relatively uniform mammogram and its maximum link histogram.

olding algorithm described in [19].)

3. Check the size, intensity characteristics, and shape of each remaining object. Extract objects that are less than the specified size (in our case 1/10 of the total image size), have higher values than the image mean, and have a relatively circular shape (we have used the measure of compactness). These objects are potential nodules.

We have employed simple reasoning in the third step; more sophisticated considerations can eliminate most of the false alarms.

4. Performance Evaluation

Performance evaluations were carried out using: (i) synthetically generated objects superimposed on normal mammograms and (ii) mammogram images. The experiments with synthetically generated objects were carried out on two different backgrounds (normal mammograms), and the each object was placed at five or more locations in the image, and the results were averaged for different locations. Total of 89 real mammograms were used for the evaluation; 50 of the mammograms were normal, 27 contained microcalcifications, and 12 contained nodules. All images were processed by subdividing a mammogram into non-overlapping windows of size 256×256 and integrating the individual results. The specific experiments and results are described in the following. First, Section 4.1 describes synthetic object generation, and Sections 4.2 and 4.3 summarize the results for detection of microcalcifications and nodules, respectively.

4.1 Synthetic Image Generation

The superposition of synthetically generated objects on real mammograms provides for an objective study of capabilities of our method regarding contrast, size, and shape of objects. The error estimation in this case is accurate since the truth images are known precisely.

Normal mammograms of varying texture complexity were used as the background for the study. The complete sets of experiments were carried out using two mammograms, shown in Figure 3, as the background. These two mammograms were chosen because they represent extremes in complexity of generic textures in our sample set of images. The mammogram shown in Figure 3(a) is characterized by limited variation in intensity, while the mammogram shown in Figure 3(b) is highly textured and a more challenging background for the tests.

Two sets of experiments were carried out. The first set pertains to establishing the capability of the proposed method to detect microcalcification, and the objective of the second set was to evaluate the performance when detecting larger low contrast objects, simulating nodules (benign and malignant). In both cases the objects

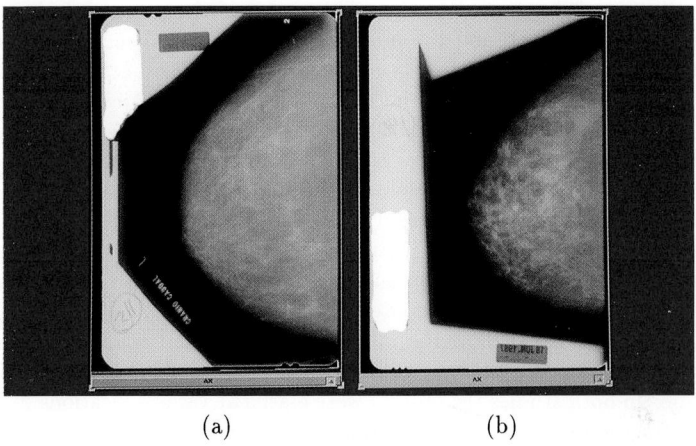

Figure 3: Two normal mammograms that were used as the background for superimposing synthetic objects: (a) low textured background, (b) highly textured background.

were modeled in the same way, and by using different placement rules and specific parameters different classes of objects were generated.

Object Model

An object in all experiments was modeled by an ellipse with a specified major axis, minor axis, and the angle ω between the major axis and the x-axis (horizontal axis). By varying the ratio of the two axes the objects could vary from circular to very elongated ellipses of varying ω centered at the same point. A star-like structure encountered in some nodules, was generated by a number of elongated ellipses of varying ω. Microcalcifications were modeled by a pattern of small circular objects placed in a spiral fashion around a specified center (the number of objects was varied).

Object Edges

In order to allow natural variation in edge location, edges of each object were deformed using a random number generator (and a specified seed); pixels were either removed or added to the individual edge locations depending on if the number returned by the random number generator was odd or even. By repeatedly performing edge deformation, an object was deformed as desired.

Edge Profiles

Generally, objects of interest in mammograms do not have sharp edges and blend with the surrounding area. Therefore, we have chosen to model object edges using the ramp edge model, in contrast to the step edge model. The ramp edge model allows a gradual transition of intensities and a blending of objects and backgrounds.

An object was assigned a chosen intensity, i, and the object edge profiles were changed into ramps of specified profile. The center of the ramp was placed on the physical edge of the object, and the intensities gradually changed starting from the inside of the object. (Clearly, there is a relationship between object size (in particular minor axis) and possible width of the ramp.) Finally, the object is superimposed on the chosen background. It should be noted that the true edge locations remain unchanged relative to the step edges since the ramp is centered at the step edge. Therefore, the truth images correspond to the step edge model. An object may be subjected to Gaussian noise of specified mean and standard deviation prior to being superimposed onto the background image.

By changing the intensity, i, incrementally identical images with varying object contrast were generated for the purpose of studying the sensitivity of the proposed method to contrast. By keeping the intensity the same and changing the values of the major and minor axes, we have studied the sensitivity of the proposed method to object shape. In both studies the objects were placed at various locations in the same image, and the errors were averaged for different placements in order to countereffect the impact of specific background intensities.

4.2 Detection of Microcalcifications

It is well established that microcalcifications are one of the earliest signs of potential cancerous changes in breast tissue [15]. Physically microcalcifications have dimensions between .1-1. mm (in mammograms), implying that they are guaranteed to be correctly digitized when using a resolution of at least $50\mu m$. Mammograms digitized at lower resolutions may still show the presence of microcalcifications; however, the contrast between the microcalcifications and the surrounding tissue is much lower, and in some cases, depending on resolution, the microcalcifications are blended into surrounding tissue (through digitization) and are not detectable in the digitized images. In the following we describe the results obtained when applying the fuzzy pyramid linking algorithm (Section 3.2) to synthetic microcalcifications and real microcalcifications.

Synthetic microcalcifications

A limited number of available mammograms containing microcalcifications has motivated us to perform these experiments. In addition, some of the available mammograms were of lower resolution than required; therefore, we could not draw any reliable conclusions based on them. The primary objective of our experiments was to determine the lowest contrast for which the method was able to correctly detect the synthetic objects. The experiments were carried out by generating clusters of objects ranging individually in diameter from 1 to 3 pixels and placing identical clusters over a normal mammogram at different locations. Different locations were chosen in order to avoid the impact of neighbouring intensities that may make detection easier in some cases. The results were averaged for different locations. The contrast of a cluster of objects was varied relative to the mean of the image region in predetermined steps.

The performance of the method varied with the complexity of the texture background. The method was able to correctly detect objects placed on the background in Figure 3(b) up to a contrast difference of 15 (between the region mean and the objects). By further lowering the contrast, the number of pixels that the method could not detect increased, and finally at contrast difference 10 only 60% of pixels were correctly detected. The average standard deviation of the background was in this case 9.5. In the case of the background shown in Figure 3(a), which is less textured, the method was able to detect the synthetic objects correctly for contrasts up to 10. By decreasing contrast to 9, the number of correctly detected pixels was reduced to 80%. The average standard deviation of the background was in this case 5.3. In either of the cases, the method did not detect any false positives. Two examples of superimposed objects, the truth images, and the obtained results are shown in Figure 4.

The superposition of synthetic objects allowed evaluating the method's capabilities to detect objects that are small and have specific contrast; however, the background in our experiments differs from the case of detecting microcalcifications in high resolution mammograms in that the latter is expected to show more variations in the intensities of the normal tissue. However, the expected variations are relatively small and, as discussed in Section 2.2.3, are unlikely to significantly impact the results.

Real Microcalcifications

The performance of the method was evaluated on two sets of images. The first set contained 17 mammograms containing microcalcifications and 50 normal mammograms. This set was supplied by the University of South Florida and was accompanied by the corresponding truth images. These images were of considerably lower resolution than required by the sampling theorem and physical size of individual microcalcifications. The results on these images are as follows:

- The method has detected the presence of microcalcifications in 13 images (out of 17) in the same regions as in the accompanying truth images.

- The method has detected fewer individual microcalcifications than the truth images point at in the cluster regions. (On average, one out of four individual microcalcifications indicated in the truth images was missed.)

- No false positives were detected in any of the normal mammograms.

- No microcalcifications were detected in 4 images (out of 17) labelled as containing microcalcifications, and in another image (out of the remaining 13) no microcalcifications were detected in one of the regions pointed at by the truth image.

It should be noted that in cases where no microcalcifications were detected, careful examination on pixel level shows no presence of visible small bright objects.

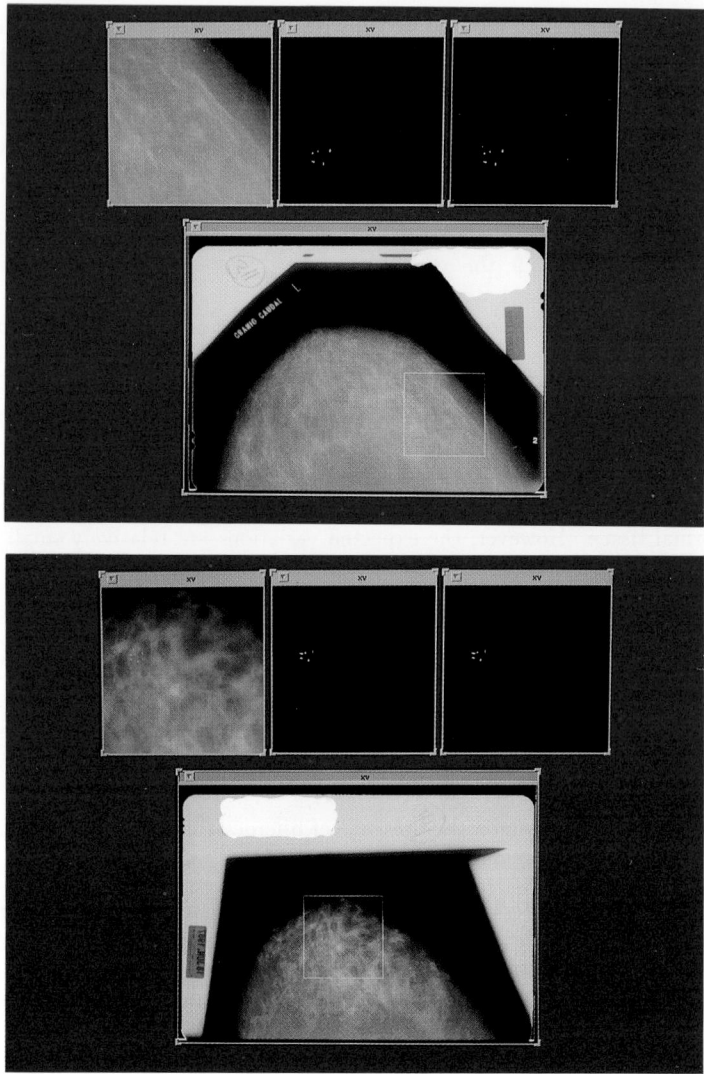

Figure 4: Two examples of superimposed synthetic microcalcifications on normal mammograms. The regions where the objects were superimposed are shown enlarged, together with the truth images and the segmentation results (left to right).

The second set of mammograms consisted of 10 images digitized at resolution of .1 mm. In order to achieve required resolution the mammograms were digitized in parts. Each digitized mammogram was verified by the medical expert to contain both macrocalcifications and microcalcifications. The diameter of macrocalcifications varied from 4 to 6 pixels (area varied 12−25 pixels); the diameter of microcalcifications was 1 − 2 pixels (area varied 1 − 3 pixels). The results are as follows:

- The presence of macrocalcifications was correctly detected in all cases.
- The presence of some microcalcifications was detected in all cases.
- An average of 2 false positives (2 pixels) were detected in cases when microcalcifications are present in an image.
- Up to 50% of individual microcalcifications were missed if
  - contrast, relative to the neighbouring pixels, was below 15
  - an individual microcalcification was adjacent to a small dark region on only one of its sides.

It should be noted that the contrast of 15 between microcalcifications and the neighbouring pixels is in agreement with our findings for synthetic images. A bright pixel neighbouring with an individual dark pixel is perceived as a gray region at lower resolution. If the mean of this region is close to the mean of the larger neighborhood, the bright pixel, i.e., the microcalcification, may be missed. In summary, the method detects all calcifications of area larger than 2 pixels, and about 50% of the smaller calcifications. Also, the method detects no false positives in images where no microcalcifications are present. Examples of detected microcalcifications are shown in Figure 5.

4.3 Detection of Nodules

As in the case of microcalcifications, we have performed two sets of experiments using synthetic objects superimposed on normal mammograms and mammograms containing irregular masses. The results are summarized in the following.

Synthetic Nodules

These experiments consisted in changing the shape, size, and contrast of objects superimposed on normal mammograms in order to establish the sensitivity of the proposed method. Generally, the method can tolerate significant variations of either size or contrast. When the contrast dropped to 10 (relative to the region mean) in cases of the average local standard deviation of 9.5 or when the minor axis dropped below 10 in the same cases, the method has failed to accurately extract objects. (The segmentation started from the level of size 8×8.) Further decrease of either contrast

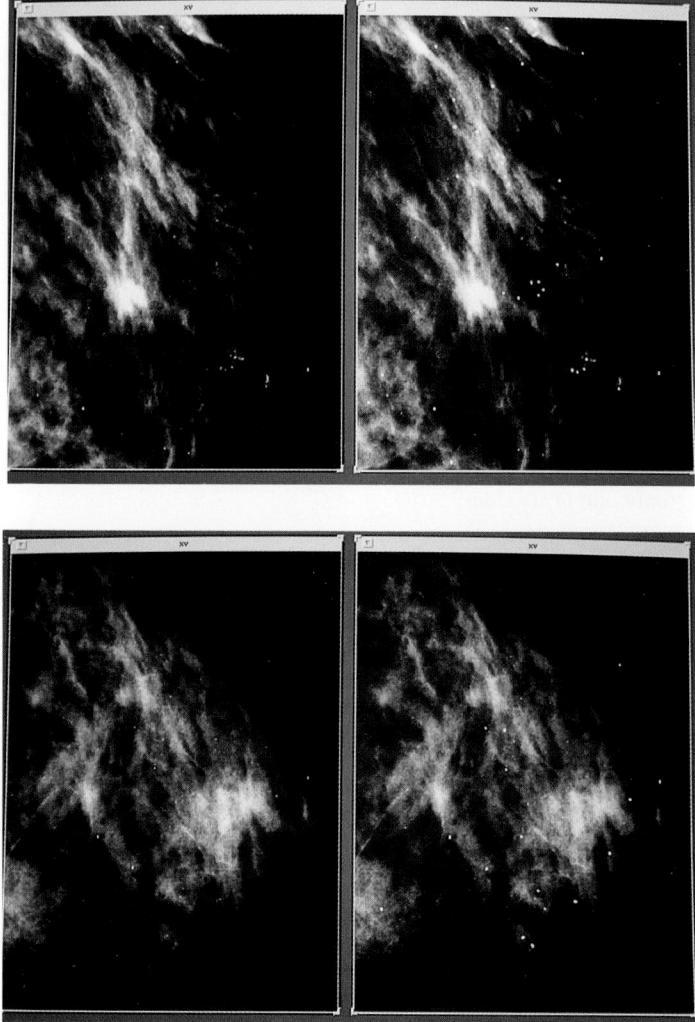

Figure 5: Two examples of mammograms containing microcalcifications. The original image is shown on the left, and the detected microcalcifications are shown enhanced on the right.

to 8 or minor axis to 9 has resulted in the method's lack of ability to detect objects of interest.

Also, the method has shown sensitivity to shape, and in cases of star-like objects its accuracy was lower than in the case of round objects. However, the method has failed for the same contrasts. (The size experiments do not apply to this case due to the nature of the object.)

Real Nodules

A total of 12 images, supplied by the University of South Florida and labelled irregular mass, were available for this study. The results are as follows:

- In 8 cases the method has detected nodules in agreement with the truth images. Except for the edge location, the agreement is on pixel to pixel basis.
- Regarding the edge location, there is an average disagreement for up to ±3 pixels per object.
- In the remaining 4 mammograms the method has detected only the rudiments of the nodules, and more than 50% of object's pixels were missed.
- The method has detected false positives in 5 out of 50 normal mammograms.

The incidence of false positives can be reduced by post-processing that examines the shape and intensity characteristics of the extracted objects. Examples of two detected nodules, the corresponding truth images, and the obtained results are shown in Figure 6.

4.4 Advantages of the proposed method

Mammograms vary in density and complexity of texture background and therefore require adaptive image processing methods. The proposed method shows unique capability to detect objects that vary in size, shape and contrast. This is best illustrated by the fact that the same method can be adapted for detection of both microcalcifications and nodules. The method is proven to be a generalization of the standard linking methods. In general, it outperforms the hard-linking methods when the objects of interest do not have clearly defined boundaries [5],[24]. It is adaptive and its sensitivity (with respect to intensity/texture variations and object size) depends on the choice of the fuzzy linking function parameters and the choice of the threshold value that allows replacement of a pixel value by the pixel value above. However, the relationship between parameters and performance is robust, and a chosen set of parameter guarantees particular level of performance.

We have compared the performance of the proposed method to gray scale morphology [23] when detecting microcalcifications. The fuzzy pyramid linking yields in general much lower rate of false positives, and in particular it does not detect false positives in mammograms when no microcalcifications are present, in contrast

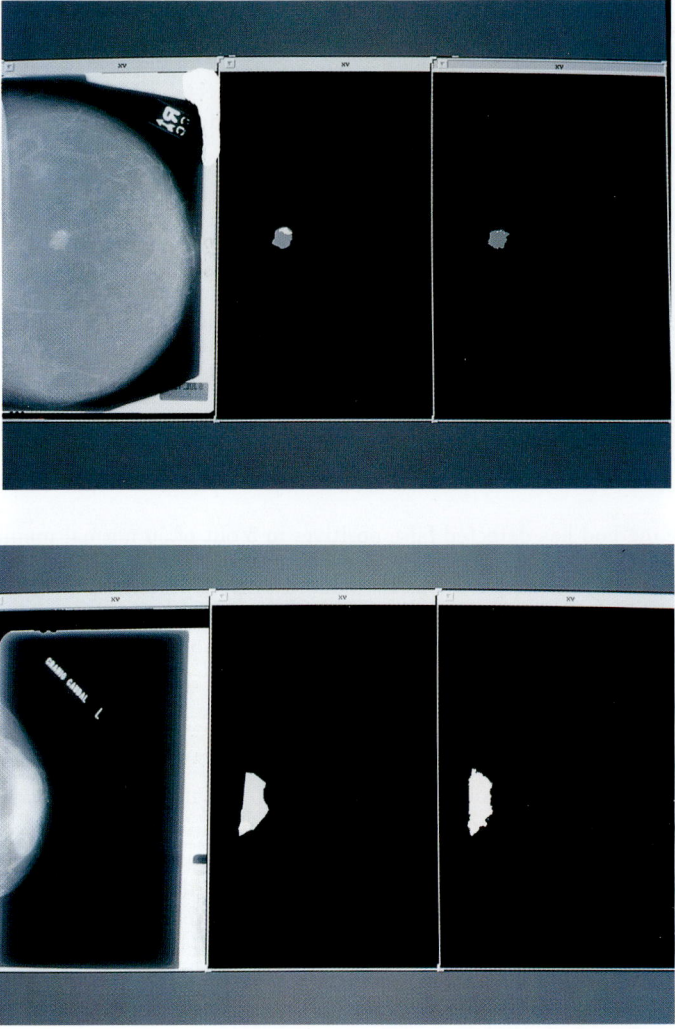

Figure 6: Two examples of mammograms containing irregular masses. From left to right: mammogram, truth image, and segmentation results. The top images contains the results obtained by combining outputs of the detected microcalcifications and nodules, since this mammogram contains both (as shown by the truth image).

to morphological operators. Also, we have considered performance of region-growing and local thresholding methods when detecting nodules. Both of the approaches generate a large number of regions, and are of little use in dense mammogram analysis.

The most important advantage of the proposed method lies in the fact that the parameters can be chosen to detect desired contrast and object size. Furthermore, the parameters can be automatically adjusted to texture background. It is possible to combine the outputs obtained with different parameters and assign confidence to the final results based on the changes induced by different parameters of the fuzzy linking function. When varying only the segmentation parameters, the pyramid needs to be generated only once, and the therefore the number of required computations is small.

5. Conclusions

This paper describes an adaptive image segmentation method that uses multiresolution processing. The primary objective of this method is to pre-screen mammograms and separate them into two groups: those containing potential cancerous signs and those containing no suspicious regions. The primary concerns in designing this method were to detect very subtle region changes indicative of cancer, while minimizing the number of false alarms. Since only a limited number of low resolution mammograms was available for testing, we have also used synthetically generated objects superimposed on normal mammograms to evaluate the method's performance.

The performance evaluation indicates that the method has the potential to be used in massive mammogram screenings. Generally, the method is capable of detecting changes in mammograms, when they are visually present. Moreover, a very low rate of false alarms is reported by this method. It should be noted that a different selection of parameters can make the method more sensitive to intensity changes. However, in that case the number of false positives would increase significantly. At present we experimenting with increased sensitivity while a incorporating decision rules to reduce the number of false alarms. The decision rules are based on reasoning employed by medical experts.

References

[1] H. J. Antonisse, "Image Segmentation in Pyramids," *Computer Graphics and Image Processing*, **19** (1982) 367-383.

[2] S. M. Astley and C.J. Taylor, "Combining Cues for Mammographic Abnormalities," Proc. of the British Machine Vision Association Conference, Oxford, England (1990) 253-258.

[3] J.C. Bezdek, "A Convergence Theorem for Fuzzy ISODATA Clustering Algorithm," *IEEE Trans. on Pattern Analysis and Machine Intelligence,* **2** (1980) 1-8.

[4] C.C. Boring, T.S. Squires, T. Tong, "Cancer Statistics 1991," *CA-A Cancer Journal for Clinicians*, **41** (1991) 19-51.

[5] D. Brzakovic, H. Beck and N. Sufi, "An Approach to Defect Detection in Materials Characterized by Complex Textures," *Pattern Recognition*, **23** (1990) 99-107.

[6] D. Brzakovic, X.M. Luo, and P. Brzakovic, "An Approach to Automated Detection of Tumors in Mammograms," *IEEE Trans. on Medical Imaging*, **9** (1990) 232-241.

[7] P.J. Burt, and E.H. Andersen, "The Laplacian Pyramid as a Compact Image Code," *IEEE Trans. on Commun.*, **31** (1983) 532-540.

[8] P.J. Burt, "Fast Filter Transforms for Image Processing," *Computer Graphics and Image Processing*, **16** (1981).

[9] H.P. Chan et al., "Image Feature Analysis and Computer-aided Diagnosis in Digital Radiography. 1. Automated Detection of Microcalcifications in Mammography," *Med. Phys.*, **14** (1987) 538-548.

[10] J.H. Davies, D.R. Dance, and C.H. Jones, "Automatic Detection of Microcalcification in Digital Mammograms Using Local Area Thresholding Techniques," Proc. SPIE, Med. Imaging III: Image Processing, **1092** (1989) 153-159.

[11] A.P. Dhawan, Buelloni, and R. Gordon, "Enhancement of Mammographic Features by Optimal Adaptive Neighborhood Image Processing," *IEEE Trans. on Medical Imaging,* **5** (1986).

[12] A.I. Holleb, editorial "Breast Cancer: Change and Challenge," *CA-A Cancer Journal for Clinicians,* **41** (1991) 69-70.

[13] S. Kasif, and A. Rosenfeld, "Pyramid Linking is a Special Case of ISODATA," *IEEE Trans. on Systems, Man, and Cybernetics,* **13** (1983) 84-85.

[14] S. Lai, X. Li, and W.F. Bischof, "On Techniques for Detecting Circumscribed Masses in Mammograms," *IEEE Trans. on Medical Imaging,* **8** (1989) 377-386.

[15] J.L. Lamarque, *An Atlas of the Breast Clinical Radiodiagnosis*, (London, England: Wolfe Medical Publications Ltd., 1981).

[16] I.E. Magnin, M. E. Alaoui and A. Bremond, "Automatic Microcalcification Pattern Recognition from X-ray Mammographies," Proc. of SPIE **1137**, (1989) 170-175.

[17] M.E. Morra and B.D. Blumberg, "Women's Perceptions of Early Detection of Breast Cancer: How are we Doing?" *Seminars in Oncology Nursing*, **7** (1991) 151-160.

[18] W.M. Morrow, et al., "Region-based Contrast Enhancement of Mammograms," *IEEE Trans. on Medical Imaging*, **11** (1992) 392-406.

[19] N. Otsu, "A Threshold Selection Method from Gray-Level Histograms," *IEEE Trans. on System, Man and Cybernetics*, **9** (1979) 62-66.

[20] W. Qian, M. Kallergi, L.P. Clarke, K. Woods, and R.A. Clark, "Application of Nonlinear Filtering in Mammograms," Proc. of Medical Imaging VI: Image Processing, Newport Beach, Ca, (1992) 660-667.

[21] L. Shuk-Mei and W.F. Bischof, "On Techniques for Detecting Circumscribed Masses in Mammograms," *IEEE Trans. Medical Imaging*, **8** (1989) 377-386.

[22] W. Spiesberger, "Mammogram Inspection by Computer," *IEEE Trans. on Biomedical Engineering*, **26** (1979) 213-219.

[23] S.R. Sternberg, "Grayscale Morphology," *Computer Vision, Graphics, and Image Processing*, **35** (1986) 333-355.

[24] N. Sufi, Pyramid Based Segmentation of Texture Images, (MS Thesis, University of Tennessee, 1988).

[25] P.G. Tahoces, J. Correa, M. Souto, C. Gonazelz, L. Gomez and J.J. Vidal, "Enhancement of Chest and Breast Radiographs by Automatic Spatial Filtering," *IEEE Trans. on Medical Imaging*, **10** (1991) 330-335.

[26] K. Woods, L.P. Clarke, P. Laurence, R. Velthuizen, "Enhancement of Digitized Mammograms Using a Local Thresholding Technique," Proc. of the 13th Annual Inter. Conf. of the IEEE Eng. in Medicine and Biology Society, Orlando, Fl, (1991), 114-115.

[27] L.A. Zadeh, "Fuzzy Sets," *Information and Control*, **8** (1965) 338-353.

Acknowledgement

Part of the images used in this research were provided courtesy of the Center for Engineering and Medical Image Analysis and the H. Lee Moffitt Cancer Center and Research Institute at the University of South Florida.

The authors greatly appreciate the help from Dr. P. Brzakovic, Ph.D., M.D., in identifying important characteristics of mammograms.

FEATURE EXTRACTION FOR COMPUTER-AIDED ANALYSIS OF MAMMOGRAMS

Håkan Bårman   Gösta Granlund   Leif Haglund
Computer Vision Laboratory, Linköping University
S-581 83 Linköping Sweden

Abstract

A framework for computer-aided analysis of mammograms is described. General computer vision algorithms are combined with application specific procedures in a hierarchical fashion. The system is under development and is currently limited to detection of a few types of suspicious areas.

The image features are extracted by using feature extraction methods where wavelet techniques are utilized. A low-pass pyramid representation of the image is convolved with a number of quadrature filters. The filter outputs are combined according to simple local Fourier domain models into parameters describing the local neighbourhood with respect to the model. This produces estimates for each pixel describing local size, orientation, Fourier phase, and shape with confidence measures associated to each parameter.

Tentative object descriptions are then extracted from the pixel-based features by application-specific procedures with knowledge of relevant structures in mammograms. The orientation, relative brightness and shape of the *object* are obtained by selection of the pixel feature estimates which best describe the object.

The list of object descriptions is examined by procedures, where each procedure corresponds to a specific type of suspicious area, e.g. clusters of microcalcifications.

Keywords: Computer vision, feature extraction, image processing, mammography, microcalcifications, wavelets.

1 Background

Breast cancer is one of the more common types of cancer. Scientific studies have shown that the mortality in breast cancer is decreased by early detection and treatment. It is well known that mammography is the best method for detection of small breast tumors. This makes it desirable to use mammography in mass screening programmes to reduce the mortality in breast cancer [1]. A mass screening program requires a large number of radiologists with special training in mammography and this involves problems such as high costs, shortage of qualified personnel, and visual fatigue.

Computer-aided analysis could be a solution to the problems mentioned above. Consequently, many efforts have been made to incorporate image processing. However, the methods developed have not been sufficient to introduce computer-aided analysis in clinical use. A survey of the area can be found in [8].

2 Overview

The digital mammogram is analyzed with a combination of general image processing and computer vision algorithms in combination with procedures which have been specially designed for the application. The following steps are carried out, where steps 1–3 are general algorithms and steps 4–6 are application specific algorithms.

1. A low-pass pyramid representation of the image is produced by low-pass filtering combined with resampling of the image.

2. Local feature extraction algorithms are used on the different layers of the low-pass pyramid to produce estimates of orientation, Fourier phase and energy.

3. The feature estimates are combined over scale, and local estimates of size (spatial frequency) are computed [11].

4. The combined phase estimates are used to guide the extraction of image objects. The phase describes the relative grey value, i.e. whether or not the pixel is darker or lighter than the surround. Brightness maxima are used as seed points for the object extraction.

5. The feature estimates of the pixels belonging to objects are used to compute parameters describing the objects. The current relatively crude implementation only includes parameters describing position, size, orientation and 'roundness'.

6. The object list is examined by search procedures, where each procedure has knowledge of the appearance of one type of suspicious area.

Each of these steps are now described in detail.

3 The Low-Pass Pyramid

The logarithmic partitioning of the frequency domain used in wavelet theory [20] can be obtained either by scaling/translation of the filter function or by constructing a low-pass pyramid of the image. The latter alternative is preferable with respect to computational complexity. The pyramid is obtained by a low-pass filtering to eliminate the high frequencies followed by a subsampling to move the remaining spatial frequencies 'towards' the frequency function of the wavelet filter, e.g. a subsampling factor of two moves the spatial frequency $\pi/2$ to π. The low-pass filter should, according to the theory, be an ideal low-pass filter. Ideal low-pass filters introduce 'ringing', i.e. false edges, in the filtered images. Edges and similar structures play an important role in the later processing stages. For that reason a Gaussian filter function is used.

The current implementation has 1 octave between the layers, i.e. the subsampling factor is two. The frequency function of the Gaussian filter is given by

$$G(\mathbf{u}) = \exp(\frac{-(u_1^2 + u_2^2)}{2\sigma^2}) \tag{1}$$

and the corresponding spatial function is

$$g(\boldsymbol{\xi}) = \sqrt{2\pi}\, \sigma \exp(-(\xi_1^2 + \xi_2^2)\sigma^2/2) \tag{2}$$

with $\sigma = \pi/4$. The maximum spatial frequency [5] is normalized to π. The frequency and spatial coordinates are denoted u and ξ.

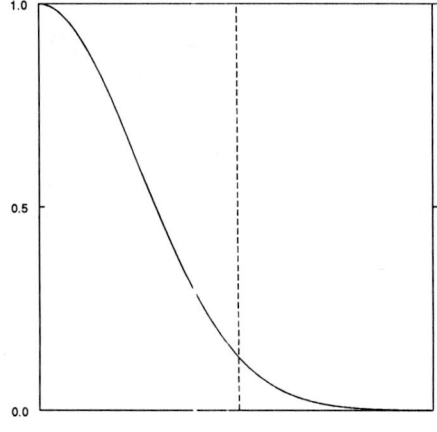

Figure 1: *The frequency function of the Gaussian filter. The dashed line indicates the ideal cutoff frequency $\pi/2$.*

This filter will not introduce any edge artifacts but will suppress the highest frequencies below $\pi/2$ and will not entirely remove frequencies above $\pi/2$ (the filter has a value of about 13.5 % of its top value at the frequency $u = \frac{\pi}{2}$). Figure 1 illustrates the difference between the ideal filter and the Gaussian filter.

Filtering and resampling is done simultaneously with an even sized filter (8×8) with its centre displaced by half a pixel unit in both ξ_1 and ξ_2, i.e. the centre is located in the middle of four pixels. The resampling is done by retaining only every other column and every other row in the filtered image. The process is schematically illustrated in Figure 2.

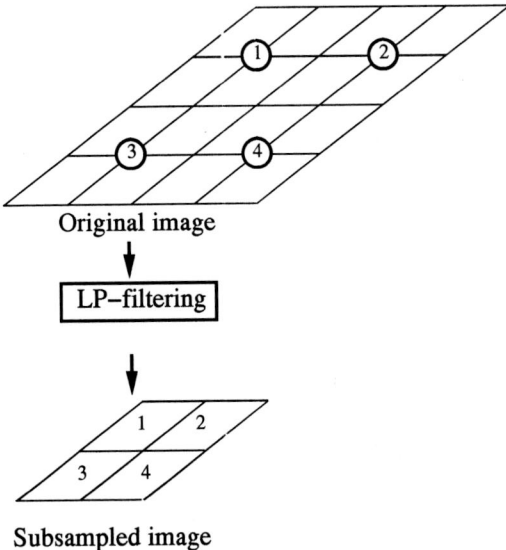

Figure 2: *Illustration of the subsampling process. The circles indicate the centre positions for the Gaussian filter. The numbers refer to the outputs from these filters.*

4 Layer Feature Extraction

The feature extraction is carried out on each of the image layers using *quadrature filters*. The quadrature filter concept forms a basis for minimizing the sensitivity to phase changes in the signal [15, 4, 11]. A number of features are obtained by combining the filter outputs according to simple local Fourier domain models. The features are local orientation, energy and phase, all estimated by convolution with four quadrature filter pairs.

The quadrature filters used are defined by polar separable frequency functions. The radial frequency function H_ρ should fulfill the wavelet requirements. The lognormal filter

$$H_\rho(\rho) = \exp(\frac{-4}{\ln 2} B^{-2} \ln^2(\rho/\rho_c)) \quad , \quad \rho \in [0\ldots\pi]. \tag{3}$$

where ρ_c is the centre frequency and B is the 6 dB sensitivity bandwidth, is suitable if ρ_c and B have reasonable values.

Choosing $\rho_c = \pi/4$ and $B = 2$ gives:

$$H_\rho(\rho) = \exp(\frac{-1}{\ln 2} \ln^2(4\rho/\pi)) \quad , \quad \rho \in [0\ldots\pi]. \tag{4}$$

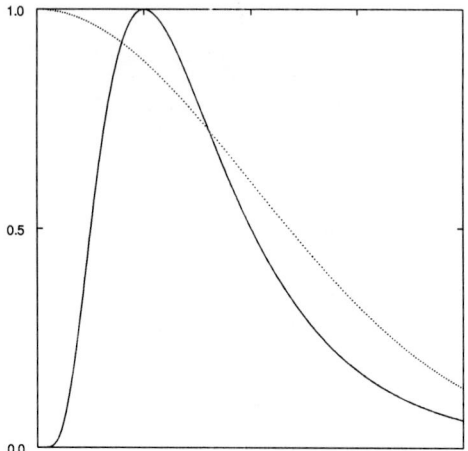

Figure 3: *The lognormal filter (solid line) given by Eq. 4 compared with the Gaussian spectrum (dashed line) obtained with the low-pass+resampling procedure.*

This choice of centre frequency places the filter in the part of the frequency spectrum where the compromise of using a Gaussian instead of an ideal low-pass filter is negligible [11] (see Figure 3). Using this filter on the subsampled images corresponds to filtering with lognormal filters with centre frequencies of $\pi/8$, $\pi/16$, $\pi/32$, ...etc. Filter sets with $\rho_c = \pi/2$ and $\rho_c = \pi$ are used on the full resolution image to give additional coverage of the high spatial frequencies.

The angular frequency function specifies the orientation selectivity of the quadrature filter. Each filter set consists of four quadrature filters with the angular frequency function:

$$H_{\varphi k}(\varphi) = \cos^2(\varphi - \varphi_k) \quad , \quad \varphi_k = \pi/8, \ 3\pi/8, \ 5\pi/8, \ 7\pi/8 \tag{5}$$

where φ_k defines the direction of the filter.

Filters with the frequency function specified by Eq. 3 and 5 can be synthesized by:

$$H(\rho, \varphi) = a_0 B_{00} + \sum_{n=1}^{3} a_r \left[B_{n0} \cos(n\varphi_k) + B_{n1} \sin(n\varphi_k) \right] \tag{6}$$

where the basis filters B_{ij} are defined by:

$$\begin{aligned} B_{n0}(\rho, \varphi) &= H_\rho(\rho) \cos(n\varphi) & n = [0\ldots 3] \\ B_{n1}(\rho, \varphi) &= H_\rho(\rho) \sin(n\varphi) & n = [1\ldots 3] \end{aligned} \tag{7}$$

and the weight vector $\mathbf{a} = (\ a_0 \quad a_1 \quad a_2 \quad a_3\ )^T$ (obtained by the theory of digital

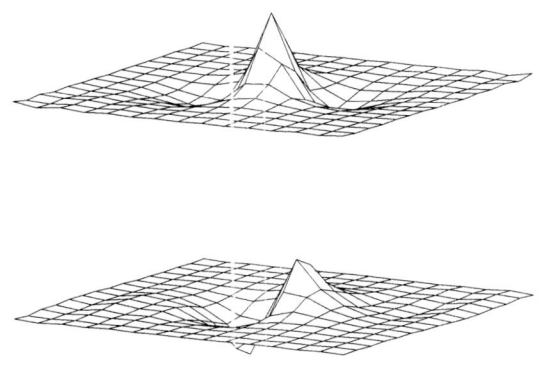

Figure 4: *One of the lognormal quadrature filters with centre frequency $\pi/4$ and a bandwidth of 2 octaves.*

prolate spheroidals [18, 24, 22, 23, 26]) is given by:

$$\mathbf{a} = \begin{pmatrix} 0.23675 \\ 0.39357 \\ 0.21692 \\ 0.06524 \end{pmatrix} \tag{8}$$

This approach (described in [2]) has a slight computational advantage and gives rotational invariant estimates of the local phase (Eq. 13).

The spatial representation of a quadrature filter is complex-valued with the real-valued part corresponding to a line filter and the imaginary part of the filter corresponding to an edge filter. Figure 4 contains a mesh surface plot of one the synthesized filters.

A benefit of choosing Eq. 5 as angular function is that the local orientation estimate can be estimated by the vector sum:

$$V = \sum_k q_k \exp(2\varphi_k i) \tag{9}$$

where q_k denotes the magnitude of the (complex) filter response $\mathbf{q}_k = e_k + io_k$ of the filter pair k [15]. The local orientation estimate is represented with the 'double angle' representation [10], i.e. the argument of the 2D vector V equals 2ϕ, where ϕ corresponds to the gradient direction. The magnitude of the vector is a certainty measure. The double angle representation has the advantage that it is continuous which makes local averaging a meaningful operation.

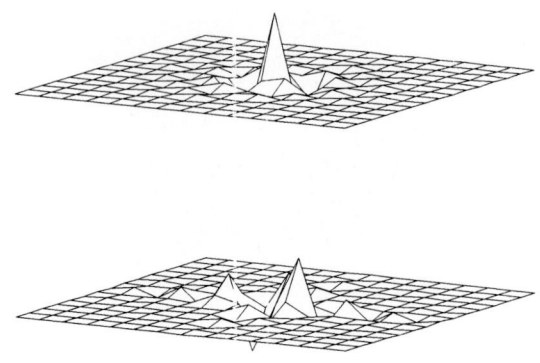

Figure 5: *'Extra' lognormal quadrature filters used on the full resolution image with a centre frequency of π and a bandwidth of 2 octaves.*

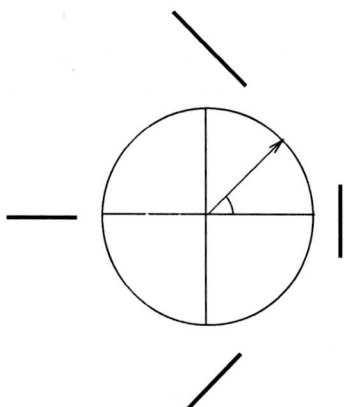

Figure 6: *The double angle representation of orientation. Taking the average of two lines, one oriented as $\phi = 0 + \epsilon$ and one as $\phi = \pi - \epsilon$, does not give the expected result if a single angle representation is used, while the double angle gives the correct answer.*

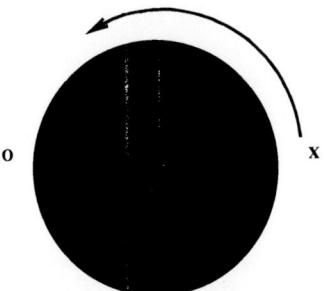

Figure 7: *Circle illustrating the edge discontinuity. The phase changes sign somewhere on the path on the edge indicated by the arrow.*

The estimation of the local energy is even simpler:

$$M = \frac{1}{2} \sum_k q_k. \tag{10}$$

This gives an estimate of the local Fourier domain energy spectrum weighted with the radial frequency function of the filter set.

The quadrature filter phase, i.e. the relation between the even and the odd filter, can be used to obtain a description of local contrast. The information resembles the information obtained by computation of local contrast or bandpass filtering, but the phase estimate gives additional information of the local image structure.

The local phase is in principle given by:

$$P = \sum_k e_k + i \sum_k o_k. \tag{11}$$

The argument of the vector P represents the local brightness with $\arg(P) \approx 0$ for lines and blobs brighter than the surroundings, $\arg(P) \approx \pi$ for lines and blobs darker than the surroundings, and $\arg(P) \approx \pi/2$ for edges. The sign cannot be determined without the orientation of the edge.

The phase sign gives problems with respect to both estimation and representation. The problem is examplified in Figure 7. The sign of the edge can, for example, be defined as positive at 'x' and negative at 'o'. This implies that the phase abruptly changes its sign somewhere on the edge between the two points. A remedy is to incorporate the (edge) orientation in the phase description,

$$\mathbf{p} = \begin{pmatrix} \cos\phi\sin\theta & \sin\phi\sin\theta & \cos\theta \end{pmatrix}^T \tag{12}$$

where $\theta = \arg(P)$ and ϕ is the gradient direction. This modification of Eq. 11 makes the representation continuous, a necessary requirement for the algorithm described in the next section. Appendix A verifies that **p** can be estimated by:

$$\mathbf{p} = \sum_k \left(\frac{2a_0}{a_1} o_k \begin{pmatrix} \cos\varphi_k & \sin\varphi_k & 0 \end{pmatrix}^T + e_k \begin{pmatrix} 0 & 0 & 1 \end{pmatrix}^T \right). \tag{13}$$

5 Scale Feature Extraction

The estimates of orientation, energy and phase are combined over scale to find 'events', i.e. adjacent scale layers describing the same image structure. The algorithm handles nested objects, i.e. a pixel can contain one or more events, and is implemented as a pixelwise operation, where the feature estimates of all scales are examined with consistency measures to extract the events of the pixel. Information of the appropriate scale for description of the event and an explicit measure of the local spatial frequency is also obtained.

The implementation of the scale analysis as a pixelwise operation requires that the feature estimates of the different scale layers have identical size. This is done by resampling the layers of the feature description pyramids to the original image size. The resampling is done with a scheme very similar to the one described in section 3; nearest neighbour expansion followed by averaging with a 7×7 Gaussian filter specified by Eq. 2.

Note that averaging of the phase estimate would give unpredictable results if the phase estimate of Eq. 11 is used, while the representation of Eq. 13 is well-behaved. The local phase estimate (Eq. 11) is examined using an 1D-search in the scale (layer) dimension to find the number of 'events' described by the feature estimates of the pixel. Abrupt changes of the phase vector create new events. A scalar product is used as criterion:

$$\mathbf{p}_l \cdot \sum_{k}^{l-1} \mathbf{p}_k > \epsilon \tag{14}$$

i.e. layer l is incorporated in the event if the scalar product of the layer phase vector and the phase vector sum of the event is positive.

The dominant spatial frequency (size) of the event is estimated by:

$$F = \sum_l \delta_l M_l \exp(\frac{2\pi l i}{L}) \tag{15}$$

where L is the total number of layers, and δ_l is 1 if the layer is part of the event and 0 otherwise. The frequency estimate (the argument of the vector F) is unbiased, and the certainty measure (the magnitude of the vector F) is invariant to the frequency value in the range $[2c_b..\pi/2]$, where c_b is the centre frequency of the feature estimation filter used at the top of the low-pass pyramid [11]. Note the wraparound area in the vicinity of 2π corresponding to neighbourhoods with a mix of low and high frequencies.

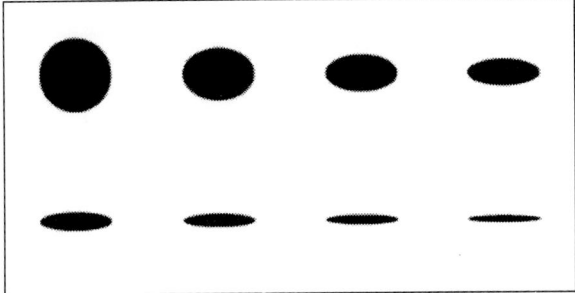

Figure 8: *Synthetic test image for evaluation of Eq. 17.*

6 Object Extraction

The extraction of image objects from the feature pyramid can be done in a number of ways, e.g. by edge contour following etc. The method used utilizes that microcalcifications are small and brighter than the surrounding tissue. It is very likely that the object extraction procedures must be extended to incorporate dectection of other types of suspicious areas.

The local phase and frequency are suitable features for selection of small and bright objects. The individual layers of the local phase pyramid are used to locate the local maxima of brightness using the maxima criterion:

$$\begin{pmatrix} 0 & 0 & 1 \end{pmatrix} \mathbf{p} > \max_{S} \begin{pmatrix} 0 & 0 & 1 \end{pmatrix} \mathbf{p}_s \qquad (16)$$

where S denotes the eight adjacent pixels. Local maxima accompanied by frequency estimates indicating that the local structure is better described at another layer are disregarded. The remaining maxima are candidate objects.

The candidate object description consists of certainty (from the phase estimate), position (pixel coordinates), size (spatial frequency) and a *shape* measure computed by:

$$S = M \exp(\sqrt{1 - \mathrm{mag}(V)/M}\ \pi i). \qquad (17)$$

V and M are computed by Eq. 9 and 10 on the scale layer where the brightness maximum was extracted. An argument of 0 corresponds to linear shape and π corresponds to circular shape. This measure have been used as context information in image enhancement applications [14]. Similar ideas has been used to disregard false calcification candidates originating from linear structures such as blood vessels (e.g. [17, 12]). One advantage of using Eq. 17 is that the shape estimation is done within the same feature extraction framework and no extra convolutions are required. The shape estimate has a reasonable scale invariance as indicated by Figures 8 and 9.

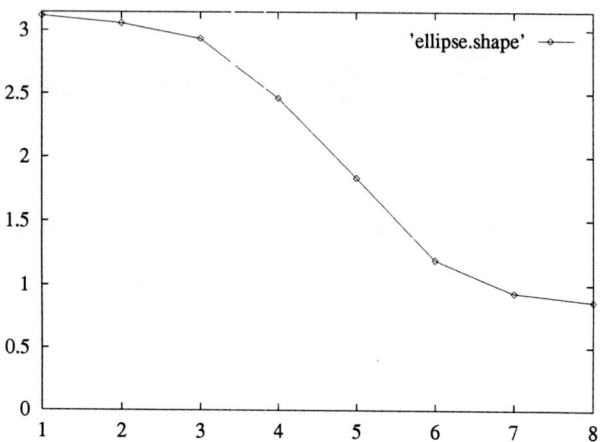

Figure 9: *The result of using Eq. 17 on Figure 8. The argument of the vector S is plotted with the estimate from the circular shape leftmost.*

7 Search Procedures

Objects with phase, frequency and shape corresponding to micro-calcifications are extracted from the object candidate list. The following steps are carried out to find clusters in the list of tentative micro-calcifications.

1. The certainty values of the tentative micro-calcifications are inserted at the object's position in an 'empty' image. The image is filtered with two filters, one Gaussian filter $a(\boldsymbol{\xi})$ and one complex-valued filter:

$$d(\boldsymbol{\xi}) = a(\boldsymbol{\xi})\exp(i\arg(\xi_1 + i\xi_2)) \qquad (18)$$

   The quotient of the two filter outputs calculates the distance and direction to the centre of mass of the neighbourhood.

2. Local distance minima are used as seed points for cluster centres. The distances to the cluster centres are computed for all tentative micro-calcifications. A micro-calcification is assigned to the nearest cluster if the distance is shorter than a threshold R. Unassigned calcifications are removed.

3. Micro-calcifications with more than one cluster centre on shorter distance than R are used to compute 'merge-values' for pairs of clusters. The calcifications

with short distances to both cluster centres are used to compute a sum, where the contribution from an individual calcification is $c_\xi\, a(\mathbf{r}_2)$, where c_ξ is the certainty value of the calcification, $\mathbf{r}$ is the distance to the adjacent cluster and a is the Gaussian function used to specify the averaging filter in the centre of mass computation above. Two clusters are marked for merging if the sum is larger than a threshold T_m.

4. Clusters marked for merging are merged and the certainties of the cluster members are summed, $C = \sum c_\xi$. Clusters with low certainty $C < T_c$ or are disregarded. Similar relaxation approaches can be found in e.g. [7, 12].

5. The cluster centres are recomputed using

$$\mathbf{m}_c = \frac{\sum c_\xi \boldsymbol{\xi}}{\sum c_\xi} \qquad (19)$$

and the shape and orientation of the cluster is measured by computation of the eigenvalues and eigenvectors of the matrix [9]

$$\frac{\sum c_\xi \boldsymbol{\xi}\boldsymbol{\xi}^T}{\sum c_\xi} - \mathbf{m}_c \mathbf{m}_c^T \qquad (20)$$

8 Results

The USF database of digitised mammograms contains a number of images with malignant microcalcifications. However, the spatial resolution of the images is far from the recommended 25 μm^2/pixel [1] and the calcifications are not clearly visible on all of the images. A part of the image 'mam096' with visible calcifications is displayed in Figure 10.

The framework described in this paper is used on this image. The result from the object extraction (49 tentative calcifications) is visualized as white pixels in Figure 11. Five cluster centre candidates were found using step 1-2 described in section 7. All but four of the microcalcification candidates were assigned a cluster after the distance computation (the candidate on the top row and the three tentative calcifications at the bottom) with the threshold $R = 100$. Three of the clusters shared members and were merged into one single cluster. The smallest cluster, consisting of the three candidates at the upper right, failed to fulfill the certainty criterion of step 4. This cluster is located outside the breast area with the candidates originating from digitisation errors. The addition of a region-of-interest criterion guided by e.g. contour following of the breast contour would also eliminate the cluster [21]. The cluster centres are recomputed and the shape of the clusters are estimated using Eq. 19-20. The result is superimposed on Figure 11 as black ellipses. Note that the ellipses describe the *shape and orientation* of the clusters and not the cluster border.

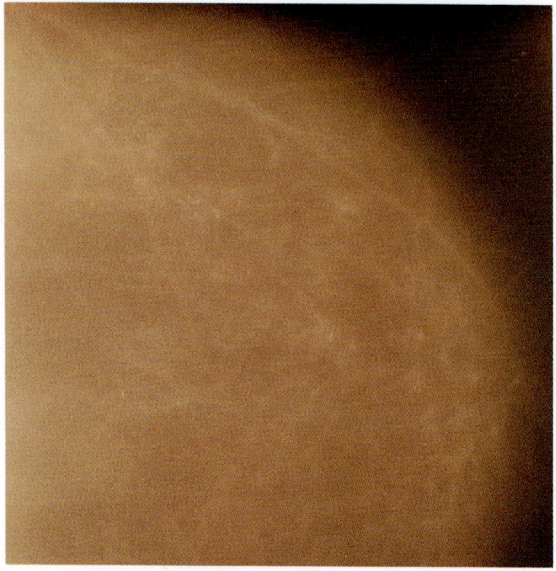

Figure 10: *A part of 'mam096' with malignant microcalcifications.*

A part of a mammogram digitised with a high resolution scanner is displayed in Figure 12. Two suspicious clusters of micro-calcifications can be found. The objects classified as tentative micro-calcifications are presented together with the cluster shapes in Figure 13.

The H. Lee Moffitt Cancer Center and Research Institute at the University of South Florida have lately uppdated the USF database with 24 mammograms digitised at 70 μm. The algorithms described in this paper were tested on seven images with clustered calcifications to get an indication of the method's performance. Box-classification with different values of the threshold parameters resulted in a sensitivity of 90.3 % (187/207). Most of the 20 undetected calcifications were faint and located within detected cluster. Most of the false alarms originated from background structure in detected clusters. One false cluster was 'created' by the classification. The total of 26 false alarms gives an accuracy of 87.8 % (187/213) in the classification.

9 Discussion

The hierarchical framework for computer-aided analysis of mammograms described in this paper consists of two parts, one part with general image processing and computer vision algorithms arranged in a wavelet inspired fashion, and one application specific part where 'objects' are extracted from the pixel-based information obtained in the

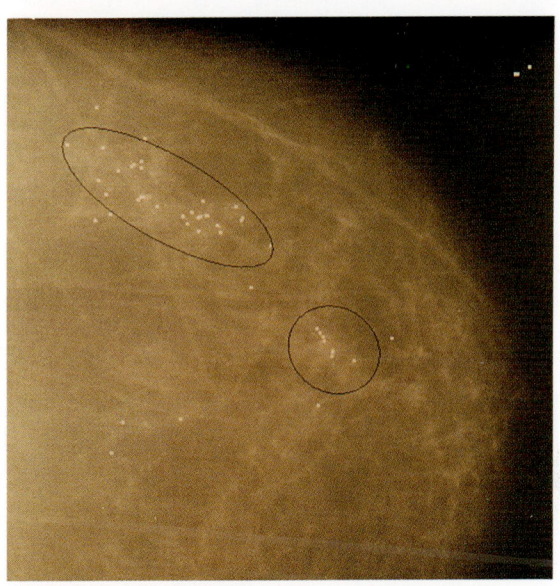

Figure 11: *The result of the calcification algorithms superimposed on the image. Tentative calcifications are white and the clusters centre, shape and orientation are represented with black ellipses.*

Figure 12: *Detail of high resolution mammogram with clusters of micro-calcifications*

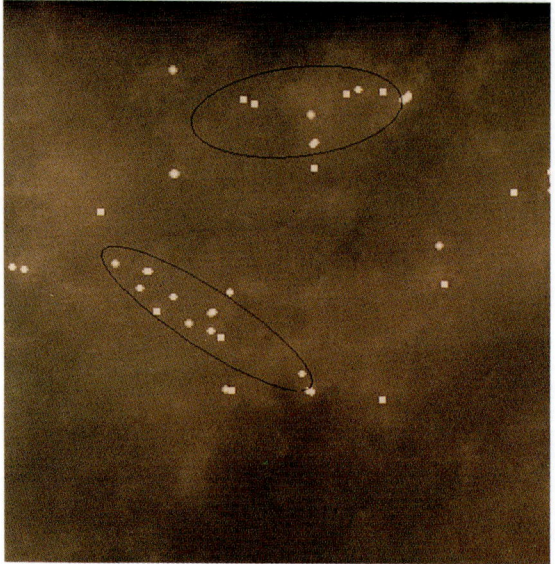

Figure 13: *The result of the calcification algorithms superimposed on the image.*

first part and specialized procedures searches for suspicious areas in the object list.

The system is currently under development and is still lacking in the domain specific features, i.e. the procedures with knowledge of the appearance of suspicious areas. New search procedures will be added, and the existing search procedures will be modified to incorporate more of the information from the feature pyramid and exchange the thresholding with more sophisticated and fully automated methods. Additions will also be made to the general image processing algorithms, e.g. hierarchical estimation of stellar patterns.

The current implementation uses a number of thresholds. Only tentative microcalcifications with certainty $c_\xi > c_T$ are included in the object list. This threshold should be set to a level close to but above the film noise. The threshold R determines whether or not a tentative calcification is part of a cluster, and is typically set to the size of the filters used in the centre of mass computation, a size that is determined from the spatial resolution of the mammogram. The thresholds for merging clusters, T_m, and disregarding clusters, T_c, are more cumbersome. Learning methods and heuristics are going to be used to automate the method.

Acknowledgement

The authors wishes to thank Hans Knutsson and Mats T. Andersson at the Computer Vision Laboratory for discussions and design of some of the algorithms; Neil Roberts and Dibendu Betal at the Magnetic Resonance Research Centre, University of Liverpool, for discussions and exchange of images; Gunilla Svane and Edward Azavedo at the Department of Radiology, Karolinska Hospital, for comments on the results; and Öjvind Sundvall at MoDo Development Centre for scanning mammograms with a high resolution scanner.

Images used were provided courtesy of the University of Liverpool; Karolinska Hospital, Stockholm; the Center for Engineering and Medical Image Analysis and the H. Lee Moffitt Cancer Center and Research Institute at the University of South Florida.

This work was sponsored by NUTEK, the Swedish National Board for Industrial and Tecnical Development. Part of the work was carried out at the Centre for Image Analysis, Uppsala University, headed by Ewert Bengtsson.

A Proof of Eq. 13

Assume for simplicity that the quadrature filters are directed as $\varphi_0 = 0$, $\varphi_1 = \pi/4$, $\varphi_2 = \pi/2$ and $\varphi_3 = 3\pi/4$.

The even part of a quadrature filter synthesized by Eq. 6 consists of the even parts B_{00}, B_{20} and B_{21}, i.e.:

$$E_k(\rho, \varphi) = a_0 B_{00} + a_2 (B_{20} \cos 2\varphi_k + B_{21} \sin 2\varphi_k) \qquad (21)$$

which in terms of filter responses gives:

$$e_k = a_0 b_{00} + a_2 (b_{20} \cos 2\varphi_k + b_{21} \sin 2\varphi_k) \tag{22}$$

where b_{ij} is the response of the filter B_{ij}. Eq. 7 gives:

$$\begin{aligned} e_0 &= h_r(a_0 + a_2 \cos 2\phi) \\ e_1 &= h_r(a_0 + a_2 \sin 2\phi) \\ e_2 &= h_r(a_0 - a_2 \cos 2\phi) \\ e_3 &= h_r(a_0 - a_2 \sin 2\phi) \end{aligned} \tag{23}$$

where r and ϕ are spatial coordinates. The contribution to Eq. 13 is:

$$p_3 = \sum e_k = 4 a_0 h_r \tag{24}$$

The odd part of a quadrature filter synthesized by Eq. 6 consists of the odd parts B_{10}, B_{11}, B_{30} and B_{31}, i.e.:

$$O_k(\rho, \varphi) = a_1 (B_{10} \cos \varphi_k + B_{11} \sin \varphi_k) + a_3 (B_{30} \cos 3\varphi_k + B_{31} \sin 3\varphi_k) \tag{25}$$

which in terms of filter responses gives:

$$o_k = a_1 (b_{10} \cos \varphi_k + b_{11} \sin \varphi_k) + a_3 (b_{30} \cos 3\varphi_k + b_{31} \sin 3\varphi_k) \tag{26}$$

Insertion of the φ_k values gives:

$$\begin{aligned} o_0 &= h_r(a_1 \cos \phi + a_3 \cos 3\phi) \\ o_1 &= h_r/\sqrt{2} \; [a_1(\cos \phi + \sin \phi) + a_3(-\cos 3\phi + \sin 3\phi)] \\ o_2 &= h_r(a_1 \sin \phi - a_3 \sin 3\phi) \\ o_3 &= h_r/\sqrt{2} \; [a_1(-\cos \phi + \sin \phi) + a_3(\cos 3\phi + \sin 3\phi)] \end{aligned} \tag{27}$$

The contribution to Eq. 13 is:

$$\begin{aligned} p_1 &= \sum \cos \varphi_k \, o_k = \frac{2 a_0}{a_1} h_r \; [a_1 \cos \phi + a_3 \cos 3\phi \\ & \quad + a_1/2 \; (\cos \phi + \sin \phi) + a_3/2 \; (-\cos 3\phi + \sin 3\phi) \\ & \quad + 0 \\ & \quad - a_1/2 \; (-\cos \phi + \sin \phi) - a_3/2 \; (\cos 3\phi + \sin 3\phi)] \\ &= 4 a_0 h_r \; \cos \phi \end{aligned} \tag{28}$$

and:

$$\begin{aligned} p_2 &= \sum \sin \varphi_k \, o_k = \frac{2 a_0}{a_1} h_r \; [0 + \\ & \quad a_1/2 \; (\cos \phi + \sin \phi) + a_3/2 \; (-\cos 3\phi + \sin 3\phi) \\ & \quad + a_1 \sin \phi - a_3 \sin 3\phi \\ & \quad + a_1/2 \; (-\cos \phi + \sin \phi) + a_3/2 \; (\cos 3\phi + \sin 3\phi)] \\ &= 4 a_0 h_r \; \sin \phi \end{aligned} \tag{29}$$

This implies that $p_1 + ip_2$ is directed in the edge direction and that the even and odd parts have identical amplification ($4a_0$), viz:

$$\arg(P) = \arg(p_3 + i\sqrt{p_1^2 + p_2^2}) \qquad (30)$$

References

[1] Mammografi screening. Uppföljning och kvalitetssäkring. Allmänna råd från socialstyrelsen 1990:3. Allmänna Förlaget, Kundtjänst, 106 47 Stockholm. In Swedish.

[2] M. T. Andersson. *Controllable Multidimensional Filters in Low Level Computer Vision*. PhD thesis, Linköping University, Sweden, S-581 83 Linköping, Sweden, September 1992. Dissertation No 282, ISBN 91-7870-981-4.

[3] Sue Astley, Ian Hutt, Stephen Adamson, Peter Miller, Peter Rose, Caroline Boggis, Chris Taylor, Tim Valentine, Jack Davies, and Janette Armstrong. Automation in mammography: Computer vision and human perception. In *Proc. of the 1993 SPIE Conference on Biomedical Image Processing and Biomedical Visualization*. SPIE, 1993.

[4] H. Bårman. *Hierachical Curvature Estimation in Computer Vision*. PhD thesis, Linköping University, Sweden, S-581 83 Linköping, Sweden, September 1991. Dissertation No 253, ISBN 91-7870-797-8.

[5] R. Bracewell. *The Fourier Transform and its Applications*. McGraw-Hill, 2nd edition, 1986.

[6] D. Brzakovic, P. Brzakovic, and M. Neskovic. An approach to automated screening of mammograms. In *Proc. of the 1993 SPIE Conference on Biomedical Image Processing and Biomedical Visualization*. SPIE, 1993.

[7] Heang-Ping Chan, Kunio Doi, Simranjit Galhotra, Carl J. Vyborny, Heber MacMahon, and Peter M. Jokich. Image feature analysis and computer-aided diagnosis in digital radiography. i. automated detection of microcalcifications in mammography. *Medical Physics*, 14(4):538–548, Jul/Aug 1987.

[8] Maryellen L. Giger. Computer-aided diagnosis. In A. Haus and M. J. Yaffe, editors, *Syllabus: Categorical Course in Physics. Technical Aspects of Breast Imaging*, pages 257–270. Radiological Society of North America, 1992.

[9] Rafael C. Gonzalez and Paul Wintz. *Digital Image Processing*. Addison-Wesley, second edition, 1987.

[10] G. H. Granlund. In search of a general picture processing operator. *Computer Graphics and Image Processing*, 8(2):155–178, 1978.

[11] L. Haglund. *Adaptive Multidimensional Filtering*. PhD thesis, Linköping University, Sweden, S–581 83 Linköping, Sweden, October 1992. Dissertation No 284, ISBN 91–7870–988–1.

[12] Nico Karssemeijer. Stochastic model for automated detection of calcifications in digital mammograms. *Image and Vision Computing*, 10(6):369–375, July/August 1992.

[13] Nico Karssemeijer. Recognition of clustered microcalcification using a random field model. In *Proc. of the 1993 SPIE Conference on Biomedical Image Processing and Biomedical Visualization*. SPIE, 1993.

[14] H. Knutsson, R. Wilson, and G. H. Granlund. Anisotropic non-stationary image estimation and its applications — part I: Restoration of noisy images. *IEEE Trans on Communications*, COM-31(3):388–397, March 1983. Report LiTH–ISY–I–0462, Linköping University, Sweden, 1981.

[15] Hans Knutsson. *Filtering and Reconstruction in Image Processing*. PhD thesis, Linköping University, Sweden, 1982. Diss. No. 88.

[16] Robert M. Nishikawa, Maryelllen L. Giger, Kunio Doi, Carl J. Vyborny, Robert A. Schmidt, Charles E. Mentz, Yuzheng Wu, Fang-Fung Yin, Yulei Jiang, Zhimin Huo, Ping Lu, Wei Zhang, Takihiro Ema, Ulrich Bick, John Papaioannou, and Rufus H. Nagel. Computer-aided detection and diagnosis of masses and clustered microcalcifications from digital mammograms. In *Proc. of the 1993 SPIE Conference on Biomedical Image Processing and Biomedical Visualization*. SPIE, 1993.

[17] Birger Olander. Detection of microcalcifications in mammography images using the gop-300 image processing system, 1987.

[18] A. Papoulis. *Signal Analysis*. McGraw–Hill, New York, 1977. ISBN: 0-07-048460-0.

[19] Wei Qian, Laurence P. Clarke, Maria Kallergi, Huai-Dong Li, Robert Velthuizen, Robert A. Clark, and Martin L. Silbiger. Tree-structured nonlinear filter and wavelet transform for microcalcification segmentation in mammography. In *Proc. of the 1993 SPIE Conference on Biomedical Image Processing and Biomedical Visualization*. SPIE, 1993.

[20] O. Rioul and M. Vetterli. Wavelets and signal processing. *IEEE Signal Processing Magazine*, pages 14–38, October 1991.

[21] John L. Semmlow, Annapoorin Shadagopappan, Laurens V. Ackerman, William Hand, and Frank S. Alcorn. A fully automated system for screening xeromammograms. *Computers and Biomedical Research*, 13:350–362, 1980.

[22] D. Slepian. Prolate spheroidal wavefunctions, Fourier analysis and uncertainty - IV. *Bell Syst. Tech. J.*, 43(6):3009–3058, 1964.

[23] D. Slepian. Prolate spheroidal wavefunctions, Fourier analysis and uncertainty - V, The discrete case. *Bell Syst. Tech. J.*, 57(5):1371–1430, 1978.

[24] D. Slepian and H. O. Pollak. Prolate spheroidal wavefunctions, Fourier analysis and uncertainty - I. *Bell Syst. Tech. J.*, 40(1):43–64, 1961.

[25] Wolfgang Spiesberger. Mammogram inspection by computer. *IEEE Transactions on Biomedical Engineering*, BME-26(4), April 1979.

[26] R. Wilson. Finite prolate spheroidal sequences and their applications i: generation and properties. *IEEE Trans. on Pattern Analysis and Machine Intelligence*, PAMI-9(6):787–795, Nov. 1987.

[27] Kevin S. Woods, Jeffrey L. Solka, Carey E. Priebe, Christopher C. Doss, Kevin W. Bowyer, and Laurence P. Clarke. Comparative evaluation of pattern recognition techniques for detection of microcalcifications. In *Proc. of the 1993 SPIE Conference on Biomedical Image Processing and Biomedical Visualization*. SPIE, 1993.

ADAPTIVE NOISE EQUALIZATION AND RECOGNITION OF MICROCALCIFICATION CLUSTERS IN MAMMOGRAMS

Nico Karssemeijer

Department of Diagnostic Radiology
University Hospital Nijmegen
The Netherlands

Abstract: A statistical method is described for detection of microcalcifications in digital mammograms. It is shown that the detection performance depends strongly on a preprocessing step, in which the images are rescaled to equalize image noise. A robust algorithm is proposed for rescaling, which can be used to determine a proper scale conversion from a phantom recording. The same algorithm, however, can also be applied to the image to be processed itself. Such an adaptive approach, in which noise characteristics are estimated from the image at hand, appeared to be the basis for far better results than could be obtained by using a fixed scale conversion. The method used for detection is based on Bayesian techniques. A random field model is used to model spatial relations between the labels in an iterative segmentation process. Results of an experimental study using a set of 65 mammographic images digitized at 2048 × 2048 are presented.

1 Introduction

Computer aided detection of microcalcifications has been studied by a number of researchers [1-4]. Although clinically acceptable error rates have not yet been reported, there is some evidence that the performance of radiologists detecting subtle microcalcifications can be increased by providing them with the output of a computer program marking suspicious areas [5]. Moreover, automated detection is an important step towards computer aided characterization of different types of clusters, which often is much more difficult for a radiologist than detection.

A method has been developed for detection of microcalcifications based on the use of statistical models and the general framework of Bayesian image analysis. Starting from an initial segmentation the labeling is optimized by applying an iterative rule for updating pixel labels. In this labeling process the image data is represented by filtered versions of the original mammogram, each depicting a local image feature thought to be important to distinguish microcalcifications from other structures. In addition to these features, a random field defined on the pixel labels models the fact that microcalcifications occur in clusters. A principal advantage of this approach is that all information available, i.e. the image data, the current labeling and prior beliefs, is exploited simultaneously. In an early stage of its development this detection method has been described in [4]. In this investigation its performance was tested on a set 40 digitized mammograms, using a different set of 25 mammograms for learning. An improved set of local image features was used and experiments with different choices of the random field model were performed.

It was found that the use of a rescaling procedure for equalizing image noise prior to processing is extremely important to obtain good overall results. It appeared that the use of a fixed scale transform for noise equalization, as suggested previously [6], could not deal sufficiently with variation of the noise characteristics over the images, despite the highly standardized mammographic imaging process and the fixed protocol for digitization which was applied. To overcome this problem an algorithm for adaptive noise equalization was developed, which estimates the noise characteristics from the image at hand. Apart from the fact that such an adaptive approach does not rely on the stability of the image formation process, it also takes tissue inhomogeneity into account as an additional noise component.

2 Images and digitization

All images used in this study were digitized from film at a size of 2048^2 with a 12 bits CCD Camera (Eikonix 1412), using a sampling aperture of .05 mm in diameter, and a 0.1 mm sampling distance. This resolution seems adequate enough for detection and interpretation of microcalcification clusters [7],[8]. The images were recorded with a Kodak MIN-R/SO177 screen/film combination using various types of equipment. A fixed calibration of the CCD camera was used, in which optical density 0.18 corresponded to the maximum output level. At this low density the signal transfer function of the film is approximately zero. The images were corrected for inhomogeneity of the light source (gordon plannar 1417) used for digitization.

A test set of 40 digitized mammographic images was used, composed of both oblique and cranio-caudal views recorded from 21 patients. Each mammogram showed one or more clusters of microcalcifications marked by expert radiologists. No mammograms without calcification clusters were included. Because the normal tissue area outside the clusters was still very large this did not seem to be necessary. The positions of individual microcalcifications were not marked. The total number of clusters in the set was 104. There was considerable variation of the visibility of the clusters. Some of the fine granular clusters included were more like faint changes of the texture pattern, only consisting of some single pixel calcifications close together, while other clusters did show up quite clear. The set was composed to give an overview of clinical cases. Most were malignant. The presence of microcalcifications was verified by histology for each case. Many clusters were also verified by magnification views. For learning a different set of 25 images was digitized in which 60 clusters were marked in the same way. [1]

To reduce processing time and to avoid artifacts caused by markers and by a sharp edge near the image boundary at the chest side, the breast tissue area was segmented first. A fixed threshold was applied for this purpose, and an edge filter to detect the chest side border of the mammogram. The latter was necessary as thresholding failed at this border because of optic flare of the CCD camera. The

---

[1]The test set of 40 images has been made available for public use. To obtain this set contact the author (Address: Department of Diagnostic Radiology, University Hospital Nijmegen, P.O. Box 9101, 6500 HB Nijmegen, The Netherlands)

tissue area was marked by selecting the biggest connected area detected. All further processing was restricted to this area, which, on average, covered 29 percent of the image matrix.

A phantom was used to estimate noise characteristics. This was a plexiglass step wedge consisting of thirteen rectangular steps of 1.5 x 12 cm in area, increasing in thickness from 0 to 6 cm with 5 mm steps.

3 Noise equalization

Detection of local image features in digital X-ray images is often hampered by the fact that noise models being assumed are too simple. Noise characteristics of, for instance, digitized films are complex and depend strongly on the grey level itself. If this dependency is not taken into account adjustment of the sensitivity of a feature detection algorithm can be very hard, if not impossible, as the noise in feature space will vary with the mean grey level at the position of the feature detector. One way to overcome this problem is to use adaptive methods, in which parameter settings change with the spatial variation of the image statistics. In regions which are more or less homogeneous such an approach may work quite well. However, problems do arise in the presence of boundaries between regions, where estimation of the image statistics is difficult. An alternative and less time consuming approach is rescaling of the pixel values, prior to feature extraction, to an iso-precision scale on which the noise level is constant [6]. Using various criteria, rescaling of image data is often applied to reduce storage requirements [9], or to optimize display [10]. For images digitized from film a logarithmic conversion is common practice.

To equalize the noise level the meaning of the term 'noise' should be defined carefully. For feature extraction it is the uncertainty in feature space which is relevant. Thus, the term noise should relate to the standard error of feature values. Unless only one feature is involved, this brings about a difficulty, because the standard error of each feature may be a different function of the grey level. If these functions differ too much it may not be possible to obtain a uniform detection sensitivity by rescaling the data. Note, however, that local features will only depend on high frequency noise components. Therefore, it seems reasonable to base rescaling on the standard error of pixel values in a high-pass filtered image, representing local contrast.

3.1 Estimation of image noise

For estimation of the high frequency noise level as a function of the grey value, one could choose to use a very straightforward method by recording a number of uniform samples at different exposures. To proceed it would be needed to process each of these samples separately. A different approach is taken here, however, which enables estimation of high frequency noise characteristics from an arbitrary image, provided that this image covers the whole range of grey values of interest and that its structure is as such that there are much more pixels in homogeneous regions than there are near boundaries.

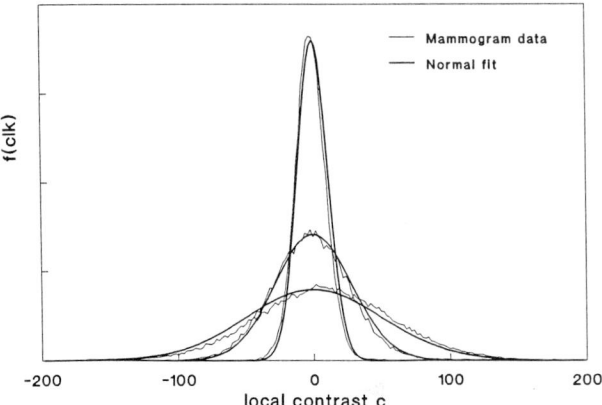

Figure 1: Normalized histograms of local contrast values calculated from a mammographic image in three different bins of the grey scale. The curves are fitted with normal densities $N(0,\sigma)$, with σ estimated by $s_c(k)$ (see Eq. 2).

Let the pixel value at site i be denoted by y_i, and let the local contrast c_i be defined by

$$c_i = y_i - \frac{1}{N}\sum_{j\in\partial i} y_j, \qquad (1)$$

with ∂i a neighborhood or window at i of size N. Independently of the test image the grey scale is divided in bins numbered $k = 1, 2, ...K$. In our application the binwidth was chosen to increase exponentially with the pixel value to obtain a more uniform distribution of the sites over the bins. By scanning the test image the probability density functions $f(c|k)$ can be estimated by normalizing the histograms of c determined within each bin k. Figure 1 shows an example calculated from a mammogram for three different bins. The mean of each density should be zero, if the noise processes involved are symmetric, and if the curve relating the pixel value to the X-ray exposure is approximately linear within each bin. In the following this will be assumed to be true, although afterwards it appeared that for mammographic image data small deviations of the mean around zero were quite usual.

Estimation of the standard deviations $s_c(k)$ is performed by

$$\hat{s}_c^2(k) = r(T) \int_{c_{min}}^{c_{max}} c^2\, \hat{f}(c|k)\, dc, \qquad (2)$$

where c_{min} and c_{max} are truncating the estimated density $\hat{f}(c|k)$ at the first value of c where it runs below a certain threshold T, starting from c=0. This threshold excludes pixels near boundaries, which have high local contrast values of low probability as they are less in number and are spread out over a large range of values. The factor $r(T)$ corrects for truncation, and was calculated by assuming $f(c|k)$ to be gaussian. By introduction of the correction factor direct dependence

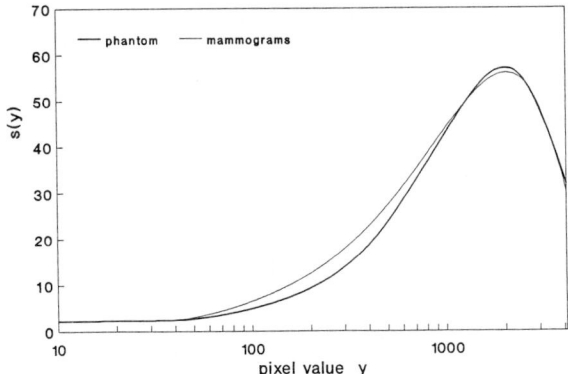

Figure 2: The standard deviation $s_c(y)$ as a function of the pixel value for a phantom recording and the mean standard deviation curve estimated from the test set of 40 digitized mammograms.

of the estimate $\hat{s}_c$ on T is avoided. This is favourable if the noise level, which will be constant after correction of the pixel value scale, is to be used as a parameter in a subsequent image analysis task. For calculation of the scale transform itself the correction factor is irrelevant, because it does not depend on k.

Having obtained estimates $\hat{s}_c(k)$ for a number of bins k, the continuous function $s_c(y)$ can be estimated by interpolation. In this paper a polynomial fit is applied for this purpose. In figure 2 the standard error $s_c(y)$ is shown for a digitized recording of a plexiglas step wedge phantom. A square neighborhood of 9 pixels in diameter was used to calculate local contrast. The average curve $\bar{s}_c(y)$ for the test set of 40 digitized mammograms is also shown in figure 2. To guide the interpolation, at $y = 4095$ fixed values of s_c and the slope of the curve had to be imposed, because in higher bins the number of pixels was often too small to estimate the noise level. These fixed values were determined from the phantom measurement.

The shape of the standard error curves $s_c(y)$ can be understood as follows. At low pixel values CCD noise is dominant, which is independent of the pixel value. For $y > 50$ the contribution of film noise becomes more important, which increases with y. For high pixel values $s_c(y)$ decreases again because the slope of the signal transfer function of the film decreases. For the larger part of the pixel value range the mean standard errors $s_c(y)$ for the set of mammograms are higher than those calculated from the phantom recording. This must be due to tissue inhomogeneity, which can be viewed as an additional noise component. At higher pixel values the difference between the two curves decreases. In this range, where tissue absorption is high, quantum noise due to the limited number of X-ray quanta dominates. At very low pixel values the difference between the two curves decreases because of the influence of CCD noise, which is the same for both.

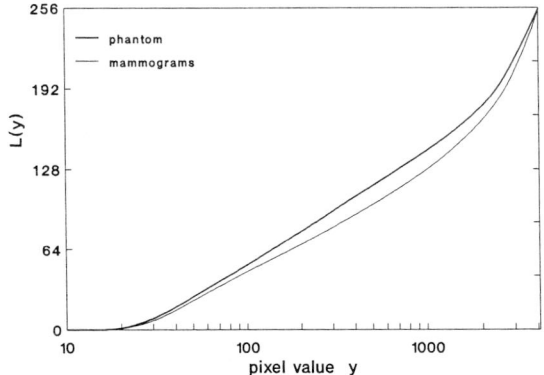

Figure 3: Iso-precision scale transform $L(y)$ calculated from a phantom recording using a 8 bit/pixel output scale, and the mean transform calculated over a set of 40 digitized mammograms.

3.2 Calculation of the scale transform

The transform $y' = L(y)$ which rescales pixel values to a scale with uniform noise level can be calculated from $\hat{s}_c(y)$ by numerically solving

$$\frac{d L(y)}{d y} = S_r \cdot \hat{s}_c^{-1}(y), \qquad (3)$$

where the constant S_r represents the noise level on the transformed scale. This constant can be used as a parameter in subsequent image processing tasks. Its value scales with the maximum of the new scale L_{max}, which is a free parameter. In this paper we will choose $L_{max} = 255$, which enables storage of the rescaled image in 8 bits/pixel.

Figure 3 shows the scale transform for the phantom image and the average transform for the set of mammograms. A minimum value of $y = 20$ was used to set the image background to zero. Variation of the diameter of the neighborhood used to compute local contrast from 5 to 25 pixels did result in a gradual increase of $s_c(y)$, but did not change the shape of $L(y)$ significantly. Also variation of the threshold T used for truncation in Eq. 2 from $T = .02$ until $T = .20$ did not notably change the estimates. In the rest of the experiments a neighborhood diameter of 9 pixels and a threshold value $T = .05$ were used. The mean value of S_r calculated for the set of mammograms was 1.98 and its standard deviation 0.08.

4 Recognition of Microcalcifications

4.1 Method

A statistical method has been developed for detection of clustered microcalcifications, based on the use Bayesian techniques and application of random field models (e.g. [11], [12]). In this method pixel labels x_i are iteratively updated by maximizing their probability, given the image data in a small neighborhood $y_{\partial i}$ of i and given the current estimate of the rest of the labeling $\hat{X}_{S\backslash i}$

$$x'_i = \max_l \left[p(x_i = l | y_{\partial i}, \hat{X}_{S\backslash i}) \right]. \qquad (4)$$

Four pixel classes are distinguished: background, microcalcifications, lines/edge, and film emulsion errors, with labels respectively numbered as $l = 1, 2, 3, 4$.

The image data $y_{\partial i}$ in the neighborhood of a given site i is represented by three local image features, the local contrast at two different spatial resolutions and the output of a line/edge detector. Extraction of these features is described in the next subsection. The values of the three features at a particular site will be denoted by the vector $\vec{\theta}_i$. Using this representation of the data and applying Bayes' relation the probability to be maximized can be written as

$$p(x_i = l | y_{\partial i}, \hat{X}_{S\backslash i}) \propto f(\vec{\theta}_i | x_i = l, \hat{X}_{S\backslash i}) p(x_i = l | \hat{X}_{S\backslash i}). \qquad (5)$$

An important step now is the approximation

$$f(\vec{\theta}_i | x_i, \hat{X}_{S\backslash i}), = f(\vec{\theta}_i | x_i), \qquad (6)$$

which restricts influence of the neighbor labels to the term $p(x_i | \hat{X}_{S\backslash i})$.

The *a priori* probability $p(x_i | \hat{X}_{S\backslash i})$ of the labels represents a random field model, which is used to impose constraints on the spatial configuration of the labels. For instance, a pixel is more likely to be part of a calcification if there are other calcifications in the neighborhood, or, a calcification connected to a film emulsion error is highly unlikely. The following model is used:

$$p(x_i = l | \hat{X}_{S\backslash i}) \propto \exp\left[-\alpha(l) + \gamma(l)[h_i(C) - h_0] - \sum_{m=1}^{4} \beta(l,m) g(m) \right], \qquad (7)$$

in which $h_i(C)$ is a function defined on the set C of pixels representing the current calcification pattern, and where $g(m)$ is the number of pixels labeled as m in a 3×3 neighborhood at i. The constants $\alpha(l)$ bias the detection sensitivity for each class. The interaction parameters γ and $\beta(l, m)$ model the *a priori* likelihood of labels to occur close to each other. The function $h_i(C)$ is defined as follows:

$$h_i(C) = \begin{cases} \sum_j \delta_j(C) f(r_{ij}) & \text{if } h_i(C) < h_{max} \\ h_{max} & \text{otherwise} \end{cases} \qquad (8)$$

where the Dirac measure $\delta_j(C)$ is equal to 1 for $j \in C$ and zero elsewhere, and where $f(r_{ij})$ is a function of the distance between the sites i and j. The constant h_{max} limits

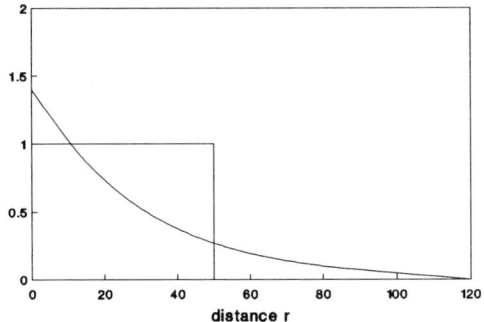

Figure 4: Two choices of the function f(r), which models long range interaction dependence on distance. The distance is measured in 0.1 mm pixels.

the magnitude of long range interaction inside dense clusters. Mostly the set C will be chosen here as a set of single pixels marking the individual microcalcifications, which can be obtained from the labeling $\hat{X}$ by thinning. In one experiment C was chosen as the set of calcification pixels itself. The long range interaction dependence on distance $f(r)$ was modeled as a rectangular or negative exponential function (figure 4).

It should be noted that evaluation of the expression in Eq. 7 requires an initial estimate of the labeling. This can be obtained by maximizing Eq. 5 with all interaction parameters set to zero. The biases $\alpha(k)$ need to be set to obtain a good starting point for the iteration. Note that clusters which are missed in the initial estimate, and which fall outside the interaction range of other clusters, will have little chance to be detected. Therefore, the values of $\alpha(k)$ must be chosen in such a way that even the faintest clusters are labeled in the initial estimate.

4.2 Feature extraction

Three different features are used to represent the image data: the local contrast at two different spatial resolutions and the output of a line/edge detector. At high resolution the local contrast is calculated by applying the operator defined in Eq. 1 to the image data. At a lower resolution the contrast is simply calculated by smoothing the result of the first operator with a 3×3 uniform filter kernel. This is equivalent to first smoothing the image and then applying the local contrast operator. In case adaptive noise equalization was applied the local contrast feature values were divided by the noise level S_r determined during the scale conversion (Eq. 3). On this relative scale the two features are corrected for variation of the noise level over different images.

The line/edge detector is designed to respond to structures which are linear within a given window size, as opposed to the blob-like microcalcifications. The use of such a feature is necessary because both thin lines and regions near strong gradients may easily give rise to false positive detections, the latter because of rippling of the local contrast at sharp boundaries. Like the line feature used in [4], the line/edge feature is calculated from the local probability density function of gradient directions $f_i(\varphi)$, which is estimated by applying the Sobel operator at each pixel in a 9 × 9 neighborhood at site i. The feature is based on the autocorrelation function of $f_i(\varphi)$ defined by

$$\phi_i(\tau) = \frac{1}{2\pi} \int_0^{2\pi} f_i(\varphi) \cdot f_i(\varphi + \tau) d\varphi. \tag{9}$$

If the autocorrelation function has a peak at $\tau = \pi$ this indicates the presence of a line, because two opposite directions dominate the the function $f_i(\varphi)$. A high value at $\tau = 0$ is obtained when the gradient direction inside the window is more or less the same at each site, indicating the presence of a boundary. On the contrary, a disk-like object inside the window generates a low value of $\phi_i(\tau)$ at any value of τ, because it gives rise to a more uniform function $f_i(\varphi)$. Using these properties the line/edge feature is defined by $\sqrt{\phi_i(0) + \phi_i(\pi)}$. The square root is taken because this made the multivariate normal model discussed in the next subsection fit better to the data.

4.3 Random field parameters and probability densities

To obtain the results presented in the next section the conditional probability density function $f(\vec{\theta}_i|l)$ was assumed to be multivariate normal. However, the line/edge feature was assumed to be class conditionally independent of the two local contrast features, which restricts the number of parameters. This assumption was verified to be true in good approximation (e.g. correlation r = 0.01 between the high resolution local contrast and line/edge features, calculated over the images in the learning set). The parameters of the probability density function were estimated from the learning set of 25 mammograms in the following way. First a reasonable initial estimate was obtained by trial and error. The parameters were adjusted in such a way that maximum likelihood (ML) segmentation of the images determined by

$$x_i = \max_l \left[\ln f(\vec{\theta}_i|l) - \alpha(l) \right] \tag{10}$$

correctly labeled the microcalcification clusters marked by the radiologist, while tissue at lines and edges was marked by the line/edge class and while clear emulsion artifacts were labeled as the rest class 4. The biases $\alpha(l)$ were chosen as in table 1. The segmentation result was subsequently processed by setting all pixels labeled as microcalcification but located outside the true cluster areas marked by the radiologists to background. These corrected segmentation results were then used to estimate the parameters from the multivariate normal model. Table 1 lists the model parameters estimated for the case of adaptive iso-precision scaling of the images. Note that $\sigma(\theta_1)$ for background is close to unity, as it should be because the local contrast feature is scaled with the noise level S_r for each mammogram.

It appears that the probability densities of local contrast values have little overlap for background and microcalcifications, which might suggest that detection

	θ_1		θ_2		θ_3		θ_1,θ_2			MRF model			
l	μ	σ	μ	σ	μ	σ	cov	α	γ	$\beta(l,1)$	$\beta(l,2)$	$\beta(l,3)$	$\beta(l,4)$
1	0.0	0.96	0.0	0.57	24.2	1.27	0.34	0.0	0.	0.	.4	0.8	0.
2	4.36	1.51	2.59	1.25	23.8	0.89	1.36	5.0	0.5	.4	0.	2.	2.
3	1.70	1.00	1.17	0.77	29.9	3.18	0.77	2.0	0.	0.8	2.	0.	0.
4	13.6	4.65	6.82	4.20	24.2	1.27	8.05	9.0	0.	0.	2.	0.	0.

Table 1: Parameters of the class conditional multivariate normal model $f(\vec{\theta}_i|l)$, and of the random field model. Labels correspond to background (l=1), calcifications (l=2), line/edge (l=3), and the rest class (l=4).

is fairly simple. One should realize, however, that the number of background pixels is overwhelmingly large compared to the number of microcalcification pixels. For instance, a threshold level at $\theta_1 = 3$ would still lead to about 2000 false positive pixels per image, assuming optimal scaling and only gaussian noise.

Suitable values of the random field parameters $\alpha(l)$, $\beta(l)$ and $\gamma(l)$ were determined experimentally. These are shown in table 1 and were used in all experiments, unless noted otherwise. For C the thinned calcification pattern the parameter h_{max} was set to 12, which means that at most 12 nearby calcifications contribute to the interaction term. For C chosen as the set of calcification pixels itself $h_{max} = 30$ and $\gamma(2) = 0.1$ were used. For changing the detection sensitivity, in experiments with spatial interaction the parameter n_0 was varied, while in case of maximum likelihood estimation the value of $\alpha(2)$ was varied.

4.4 Implementation

Because the computational burden of the method can be very high, implementation needs attention. First of all, it is important to notice that the quantity $h_i(C)$ defined in Eq. 8, which represents the number of nearby calcifications at i weighted with their distance by $f(r_{ij})$, need not be determined at each site separately. This quantity can be viewed as a feature similar to the components of $\vec{\theta}_i$, which can be computed efficiently at the end of each cycle by convolving the function $\delta_i(C)$ with $f(r_{ij})$. Although the support of $f(r_{ij})$ is quite large, the computational load of this operation is small, as the number of microcalcification sites is only small. In figure 5 the use of the matrix $h(C)$ illustrated.

During the iteration the matrix $h(C)$ can be addressed to reduce the computational load even further. Sites at which $h_i(C) = 0$ need not be processed anymore. The labels of these sites cannot be calcification and cannot be changed into calcification. Also sites with local contrast smaller than zero were not processed after being labeled as background during the first iteration cycle. Another optimization, which is common in maximum likelihood problems, was achieved by maximizing the logarithm of the expression in (5), which requires less computation. Furthermore, the probability density function $f(\vec{\theta}_i|l)$ was calculated and stored in a table before the actual processing started. It is noted that this optimization could be implemented quite easily, without using too much storage capacity, because of the

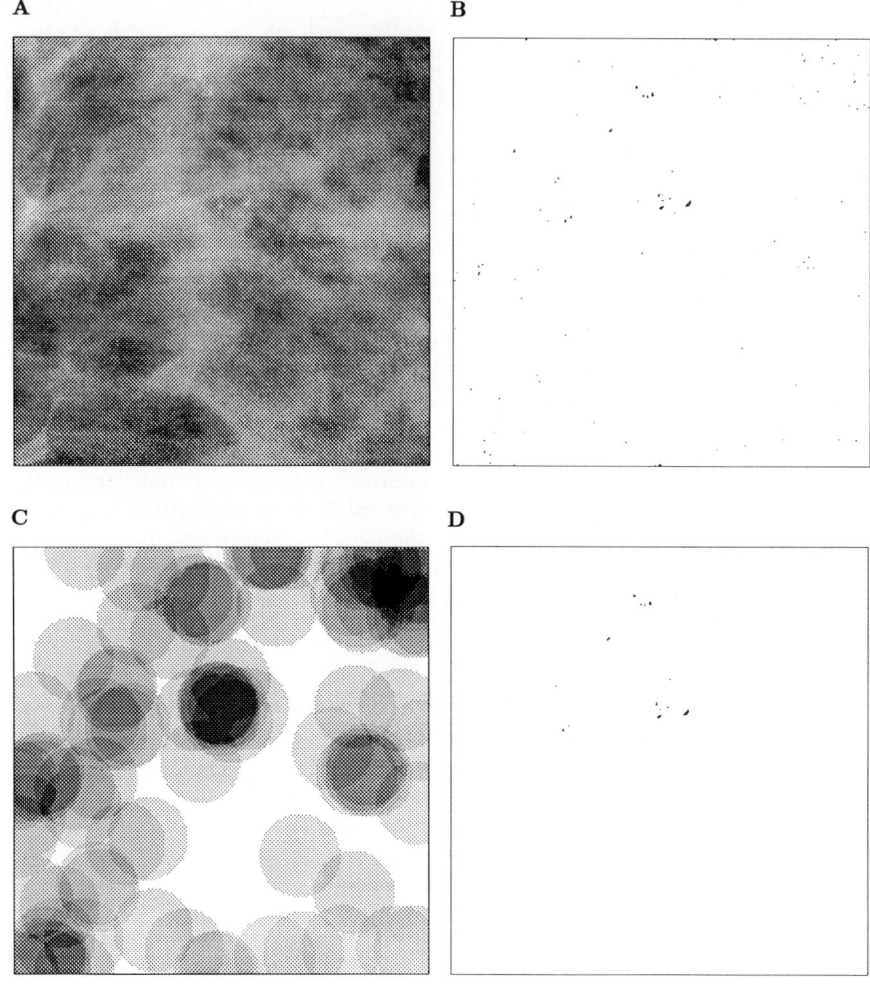

Figure 5: A 512×512 detail of a mammogram (A) and an initial estimate of the calcification pattern (B). The parameter image $h(C)$ representing a function defined on the detected microcalcifications in a certain neighborhood (C) is used to define long range interaction in a random field model. Iteratively, the segmentation converges to the pattern shown in (D).

independence of the line/edge component of the feature vector $\vec{\theta}_i$.

Storage requirements were reduced by representing $h(C)$ at a lower resolution. This also reduces the computational time of the convolution when calculating this matrix. In the experiments $h(C)$ was stored at 512×512. Also the line/edge feature was determined at a lower spatial resolution (1024×1024).

4.5 Performance evaluation

For evaluation of the detection performance the numbers of true and false positive clusters were determined for each mammogram, while the sensitivity of detection was varied. In this way the mean true positive fraction could be plotted as a function of the mean number of false positive clusters per image. Such curves are often referred to as 'free response operating characteristics' (FROC). [13],[14]. It is remarked that in a number of cases labeling of the true clusters was somewhat ambiguous, because these clusters were so close together that it was not clear whether they should be counted as one or more. For counting the number of true positives a cluster was being regarded as detected if two or more calcifications were found in the marked area covering the cluster. No verification of the individual calcifications was performed. With respect to the false positives a cluster was counted if a closed area was found in which two or more calcifications occurred, and which was enclosed by an empty region of 0.5 cm in width.

5 Results

5.1 Noise equalization

In figures 6 and 7 a digitized mammographic image is shown for which the local contrast was calculated after different scale conversions. The point patterns show the local contrast image after thresholding at some low threshold. A homogeneously distributed point pattern would be expected if the noise level is constant, unless some significant structure is present. Figure 7 shows that for logarithmic scaling the point pattern is more dense in dark areas of the film and less dense in the brightest parts. Results obtained by using the iso-precision scale are better. For the case presented, estimation of the scale transform from the image itself yields better results than estimation from the phantom image.

To enable more detailed analysis of the uniformity of the point patterns for the whole set of mammograms, the original 12 bits pixel value scale was divided in a number of intervals, where within each interval the number of marked pixels per unit area was calculated. For images scaled with the logarithmic (LOG) or fixed iso-precision (IPF) conversion fixed thresholds were used to mark the point patterns. Using adaptive iso-precision (IPA) scaling the threshold was taken relative to the noise level S_r, which was determined during calculation of the scale conversion (Eq. (3)). Mean results for the set of 40 images are given in table 2. Note that for IPA scaling the point pattern density increases in brighter parts of the images, while it decreases for the IPF transform. In the last column of table 1 the mean

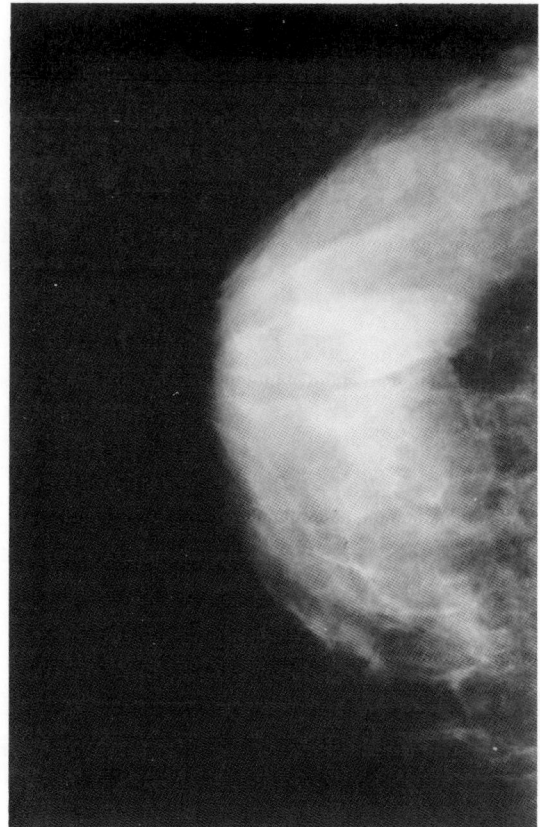

Figure 6: A digitized mammogram.

fraction of tissue pixels in each grey level interval is given.

To investigate variation of the sensitivity over different mammograms the average number of marked points per unit area N was calculated for each image. The relative variation of this number, calculated by dividing the standard deviation $s(N)$ by N, appeared to be much smaller when using the adaptive IPA transform (0.25) than when using the fixed IPF conversion (0.55). When using the logarithmic transform this relative variation was 0.58. This shows that scaling of the detection threshold with S_r significantly reduces variation.

5.2 Microcalcification detection

Maximum likelihood (ML) estimates of the microcalcification patterns for all 40 mammograms in the test set were obtained, using adaptive and fixed iso-precision scaling, and using a logarithmic conversion. The results are shown in figure 8. Using

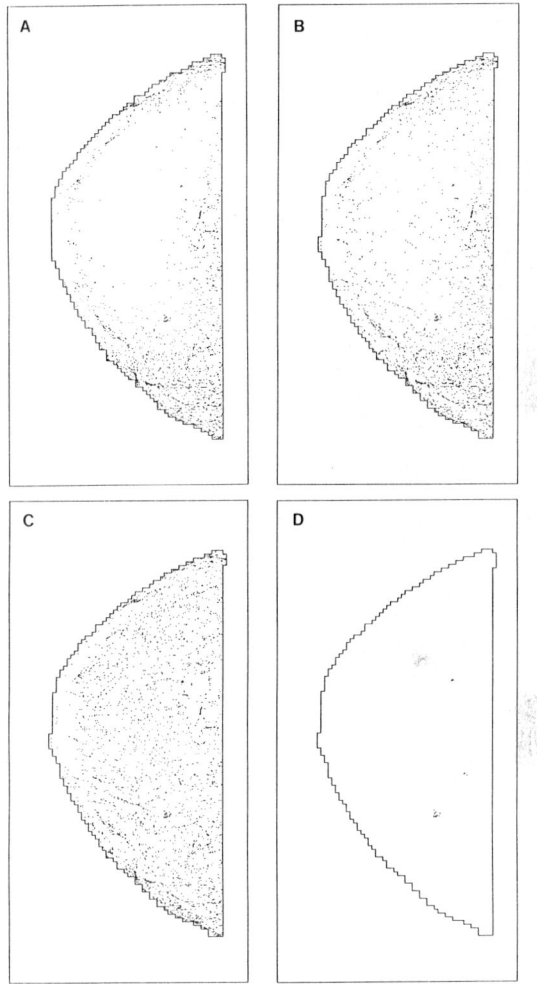

Figure 7: Thresholded local contrast of the image in figure 6, using logarithmic scaling (A) and iso-precision scaling (B and C). In B the fixed iso-precision scale conversion (IPF) determined from a phantom recording was used, whereas in C the adaptive scaling method (IPA) was applied. Image D shows verified microcalcification clusters which were automatically extracted.

Pixel value	IPF		IPA		LOG		Tissue fraction
	mean	sd	mean	sd	mean	sd	%
32 - 64	.67	.20	.61	.34	.76	.23	8
64 - 128	.65	.28	.48	.17	.77	.33	11
128 - 256	.92	.50	.45	.17	.83	.46	16
256 - 512	.86	.49	.62	.30	.71	.42	20
512 - 1024	.52	.57	.78	.57	.47	.54	24
1024 - 2048	.42	.66	1.08	1.0	.30	.59	15
2048 - 4096	.36	.39	1.17	0.8	.08	.13	2

Table 2: Mean percentages of pixels with local contrast values above a given threshold, calculated over 40 mammograms in different grey level intervals. Results are given for the fixed and adaptive iso-precision scale transforms and for a logarithmic transform. For the adaptive conversion the detection threshold was scaled for each image separately with the noise level, while for the other two conversions a fixed threshold was used.

Eq. 10 these were calculated by variation of the detection sensitivity with $\alpha(2)$, keeping the rest of the parameters fixed. For each of the three scale conversion methods new estimates of the parameters of the multivariate normal model were made from the learning set.

FROC curves for iterative detection of the microcalcification clusters using the spatial interaction model are shown in figure 9. To obtain these results noise equalization was performed adaptively. For $f(r)$ the rectangular function shown in figure 4 was used. All experiments started from an initial estimate obtained by ML at a mean false positive rate of about 20 clusters per image. A fixed number of 8 iteration cycles was used, which led to convergence of the calcification pattern for most of the images, or else came very close to it. Table 3 lists the results for each image at a 1.0 false positives per image. Many of these false positive errors could be categorized as coincidental appearances of crossing lines and line-endpoints, for which the line/edge feature is not tuned. In a number of cases it was unclear whether or not the false positive wasn't in fact a true cluster which was not marked. It is remarked that in most cases where a cluster was missed there were other clusters in the same image which were detected. The first false negative mammogram, i.e. without any cluster detected, occurred at a false positive rate of 0.25 per image (image c14o). Also shown in figure 9 are results of experiments in which the line/edge (lin) feature was not used, and in which the low resolution local contrast feature (lcs) was left out. Figure 10 shows the results of some experiments with different models of long range interaction. These were obtained by (1) using the set of calcification pixels itself to define C, instead of the thinned pattern, and by (2) using the negative exponential function $f(r)$ shown in figure 4.

The average time needed to process a $2k^2$ mammogram, using the optimizations described in section 4.4, was about 3 minutes on a HP710 workstation, including adaptive rescaling and calculation of the local contrast and line/edge parameter images.

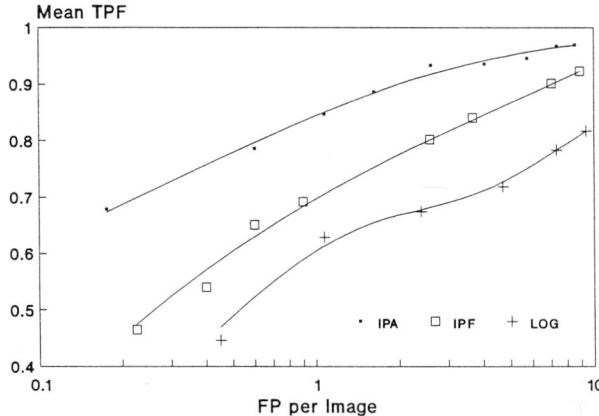

Figure 8: FROC curves for detection of microcalcification clusters for a set of 40 digitized mammograms. Three curves are shown for ML estimation (i.e. without the spatial interaction model). Images were scaled with the adaptive (IPA) and fixed (IPF) iso-precision transforms, and with a logarithmic function (LOG).

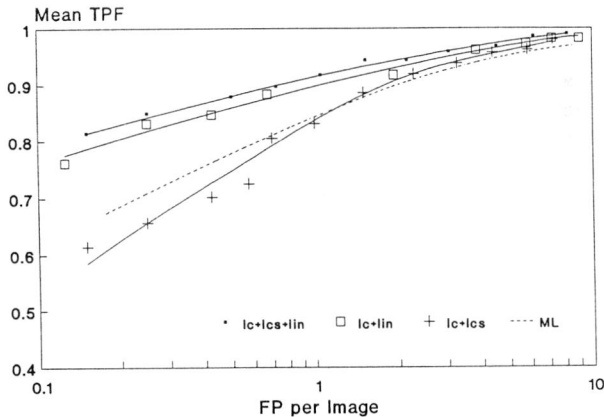

Figure 9: FROC curves for detection of microcalcification clusters using the MRF model and IPA scaling. Results are computed for the test set of 40 mammograms. The curves show the influence of the three different local image features, local contrast (lc), smoothed local contrast (lcs), and the line/edge feature (lin). The broken line represents the maximum likelihood estimate.

Image	N	TP	FP	tp	fp	Image	N	TP	FP	tp	fp
c01o	3	2	0	7	0	c11c	1	1	8	72	23
c01c	3	2	1	8	2	c12o	13	11	2	110	6
c02o	1	1	2	2	4	c12c	15	9	2	74	5
c02c	2	2	1	6	2	c13o	1	1	0	19	0
c03o	1	1	1	13	2	c13c	1	1	0	19	0
c03c	2	1	0	11	0	c14o	2	1	0	4	0
c04o	2	2	0	47	1	c14c	2	2	0	8	0
c04c	2	2	0	69	0	c15o	1	1	1	15	2
c05o	2	2	0	41	1	c15c	1	1	1	13	2
c05c	1	1	1	45	2	c16o	1	1	1	51	3
c06o	2	2	3	18	8	c16c	1	1	0	46	0
c06c	3	2	0	11	0	c17o	5	4	2	25	10
c07o	1	1	1	24	5	c17c	9	9	1	49	3
c07c	1	1	0	37	0	c18o	1	1	4	32	11
c08o	6	4	1	17	2	c18c	2	2	1	28	2
c08c	4	3	0	21	0	c18e	1	1	0	3	0
c09o	2	2	1	13	5	c19o	3	3	0	9	0
c09c	1	1	1	11	2	c19c	2	2	0	8	0
c10c	1	1	1	3	2	c20c	1	1	0	36	0
c11o	1	1	2	65	7	c21o	1	1	3	81	7

Table 3: Microcalcification detection results obtained at a false positive fraction of 1.0 per image, using adaptive noise equalization, all three components of the feature vector, and the MRF model. The number of true clusters is denoted by N. TP and FP denote the true and false positive clusters, while tp and fp are the numbers of true and false positive microcalcifications. Image names reflect oblique (o) or cranio-caudal (c) projection, or earlier screening round (e).

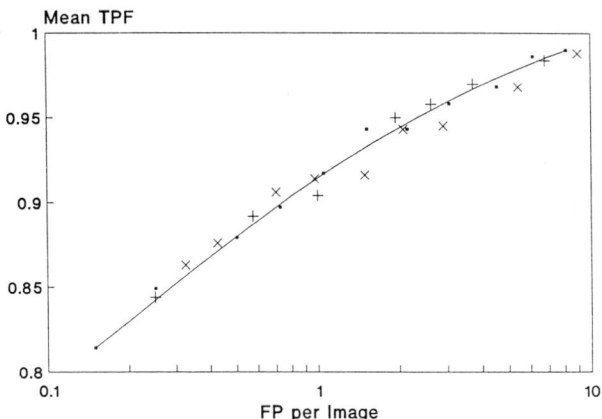

Figure 10: Detection results obtained by using different long range interaction models, defined without thinning of the microcalcification pixel mask (+) or with the weight function $f(r)$ decreasing exponentially with distance (×), compared to the result of figure 9 using thinning and $f(r)$ rectangular (·).

6 Discussion and conclusions

The results of this study demonstrate that rescaling of image data based on measured noise characteristics may significantly reduce variation of the sensitivity of local feature extraction. Image noise was estimated in two ways, from a step wedge phantom image and from a set of digitized mammograms to be processed. Differences are reflected in the scale transforms shown in figure 3. From these differences the results shown in table 2 can be understood, because the slope of the conversion function $L(y)$ scales detection sensitivity. The fact that tissue inhomogeneity is not accounted for using the phantom measurements causes the sensitivity at lower pixel values to be too high when using the fixed scale transform. On the other hand, using the adaptive transform the detection sensitivity seems to be too high at high pixel values. Probably this is due, however, to parts of the breast architecture being picked up by the algorithm, which shows up more dominant in the brighter parts of mammograms.

The maximum likelihood results in figure 8 clearly show the effect of noise equalization on the performance of microcalcification detection. Adaptive rescaling appears to yield much better results than rescaling with a fixed transform, while results of logarithmic scaling are inferior. In part the improvement of performance using adaptive noise equalization will be due to a more uniform noise level. However, also reduction of variation over the image set by scaling the local contrast for each image separately with the noise level S_r seems to play an important role. This reduction was also demonstrated in the experiment described in subsection 5.2, where the variation of the number of points per unit area marked by thresholding was determined.

Figure 9 shows that the use of the random field model improves detection performance importantly, especially in the range were the false positive rate is low. It iteratively removes clusters that are not supported strong enough by the data. It is noted that inside detected clusters the MRF results were far better than those obtained by maximum likelihood. In the latter case often only a few pixels of the cluster were marked. This difference is not reflected in the FROC curves computed for cluster detection.

From the curve computed without including the line/edge feature it can be concluded that this feature is very important in the range of low FP values, whereas also at high FP values it has a positive contribution. This feature enables the algorithm to distinguish microcalcifications from thin faint lines imaging connective tissue structures or vessels, and from artifacts at sharp boundaries. Also inclusion of the local contrast feature at a lower spatial resolution appears to result in an improvement of detection performance. Experiments with other long range interaction models did not lead to significant differences of the detection results.

The algorithm being proposed to estimate image noise appears to be robust when applied to a large set of mammographic images. It is remarked, however, that for images digitized with a CCD camera optic flare limits the accuracy of noise equalization. This flare adds an almost noiseless intensity pattern to the image, due to reflections inside the optic system of the camera, which depend on the image itself. This problem does not arise when using a laser scanner or direct digital recording with, for instance, storage phosphor receptors.

This research was supported by Siemens Medical Systems and by the Dutch Prevention Fund

References

[1] H. P. Chan, K. Doi, C. J. Vyborny, K. L. Lam, and R. A. Schmidt : Computer-Aided detection of microcalcifications in mammograms, Invest. Radiol. **23** (1988) 664-671.

[2] D. H. Davies and D. R. Dance : Automatic computer detection of clustered calcifications in digital mammograms, Phys. Med. Biol. **35** (1990) 1111-1118.

[3] S. M. Astley and C. J. Taylor : Combining cues for mammographic abnormalities, Proc. 1st. Brit. Mach. Vision Conf. (1990) 253-258.

[4] N. Karssemeijer : A stochastic model for automated detection of calcifications in digital mammograms, Proc. IPMI 91, 227-238. *Reprinted in*: Image and Vision Computing **10** (1992) 369-375.

[5] H P Chan, K Doi, C J Vyborny, R A Schmidt, C E Metz, K L Lam, T Ogura, Y Wu, and H MacMahon, Improvement in radiologist's detection of clustered microcalcifications on mammograms, Invest. Radiol. 25, (1990) 1102-1110.

[6] Karssemeijer N and van Erning L J Th O: Iso-precision scaling of digitized mammograms to facilitate image analysis, SPIE Med. Im. V, Image Processing (1990) 166-177.

[7] H. W. Nab, N. Karssemeijer, L. J. Th. O. van Erning, and J. H. C. L. Hendriks : Comparison of digital and conventional mammography: a ROC study of 270 mammograms, Med. Inform. **17** (1992) 125-131.

[8] N. Karssemeijer, J. T. M. Frieling, and J. H. C. L. Hendriks: Spatial resolution in digital mammography, Invest. Radiol. (1993) May.

[9] A. K. Jain : Fundamentals of digital image processing (Prentice-Hall, New Yersey, 1998).

[10] S. Webb : The Physics of medical imaging (Adam Hilger, Bristol, 1988).

[11] J. E. Besag : On the statistical analysis of dirty pictures, J. Royal. Statist. Soc., Ser. B **48** (1986) 259-302.

[12] R. C. Dubes and A. K. Jain : Random field models in image analysis, J. Appl. Stat. 16 (1989) 131-164.

[13] J. P. Egan, G. Z. Greenberg, and A. I. Schulman : Operating characteristics, signal detectability, and the method of free response, J. Acoust. Soc. Am. **33** (1961) 993-1007.

[14] D. P. Chakraborty and L. H. L. Winter : Free response methodology: Alternate analysis and a new observer-performance experiment, Radiology **174** (1990) 873-881.

Artificial Neural Network Based Classification Of Mammographic Microcalcifications Using Image Structure Features

Yateen Chitre, Atam P. Dhawan*, and Myron Moskowitz**

Department of Electrical & Computer Engineering
*Department of Electrical & Computer Engineering and Radiology
**Department of Radiology
University of Cincinnati, Cincinnati, OH 45221

ABSTRACT

Mammography associated with clinical breast examination and breast self-examination is the only effective and viable method for mass breast screening. Most of the minimal breast cancers are detected by the presence of microcalcifications. It is however difficult to distinguish between benign and malignant microcalcifications associated with breast cancer. Most of the techniques used in the computerized analysis of mammographic microcalcifications segment the digitized gray-level image into regions representing microcalcifications. Since mammographic images usually suffer from poorly defined microcalcification features, the extraction of microcalcification features based on segmentation process is not reliable and accurate. We present a second-order gray-level histogram based feature extraction approach which does not require the segmentation of microcalcifications into binary regions to extract features to be used in classification. The image structure features, computed from the second-order gray-level histogram statistics, are used for classification of microcalcifications. Several image structure features were computed for 100 cases of "difficult to diagnose" microcalcification cases with known biopsy results. These features were analyzed in a correlation study which provided a set of five best image structure features. A feedforward backpropagation neural network was used to classify mammographic microcalcifications using the image structure features. Four networks were trained for different combinations of training and test cases, and number of nodes in hidden layers. False Positive (FP) and True Positive (TP) rates for microcalcification classification were computed to compare the performance of the trained networks. The results of the neural network based classification were compared with those obtained using multivariate Baye's classifiers, and the k-nearest neighbor classifier. The neural network yielded good results for classification of "difficult-to-diagnose" microcalcifications into benign and malignant categories using selected image structure features.

Index Keywords: Mammographic Image Analysis, Microcalcification Classification, Texture Analysis, Neural Networks, Computerized Analysis for Breast Cancer Detection

1. INTRODUCTION

There are currently more than 50 million women over the age of 40 at risk of breast cancer in the United States. Approximately 144,000 new breast cancers are expected to be diagnosed this year. Mammography associated with clinical breast examination and breast self-examination is the only viable and effective method at present for mass-screening to detect breast cancer [1-3]. It is desirable to maintain a high positive predictive value (PPV) for suspect findings on screening. To maximize the sensitivity for minimal breast cancer detection, particularly in younger women (ages 40-49) with an incidence rate of 1.65/1000/year, clinical cases with the slightest suspicion are recommended for biopsy examinations. This causes a relatively low PPV and a high false positive rate [3].

Most of the minimal breast cancers are currently detected by the presence of microcalcifications [3-4]. It is however difficult to distinguish between benign and malignant microcalcifications associated with breast cancer. This causes a significant increase in the number of biopsy examinations. At present, the false positive call rate using microcalcification as a sign for biopsy examination is 0.88% (number of negative biopsies divided by the total number of women screened who did not have cancer) which would result in over 260,000 non-productive biopsies per year [cf. 5]. A reduction in false positive call rate will not only save a large amount of money, it will also provide women better patient care since a surgical biopsy examination is traumatic and usually leaves a scar. This could cause future complications. Reduction in the false positive rate must be achieved while maintaining the sensitivity [5-6]. Computerized analysis to help decision making for biopsy recommendation, and diagnosis of breast cancer is of significant value to improve the true positive rate of breast cancer detection. Such an image analysis system can help the physician in many different ways. One example is to develop a system that can only analyze microcalcification areas for malignancy. Computerized analysis of the microcalcifications sign alone can be considered by the physician in retrospect with other signs and history information of the patient. Alternately, such an analysis can be used by a higher-level computer analysis system which incorporates other variables in the high-level analysis.

In addition to a number of efforts to obtain good mammographic feature enhancement through specialized image processing techniques [7-12], several approaches have been used to analyze and classify mammographic microcalcifications [13-29]. In order to analyze microcalcifications, mammographic images are segmented to extract microcalcification regions. After extracting the microcalcification regions, a number of image analysis features are computed and used for further analysis. Successful extraction of microcalcification regions depends on the segmentation algorithm and the overall contrast of the image features associated with microcalcifications. Since the background in the vicinity of different microcalcification regions may vary from region to region, the extraction of microcalcification regions becomes difficult. For this reason, the general region-growing and thresholding based segmentation algorithms often fail to extract microcalcification regions effectively. Various techniques for contrast and feature enhancement have been studied in the literature to aid the segmentation process [7-12]. A common problem with most image enhancement techniques is the simultaneous enhancement of noise and other features which are not microcalcifications.

Computerized analyses have also been used for the identification of circumscribed masses [14], classification of suspicious areas, and classification of microcalcifications using conventional methods [15-20], and using expert systems [20]. In general, mammographic image analysis can be divided into three steps: (1) enhancement of mammographic features, (2) localization of suspicious areas, and (3) classification of these areas. In 1972, Ackerman and Gose [15] demonstrated the use of computers in classifying the breast lesions into four classes using the feature-based pattern classification techniques. Prior to this, Winsberg et al. [16], in 1967, had used optical scanning for the digitization of radiographic films and then analyzed digital images using a computer. Hand et al. [17] developed Bayes classification based techniques for defining suspicious areas of the breast using xeromammograms. Recently, Franklin and Angerman [22] utilized an expert system, Consult-I, for the computerized diagnosis of breast cancer. The expert system was trained using knowledge obtained from the literature and human experts. This research has shown the limitations of expert systems when the application-specific knowledge is not well defined or can not be translated into rules explicitly. Patrick et al. [20-21] utilized a probability based pattern classification approach based on a mapping created by previous observations. They utilized pattern classification and the expert system software, OUTCOME ADVISOR, to classify clusters of calcifications in digitized film-mammograms [22].

Magnin et al.[25] used a mammographic texture analysis of breast parenchyma as a method of predicting the risk of developing breast cancer. They computed local textural features to classify patients into one of 4 risk categories of developing breast cancer. Their analysis indicated that the local textural features computed are not completely satisfactory and do not lead to an actual discrimination between the different mammographic patterns. Woods et al. [26] computed selected gray-level and binary shape features on segmented suspicious regions to detect individual microcalcifications. In this study, a comparison of standard parametric methods, neural networks and the KNN(K Nearest Neighbor) method was presented. Shen and Rangayyan [27] used a multi-tolerance method for the detection of microcalcifications and extracted shape features such as moments, Fourier Descriptors and compactness values on the segmented calcification regions. Nishikawa et al. [28] used automated signal processing techniques incorporating density and microcalcification shape features to detect and classify breast masses and clusters of microcalcifications.

Most of the techniques used in the computerized analysis of mammographic microcalcifications first segment the digitized gray-level image into binary regions representing the microcalcifications. Feature analysis is then performed on such binary images. Since mammographic images are usually very poor in contrast, severely lacking in the definition of microcalcification regions, the segmentation process for extraction of such regions is not reliable and accurate. However, in the actual interpretation of mammographic microcalcifications, the gray-level values and their appearance defining the local structure in the microcalcification clusters play a significant role [29]. The grouping of microcalcification regions to define the shape of the cluster is highly dependent on the gray-level based structure and texture of the image.

The "difficult-to-diagnose" cases are those in which the microcalcificiations are not clearly defined and/or visible. Usually, a radiologist is able to mark out the suspicious region where he/she cannot make a diagnostic decision about the clinical nature of suspicious microcalcifications. The computerized segmentation of such "difficult-to-diagnose" microcalcification regions often does not provide a unique solution for extraction of boundary and shape information. This affects the description of features used in classification, and therefore causes errors in microcalcification characterization. We have started to investigate the potential of second-order histogram based image structure (texture) features in characterization of mammographic microcalcifications. The advantage of such an approach is that it does not require binary segmentation of microcalcifications.

In this paper, we present second-order gray-level histogram based features, called image structure features, for characterization of mammographic microcalcifications. The image structure features have been computed for a number of "difficult to diagnose" benign and malignant microcalcification cases with known biopsy results. We show that the image structure features provide good discrimination between benign and malignant microcalcifications. In addition, a feedforward backpropagation neural network is used as a tool to classify microcalcifications using the image structure features. A two-hidden layered feedforward neural network is used for classification because of its effectiveness in partitioning the multi-dimensional feature space into disjoint regions. Four networks representing different combinations of training and test cases, and number of nodes in hidden layers were used for comparison. False Positive (FP) and True Positive (TP) rates for microcalcification classification were computed to compare the performance of the trained networks. The results of the neural network based classification were also compared with those obtained using the multivariate Baye's classifiers, and the k-nearest neighbor classifier. Figure 1 shows the overall schematic block diagram of the presented system.

2. METHODS AND PROCEDURES

2.1. Digitization of Mammograms and Extraction of Microcalcificaion Areas

A database of more than 18,000 mammograms (developed by Myron Moskowitz, M.D.) was carefully scanned to select about 500 cases of "difficult-to-diagnose" mammographic microcalcifications. Out of this set of 500 cases, approximately 100 cases of difficult-to-diagnose" mammographic microcalcifications were selected randomly for this study. The selected "difficult-to-diagnose" mammograms with microcalcifications were digitized at a 160 microns per pixel resolution using an HITACHI (Japan) video camera and a Matrox (Canada) AT frame-grabber and image processing board housed in an IBM-PC computer. For digitization the mammograms were placed on a light box, the digital images were acquired and stored on a computer hard disk. The digitized images were displayed on a SONY (Japan) monitor. Using a cursor control, the area of microcalcifications was outlined to create a binary mask which was then used to extract a gray-level sub-image containing the microcalcifications area. The shape of the binary mask was arbitrarily chosen to encircle the microcalcifications area. In the next section, it will be shown that the shape of this binary mask of the sub-image does not affect the feature extraction and classification procedures. The extracted gray-level sub-image of the microcalcifications area was then stretched to the normalized gray-level range of 0-255. This normalized gray-level sub-image was used for feature-extraction using its second-order histogram statistics.

2.2. Second-Order Histogram Statistics

The first-order gray-level histogram is defined as the distribution of the probability of occurrence of a gray-level in the image. The second-order histogram, $H(y_q, y_r, \mathbf{d})$, represents the distribution of probability of occurrence of a pair of gray-level values separated by a given displacement vector, $\mathbf{d}$. In other words, $H(y_q, y_r, \mathbf{d})$ indicates the frequency with which particular gray-levels pairs y_q and y_r are separated by the vector $\mathbf{d}$. The second-order histogram statistics correlate well with the image structure [30-31]. This has been widely demonstrated in the literature [30] for the analysis of textured images. We selected 10 image structure features to begin our study. The definition and global interpretation of these features are as follows.

(1) Entropy of $H(y_q, y_r, \mathbf{d})$:

The entropy computed from the second order histogram provides a measure of non uniformity and is defined as:

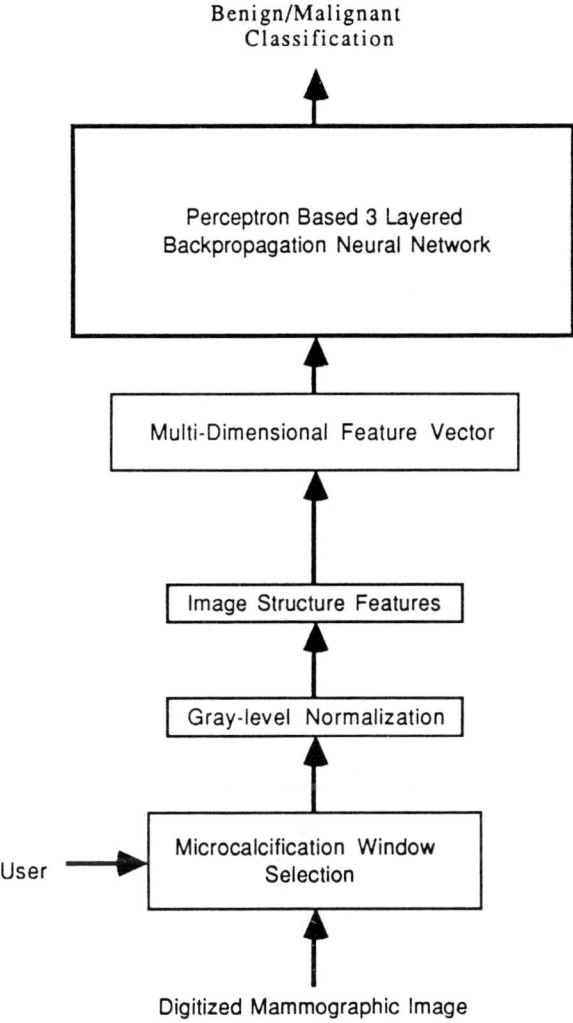

Figure 1. The schematic block diagram of the microcalfication analysis system.

$$\text{Entropy} = - \sum_{y_q=y_1}^{y_t} \sum_{y_r=y_1}^{y_t} [H(y_q,y_r,\mathbf{d})] \log[H(y_q,y_r,\mathbf{d})]$$

High values of uniformity measures will indicate less structural variations while lower values can be interpreted as indicating a higher probability of microcalcification related structures.

(2) Contrast of $H(y_q, y_r, \mathbf{d})$:

The contrast feature on the second-order histogram is defined as:

$$\text{Contrast} = \sum_{y_q=y_1}^{y_t} \sum_{y_r=y_1}^{y_t} \partial(y_q,y_r) H(y_q,y_r,\mathbf{d})$$

where $\partial(y_q,y_r)$ is a dissimilarity measure which is defined as $\partial(y_q,y_r) = (y_q - y_r)^2$.

This measure provides evidence of how sharp the structural variations in the image are.

(3) Angular Second Moment of $H(y_q, y_r, \mathbf{d})$:

The angular second moment gives a strong measure of uniformity and can be defined as:

$$\text{Angular Second Order Moment} = \sum_{y_q=y_1}^{y_t} \sum_{y_r=y_1}^{y_t} [H(y_q,y_r,\mathbf{d})]^2$$

Higher non-uniformity values provide evidence of higher structural variations.

(4) Inverse Difference Moment of $H(y_q, y_r, \mathbf{d})$:

The inverse difference moment is a measure of local homogeneity, and is defined as:

$$\text{Inverse Difference Moment} = \sum_{y_r=y_1}^{y_t} \sum_{y_q=y_1}^{y_t} \left[\frac{H(y_q,y_r,\mathbf{d})}{1+\partial(y_q,y_r)} \right] \quad \text{for } y_r \neq y_q$$

(5) Correlation of $H(y_q, y_r, \mathbf{d})$:

The correlation feature is defined as

$$\text{Correlation Measure} = \frac{\sum_{y_q=y_1}^{y_t} \sum_{y_r=y_1}^{y_t} y_q y_r H(y_q, y_r, \mathbf{d}) - \mu_{H_m(y_q, \mathbf{d})} \mu_{H_m(y_r, \mathbf{d})}}{\sigma_{H_m(y_q, \mathbf{d})} \sigma_{H_m(y_r, \mathbf{d})}}$$

where

$$H_m(y_q, \mathbf{d}) = \sum_{y_r=y_1}^{y_t} H(y_q, y_r, \mathbf{d})$$

and

$$H_m(y_r, \mathbf{d}) = \sum_{y_q=y_1}^{y_t} H(y_q, y_r, \mathbf{d})$$

are one-dimensional marginal distributions of the second-order histogram $H(y_q, y_r, \mathbf{d})$ with μ representing the mean value and σ representing the standard deviation.

The correlation feature is a measure of gray-level linear dependency of the image.

(6) Mean of $H_m(y_q, \mathbf{d})$:

The mean of $H_m(y_q, \mathbf{d})$ is defined as:

$$\text{Mean} = \sum_{y_q=y_1}^{y_t} y_q H_m(y_q, \mathbf{d})$$

This feature represents the nature of the distribution $H_m(y_q, \mathbf{d})$. Its value is small if the histogram is concentrated around $y_s = y_1$, and large otherwise.

(7) Deviation of $H_m(y_q, \mathbf{d})$:

The deviation of $H_m(y_q, \mathbf{d})$ is defined as:

$$\text{Deviation} = \sqrt{\sum_{y_q=y_1}^{y_t} \left[y_q - \sum_{y_p=y_1}^{y_t} y_p H_m(y_p, \mathbf{d}) \right]^2 H_m(y_q, \mathbf{d})}$$

This feature represents the density of the distribution of $H_m(y_q, \mathbf{d})$ about the mean. Its value is large if the histogram is concentrated around the mean.

In addition to the above seven features computed from the second-order histogram, $H(y_q, y_r, \mathbf{d})$, three features were computed from the "difference second-order histogram" statistics. The difference second-order histogram represents the probability of occurrence of differences, ($|y_q-y_r| = i$), in the gray-level values of two pixels separated by a specific distance vector **d**. It is defined as:

$$H_{diff}(i,\mathbf{d}) = \sum_{y_q=y_1, |y_q-y_r|=i}^{y_t} \sum_{y_r=y_1}^{y_t} H(y_q, y_r, \mathbf{d})$$

Three features computed from the difference second-order histogram are described below. The interpretations of these features are the same as described above for their counterparts for $H(y_q, y_r, \mathbf{d})$, except that the difference second-order histogram statistics is used. The objective behind using features computed from the difference second-order histogram statistics is to further exploit the textural properties of the image.

(8) Entropy of $H_{diff}(i,\mathbf{d})$ is defined as:

$$\text{Entropy of } H_{diff}(i,\mathbf{d}) = -\sum_{i=i_1}^{i_t} H_{diff}(i,\mathbf{d}) \log H_{diff}(i,\mathbf{d})$$

(9) Angular Second Moment (ASM) of $H_{diff}(i,\mathbf{d})$ is defined as:

$$\text{ASM of } H_{diff}(i,\mathbf{d}) = \sum_{i=i_1}^{i_t} \left[H_{diff}(i,\mathbf{d})\right]^2$$

(10) Mean of $H_{diff}(i,\mathbf{d})$ is defined as:

$$\text{Mean of } H_{diff}(i,\mathbf{d}) = \sum_{i=i_1}^{i_t} i\, H_{diff}(i,\mathbf{d})$$

It should be noted that we computed features for a particular scalar distance 'x' as the average of the features over displacement vectors $\mathbf{d} = (x, 0), (0, x), (x, x)$, and $(x, -x)$. These displacement vectors represent pixels at the same 'chessboard distance' from the reference point.

2.3. Analysis of Image Structure Features

The image structure features, described above, of the second-order histogram were computed for a set of 95 mammographic images of biopsy proven 57 benign and 38 malignant microcalcification cases. For each feature, the conditional mean and variance values of its Gaussian p.d.f.s were computed for benign and malignant categories. The efficacy of these features was studied on the basis of overlapping regions of the benign and malignant p.d.f. curves. This represents the "probability of error in classification" (PEC) using the Bayes' classification method [32]. Thus, for better features, smaller areas of the overlapping regions of the respective p.d.f. curves are desirable.

It can be shown that for the case of equal apriori probabilities, and uniform cost for normal distributions g(x, μ_1, σ_1), g(x, μ_2, σ_2) with $\sigma_1 < \sigma_2$, the PEC can be expressed as [cf. 32-34]:

$$\text{PEC} = G\left[\frac{r_2 - \mu_2}{\sigma_2}\right] - G\left[\frac{r_1 - \mu_2}{\sigma_2}\right] + G\left[\frac{r_1 - \mu_1}{\sigma_1}\right] + \left(1 - G\left[\frac{r_2 - \mu_1}{\sigma_1}\right]\right)$$

where

$$G(x) = \int_{-\infty}^{x} g(x, 0, 1)\, dx$$

and

$$g(x, \mu, \sigma) = \frac{1}{\sqrt{2\pi}\sigma} \exp^{-\left(\frac{x-\mu}{\sqrt{2}\sigma}\right)^2}$$

and r_1 and r_2 ($r_1 < r_2$), are the roots of the quadratic equation [32-34]

$$g(x, \mu_1, \sigma_1) = g(x, \mu_2, \sigma_2).$$

All features were computed for four different distances of 1,4,7 and 10. A covariance based multi-variate analysis was performed to study the correlation among the features when computed over different distances. This analysis was used for reducing the number of distances over which a specific feature could be computed.

To study the dependence of these features, a correlation coefficient, $r_{j,k}$ was computed for each feature combination at all selected distances. The correlation coefficient is expressed as follows:

$$r_{j,k} = \frac{\sum_i (x_{i,j} - \overline{x}_j)(x_{i,k} - \overline{x}_k)}{\sqrt{\sum_i (x_{i,j} - \overline{x}_j)^2} \sqrt{\sum_i (x_{i,k} - \overline{x}_k)^2}}$$

where

$$\overline{x}_j = \frac{1}{N} \sum_i x_{i,j}$$

and

$$\overline{x}_k = \frac{1}{N} \sum_i x_{i,k}$$

where N is the total number of Samples.

Correlations were computed between different distances for a specific feature. The strategy used to reduce the feature set was to dispense with features having a high correlation (approximately equal to 1.0000). It was considered that the inclusion of such features would lead to a certain amount of redundancy in the feature set.

2.4. K-Means Clustering of Image Structure Features for Classification

Cluster analysis has been employed as an effective tool in scientific inquiry. One of its most useful roles is to generate hypotheses about category structure. The 'K-Means Method' ,a non - hierarchical clustering method was used to cluster the benign and malignant cases into a single classification of 'K' clusters. The central idea in these methods is to chose some initial partition of the data units and then alter cluster memberships so as to obtain a better partition.

The K-Means Method for sorting m-data units into 'k' clusters is composed of the following steps.

1. Take the first 'k' data units in the data set as clusters of one member each.
2. Assign each of the remaining (m-k) data units to the cluster with the nearest centroid. After each assignment compute the centroid of the gaining cluster.
3. If 'd' denotes the sum of squares of the distances between the members of the jth cluster and their centroid , the method minimizes 'd' as far as possible by repeated exchanges of cluster members.

For a given combination of features , the K-Means clustering was performed on benign and malignant cases so as to classify them into 'k' clusters. An evaluation function was used to study the efficacy of the given feature set and is given by

$$f(k, x_1 x_2 \ldots x_n) = \sum_{i=1}^{k} \sum_{i \neq j}^{k} \sum_{j=1}^{k} r_{ij} m_i m_j$$

where k is the number of clusters;
$X_1 X_2 X_3 \ldots X_n$ is a combination of n features, n = 1, 2, 3 ....10;
and r_{ij} is the Euclidean distance between the ith and jth cluster centers.
In the above equation,

$$m_i = \left(\frac{n_{ib}}{n_i} - 0.5 \right)^2 n_i$$

where n_{ib} is the number of benign cases belonging to the ith cluster, and n_i is the number of cases belonging to the ith cluster.

Clearly a clustering scheme which produces homogeneous clusters with dispersed centers would give a larger value of the evaluation function. For a specified 'k', K-Means clustering was performed for all combinations of features. The scheme with the highest value of the evaluation function was considered a possible candidate of features to be used in the neural network classification scheme.

2.5. Classification of Features Using A Backpropagation Artificial Neural Network

An artificial neural network is a parallel, distributed information processing structure consisting of processing elements (called neural elements or neurons) interconnected by directional signal channels called connections. A neural element possesses a local memory and it carries out localized information processing operations. The key elements of most artificial neural network descriptions are distributed representation, local operations, and non-linear processing [35-37]. These attributes make artificial neural networks suitable for applications where only a few decisions are required from a massive amount of data, and also in applications where a complex non-linear mapping must be learned. Thus, when the expert knowledge is not explicitly defined and cannot be represented in terms of statistically independent rules, artificial neural networks may provide a better solution than expert systems. Furthermore, artificial neural networks can efficiently learn non-linear mappings through examples contained in a "training set", and use the learned mapping for complex decision making. Finally, artificial neural networks can be effectively updated to continuously learn new features while in use, without changing the structure.

The computational process envisioned with artificial neural networks is as follows. A neural element receives its input from a number of other neural elements or from an external input vector. A weighted sum of these inputs constitutes the argument of an activation function which is assumed to be non-linear [35-37]. Examples of commonly used non-linearity functions are the step, the signum, and the sigmoidal functions. The resulting thresholded value of the activation function is the output of the neural element. The output is distributed along weighted connections to other neural elements. The concept of memory of a general computer is analogous to the concept of the weight settings [36-37]. Based on the kind of non-linearity, a binary or graded response of the neural element can be obtained. An adaptation algorithm, such as an LMS algorithm, often called the Widrow-Hoff Delta Rule [35], adjusts the weights so that the output responses to the input patterns will be as close as possible to their respective desired responses. The desired response is a special signal used to train the neurons to be fed to the elements. Once the weights are adjusted and the neuron is trained, its responses can be tested by applying various input patterns to test its generalization capabilities.

A Backpropagation network with two hidden layers was used for classification of image structure features. The network architecture is presented in the next section. For each neural unit in the architecture, a sigmoid non-linearity was used. The standard backpropagation learning algorithm implemented on the ANSim software package of S.A.I.C. (California, USA) was used.

2.6 Parametric Classification Methods

Parametric multivariate methods such as linear and quadratic classifiers assuming normal density distribution of samples are widely used in statistical pattern recognition. An advantage of these methods over neural networks is that statistical parametric methods do not require the two classes be equally represented in the training set. However, they do suffer from the limitation that it takes more samples to estimate the probablilty density functions. The classifier is then selected by the conditional probability density functions used to model the sample populations. Let us assume that $f_1(x)$ and $f_2(x)$ are multivariate normal density functions with means and covariance matices μ_1 and Σ_1, and μ_2 and Σ_2 for the benign and malignant categories respectively.

$$f_i(x) = \frac{1}{(2\pi)^{p/2}|\Sigma_i|^{1/2}} \exp\left[-\frac{1}{2}(x-\mu_i)'\Sigma_i^{-1}(x-\mu_i)\right] \quad \text{for } i = 1, 2$$

Assuming that $\Sigma_1 = \Sigma_2$ the minimum expected cost of misclassification (ECM) allocation rule [34] is given by

Allocate x_0 to category 1 if

$$(\mu_1-\mu_2)'\Sigma^{-1}x_0 - \frac{1}{2}(\mu_1-\mu_2)'\Sigma^{-1}(\mu_1+\mu_2) \geq \ln\left[\frac{c(1/2)p_2}{c(2/1)p_1}\right]$$

otherwise allocate x_0 to category 2.

where $c(1/2)$ and $c(2/1)$ are the costs of misclassification and p_1 and p_2 are the prior probabilities of the two categories.

It can be shown that the classifier boundary that seperates the two classes is a hyperplane and consequently the classifier is called a linear classifier. On the other hand, the classification rules turn out to be more complicated when the population covariance matrices are unequal. If we assume that the covariance matrices and the mean vectors are different it can be shown [34] that the minimum ECM allocation rule is given by

Allocate x_0 to category 1 if

$$-\frac{1}{2}x_0'(\Sigma_1^{-1} - \Sigma_2^{-1})x_0 + (\mu_1\Sigma_1^{-1} - \mu_2\Sigma_2^{-1})x_0 - k \geq \ln\left[\frac{c(1/2)p_2}{c(2/1)p_1}\right]$$

where

$$k = \frac{1}{2}\ln\left(\frac{|\Sigma_1|}{|\Sigma_2|}\right) + \frac{1}{2}(\mu_1'\Sigma_1^{-1}\mu_1 - \mu_2'\Sigma_1^{-1}\mu_2)$$

otherwise allocate x_0 to category 2.

In this case the decision surfaces that seperate the two classes are called hyperquadrics and the classifier is called a quadratic classifier. The linear and quadratic classifiers were used with the same sets of features used with the neural network, for a specified number of training cases for each category. Maximum Likelihood estimates were used to estimate the means and covariance matrices, in the case of the linear classifier the covariance matrix was computed in a pooled manner by averaging the covariance matrices of the two classes.

2.7. K-Nearest Neighbors Classifier

The k-nearest neighbor (KNN) algorithm is a simple nonparametric rule that classifies patterns by assigning them labels most frequently represented by the nearest `k' samples. It computes the distance from a test case to every training case by selecting the `k' nearest samples to decide the category to which the test case belongs. The test sample is assigned to a class which has a majority among the `k' nearest samples. The KNN rule was used with the same sets of features used in the neural network classification scheme.

3. RESULTS AND DISCUSSIONS

A set of 95 "difficult-to-diagnose" cases of mammographic microcalcifications were selected. This set consisted of 57 biopsy proven benign and 38 biopsy proven malignant microcalcifications. After digitization, all mammograms were evaluated for extraction of sub-images containing microcalcification areas. As described above, all sub-images were normalized to the gray-level range of 0-255.

The image structure features, as described above, of the second-order histogram were computed for all microcalcification images. Figures 2-3 show, respectively, sample images of benign and malignant microcalcifications. Figures 4-5 show their respective second-order histograms using a displacement vector of (5, 0). The distinct changes in the second-order histogram are quite evident. The image structure features were computed for all microcalcification images. All features were analyzed for their use in classification of benign and malignant cases. Figures 6(a)-(d) show four features which were averaged for all cases in each category of benign and malignant microcalcifications. These features are plotted as a function of distance as the number of pixels in the direction parallel to the x-axis of the image. It is evident from these graphs, that these features can provide significant discrimination for classification of benign and malignant microcalcifications. Each feature for benign and malignant classes was computed and represented by a Gaussian distribution to analyze the error of classification as described above.

3.1 Selection of Features Based on PEC Function

Based on the PEC function (as defined above) computed from the overlapped regions of benign and malignant class distributions of the feature, the features were put in a priority order of usefulness as described above. Based on a selection threshold of PEC < 40%, only the five most useful features were selected for further analysis for the selection of input set to be used in the neural network based classification. The selected five features are ASM, ASM Diff., Deviation, Contrast, and Mean. Table 1 shows the error measure PEC for all features. All features were computed for distances of 1, 4, 7, and 10. The PEC values were computed and averaged over these distances. The average PEC value is shown in Table-1.

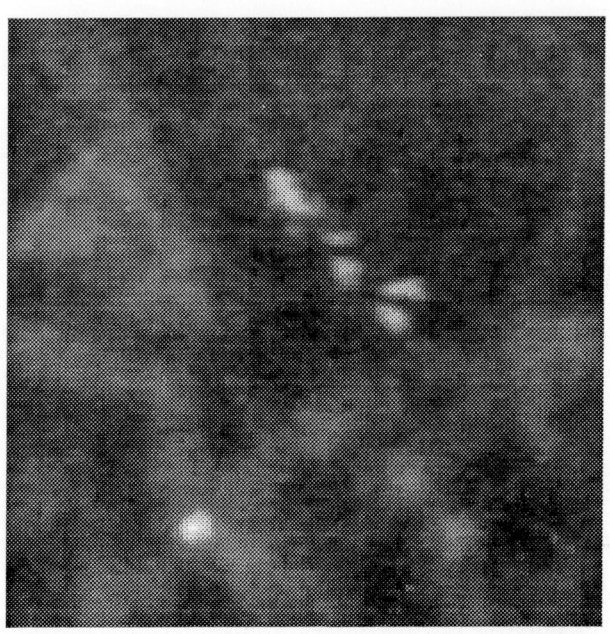

Figure 2

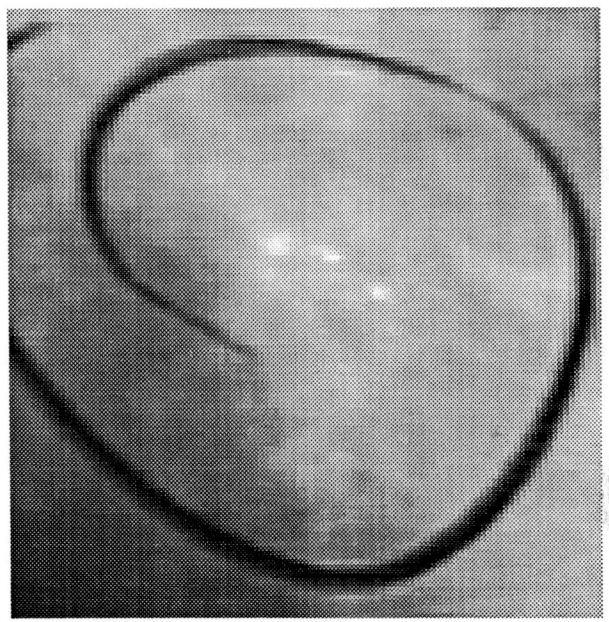

Figure 3

Figure 4

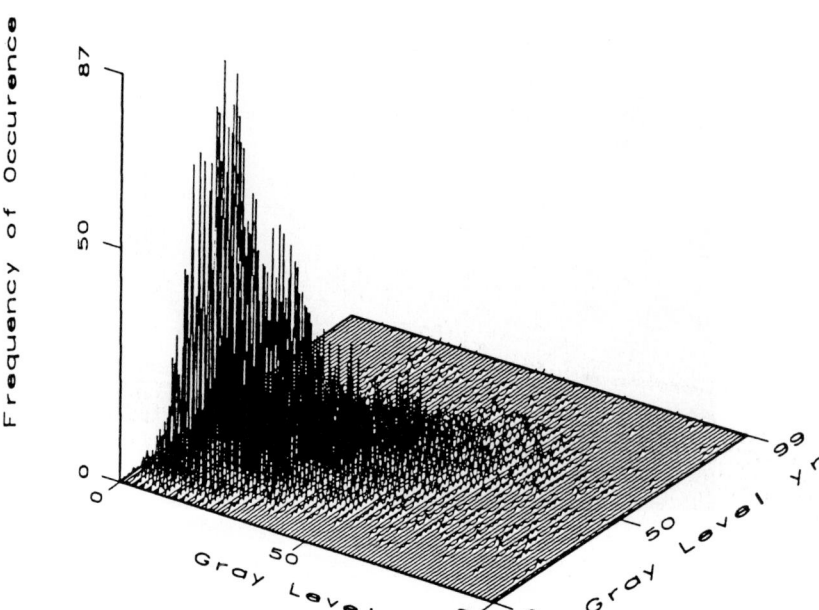

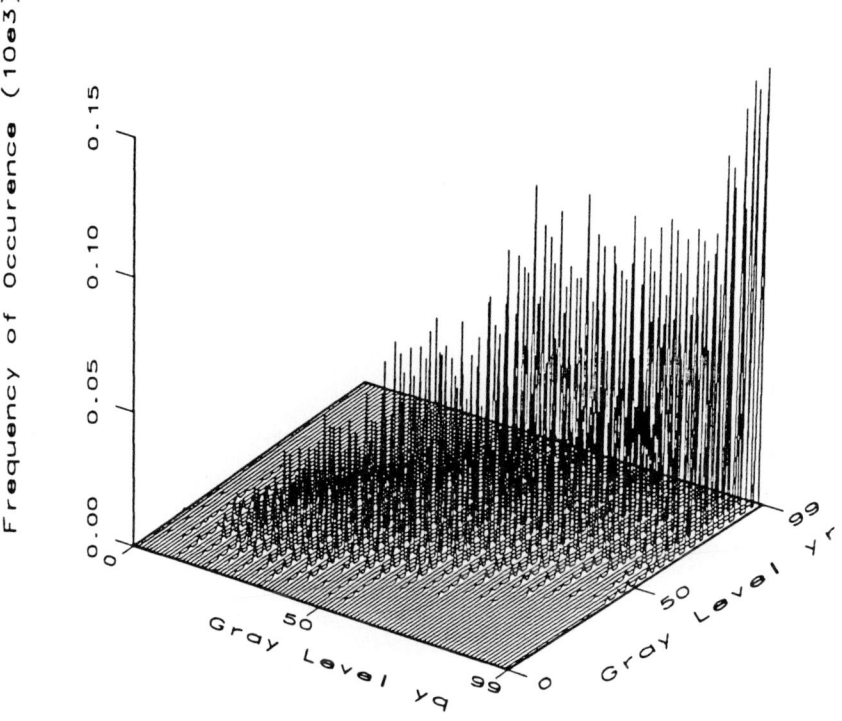

Figure 5(a)

Figure 5(b)

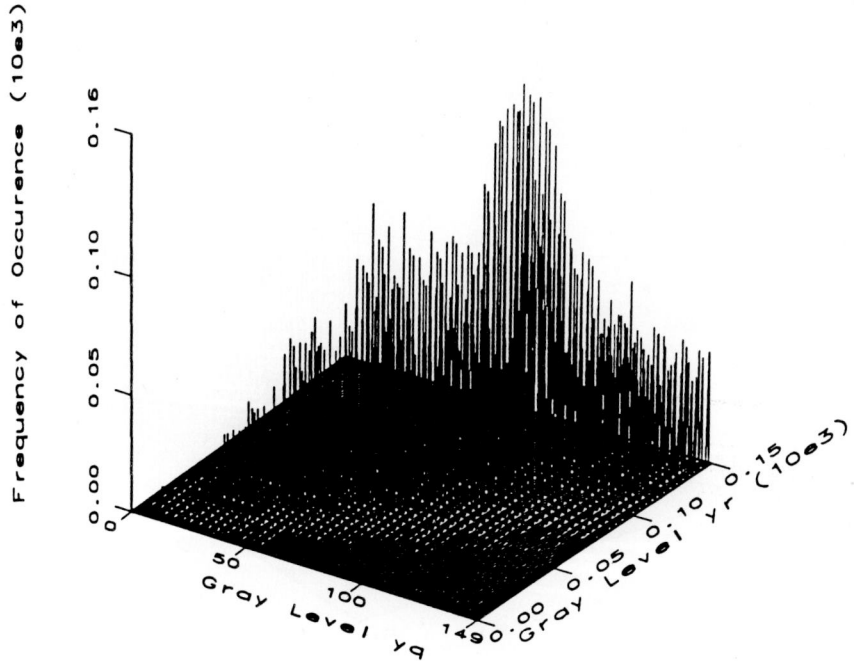

FIGURE 6(a)

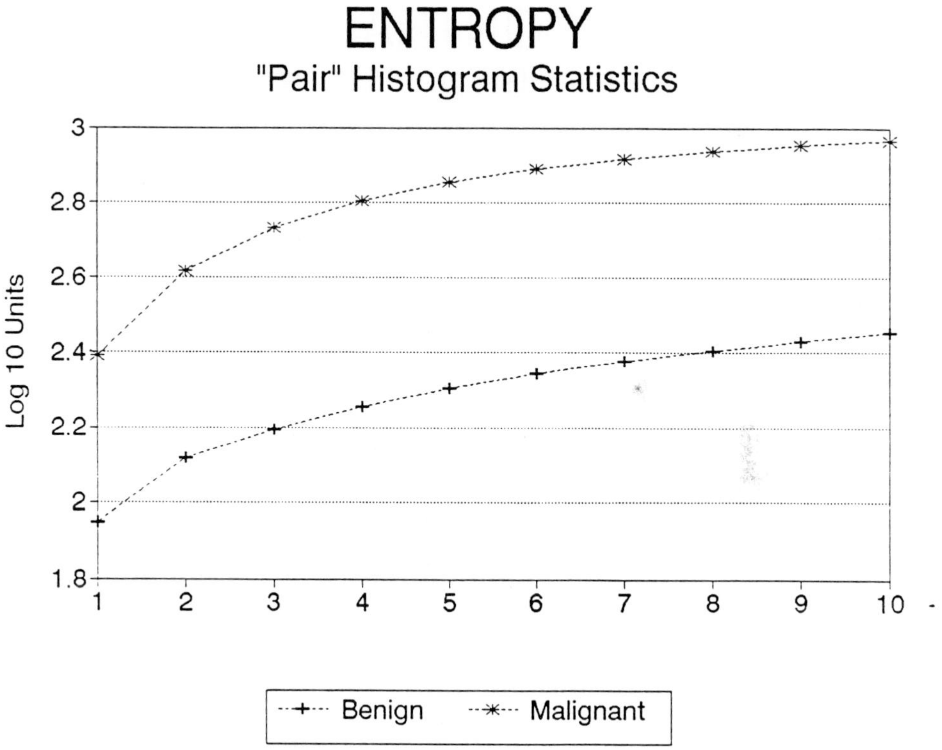
ENTROPY
"Pair" Histogram Statistics
Log 10 Units
3
2.8
2.6
2.4
2.2
2
1.8
1
2
3
4
5
6
7
8
9
10
Benign
Malignant

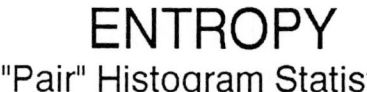

FIGURE 6(b)

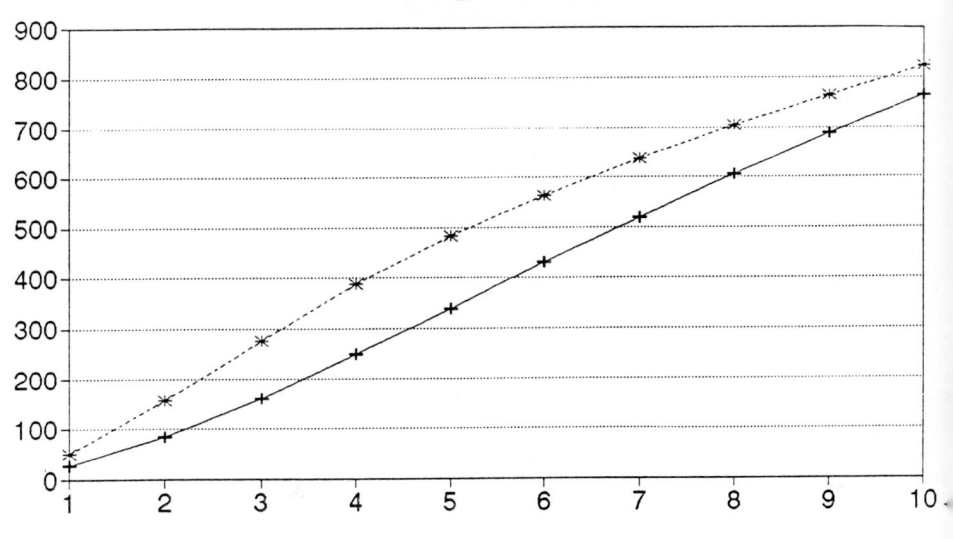

FIGURE 6(c)

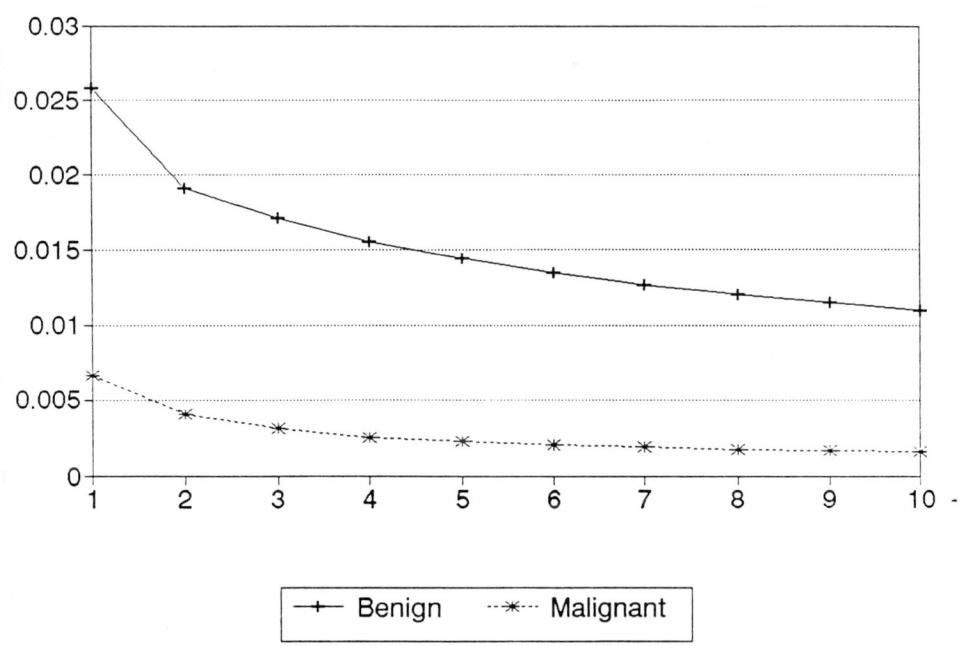

FIGURE 6(d)

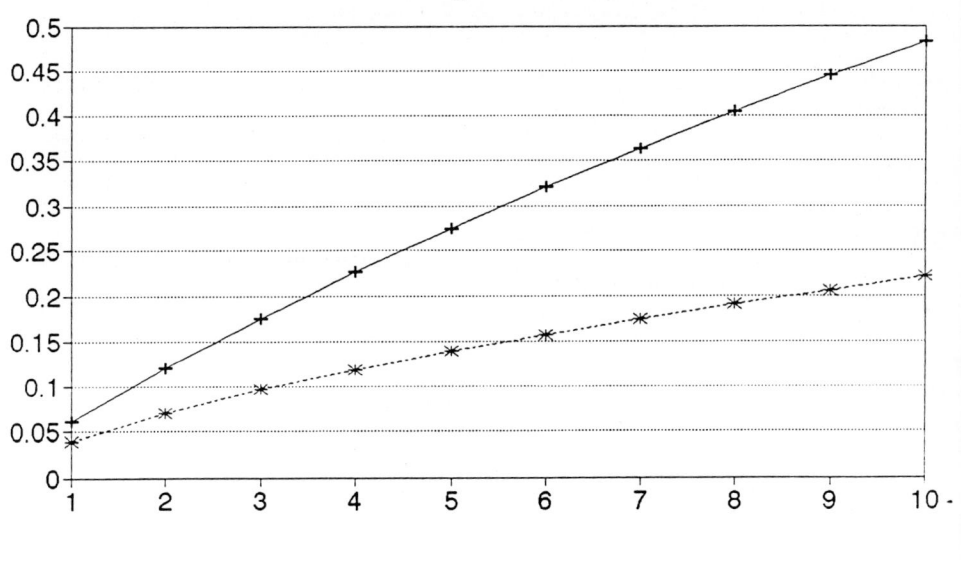

Table 1. The average PEC values for all features

Feature Identification	Average PEC Value
Angular Second Moment	0.1846
Angular Second Moment: Diff.	0.3149
Deviation	0.3469
Contrast	0.3720
Mean	0.3963
Entropy: Diff.	0.4057
Mean: Diff.	0.4099
Correlation	0.4114
Entropy	0.4161
Inverse Difference Moment	0.4602

3.2. Dependence of Image Structure Features on Distance Vector and Window Shape

We computed correlation coefficients of all features at 4 selected distances. It was observed that the image structure features computed on images of selected mammograms were not significantly dependent on distances. Therefore, in the subsequent analysis and neural network based classification, the selected features were computed for one distance only.

To study the dependence of the features on the shape of the window masks used to extract the microcalcification cluster, we computed four randomly selected features for two different shapes of windows. The area of the non-overlapping part of the two window masks was 1864 pixels for the benign cases; and 3767 pixels for the malignant class. All features were computed for two shapes of window masks over 1 benign and 1 malignant case for 2 distances (distance 4 and 7). The normalized difference of each of these features for each mask was computed as follows:

$$\text{normalized difference} = \frac{|(x_1 - x_2)|}{(x_1 + x_2)/2}$$

where x_1 and x_2 are the features computed for two different window masks.

Table 2. The effect of different masks on computation of features

Feature	Distance	Norm. Difference in Benign Case	Norm. Difference in Malignant Case
Correlation	4	0.00825	0.05773
Correlation	7	0.00000	0.00824
Mean	4	0.03484	0.01713
Mean	7	0.02481	0.01680
IDF	4	0.02371	0.12953
IDF	7	0.00672	0.12345
Entropy	4	0.01143	0.00056
Entropy	7	0.00804	0.00615

It can be seen from Table-2 that the effect of computing features over different window masks is minimal in both categories of benign and malignant microcalcifications.

3.3. K-Means Clustering and the Selection of Best Image Structure Features

The K-Means clustering method, as described above, was applied on all combinations of the 10 features computed for 95 cases. All computed features were clustered independently in two, three, four, five, six, and seven clusters. In each case, a performance measure, as described above, was computed. Based on the performance measure value, the clusters and the corresponding set of features were rated. It was observed that when two or three clusters were formed, the performance measure was very low. Therefore, in further analysis, feature sets forming four or more clusters were considered. Table-3 shows two best set of features along with their respective performance measure values in each category forming four or more clusters. Since this approach does not directly represent a non-linear classification, we analyzed Table-3 for the features which appeared repeatedly in forming clusters with high performance measure. Table-4 shows the relative frequency of occurrence of features as appeared in Table-3.

Table 3. Results of Cluster Analysis for Selection of Best Features

Number of Clusters	Set of Features	Performance Measure
4	0, 1, 2, 5, 7	56.85
4	0, 2, 3, 4, 5, 6, 7	73.16
5	0, 2, 3, 6, 7, 8	63.79
5	0, 1, 2, 3, 6, 7, 8	68.23
6	1, 2, 3, 8, 9	67.72
6	0, 2, 3, 6, 7, 8, 9	72.00
7	1, 2, 3, 5, 6, 7, 8	73.96
7	0, 1, 2, 3, 5, 6, 8, 9	74.92

Feature I.D.
0 = Contrast
1 = Correlation
2 = Deviation
3 = Entropy: Difference
4 = Mean: Difference
5 = Mean
6 = Entropy
7 = ASM
8 = Inv. Diff. Moment
9 = ASM: Difference

Table 4. The frequency-of-Occurrence List of Features from Table 3
This list was used in the selection of the best set of features.

Feature	Frequency of Occurrence in Table-3
Deviation	8
Entropy Difference	7
Contrast	6
Entropy	6
ASM	6
Inverse Difference Moment	6
Correlation	5
Mean	4
ASM: Difference	3
Mean: Difference	1

To select the best set of features for neural network based classification, we analyzed Tables 1 and 4. These two tables, respectively, represent best features in order of priority for selection based on the PEC measure, and the Frequency-Of-Occurrence list. Considering both Tables, 1 and 4, we selected the first set of best features. It can be seen that Contrast, ASM and Deviation are common in the top five candidates of both lists. The first set included these three common features and two additional features, not common to both lists with the next selection priority. Thus, the first set of features consists of Contrast, ASM, Deviation, and ASM: Difference (from Table-1), and Entropy: Difference (from Table-4). In addition, we selected a second set of features from the Frequency-Of-Occurrence list only. Thus, the second set of features consists of Deviation, Entropy Difference, Contrast, Entropy, and ASM.

3.4. Classification

As described above, two sets of selected features were used for neural network based classification. Since the variations in number of nodes in hidden layers of the feedforward neural network, and the selection of training cases may affect the performance of the network, we created four networks called A, B, C, and D. A summary of the four network architectures is shown in Table-5.

Table 5. Four network architectures used in performance comparison.

Network I.D.	# Nodes in Input Layer	# Nodes in 1st hidden Lr.	# Nodes in 2nd hidden Lr	# Nodes in Output Layer	# Training Cases	# Test Cases
A	5	5	2	1	10	85
B	5	10	2	1	10	85
C	5	8	2	1	16	79
D	5	16	2	1	16	79

All networks were trained with a sharp sigmoid activation function with -0.5 and +0.5 saturation values. The networks were trained to provide a +0.5 output value for malignant cases and a -0.5 output value for benign cases. After training each network using the backpropagation algorithm [35], the test cases were used to evaluate the performance of the network for benign and malignant classification. All four network architectures were implemented for classification using both sets of selected features. To compare the performance of classification with respect to each network architecture and set of selected feature, we computed the True Positive and False Positive rates of classification which are defined as follows.

(i) True Positive Rate: This is the ratio of number of malignant cases correctly classified to the total number of malignant cases in the test set.

(ii) False Positive Rate: This is the ratio of number of benign cases incorrectly classified to the total number of benign cases in the test set.

The classification results of four networks using two sets of selected features are summarized in Tables-6(a) and 6(b).

Table 6(a). The summary of classification results using the first set of selected features: Contrast, ASM, Deviation, ASM Difference, and Entropy Difference.

Network ID	# Benign Correctly Classified	# Benign	# Malignant Correctly Classified	# Malignant	True Positive Rate	False Positive Rate
A	9	52	30	33	91%	83%
B	9	52	30	33	91%	83%
C	28	49	21	30	70%	43%
D	28	49	20	30	67%	43%

Table 6(b). The summary of classification results using the second set of selected features. Deviation, Entropy Difference, Contrast, and ASM

Network ID	# Benign Correctly Classified	# Benign	# Malignant Correctly Classified	# Malignant	True Positive Rate	False Positive Rate
A	34	52	24	33	73%	35%
B	34	52	24	33	73%	35%
C	27	49	21	30	70%	45%
D	28	49	23	30	77%	43%

Table 7(a). The summary of classification results for the case of 5 training vectors for each category.

Feature Set	Multivariate Linear Classifier		Multivariate Quad. Classifier		K-Nearest Neighbor Classifier	
	True Positive	False Positive	True Positive	False Positive	True Positive	False Postive
Set-1	50.2%	55.1%	52.1%	51%	68.6%	52.2%
Set-2	43.3%	54.6%	43%	37.8%	64.2%	51.9%

Table 7(b). The summary of classification results for the case of 15 training vectors for each category.

Feature Set	Multivariate Linear Classifier		Multivariate Quad. Classifier		K-Nearest Neighbor Classifier	
	True Positive	False Positive	True Positive	False Positive	True Positive	False Postive
Set-1	54.8%	55.2%	46.9%	46.3%	72.4%	48.2%
Set-2	30%	61.5%	30.9%	36.8%	71.8%	48.3%

From the comparison of results shown in Tables 6(a) and (b), it can be seen that although the first set of features provided better True Positive (TP) rate of classification for both networks A and B, the corresponding False Positive (FP) rates were also high. The second set of features yielded good TP rates with low FP rates for both networks, A and B. The networks C and D did not yield any significantly better results for both sets of features. Thus, it can be concluded that the second set of features provided better results for the network architecture A.

The performance of the neural network classification was compared to standard parametric classifiers such as the linear and the quadratic classifier as well as a nonparametric classifier (KNN method). The two sets of image structure features used for the neural network classification were also used for linear quadratic, and KNN classifiers. For these classifiers, we used two different combinations of training samples. The first combination of samples has 5 training cases while the second combination has 15 training cases. The cost of misclassification and the prior probabilities were assumed to be equal for the parametric classifiers and the KNN method. In the KNN method, we used a ' k ' value of 5. These classification methods were applied to 20 randomly selected training sets for both combination as described above. The TP and FP rates were computed by averaging the results obtained from the validation sets. Tables 7(a) and 7(b), respectively, show the TP and FP rates for the parametric and the nonparametric classifiers for the combinations of 5 and 15 training vectors. It can be seen that the performance of the KNN classifier is superior to that of the linear and the quadratic classifiers. A comparison of Tables 6 and 7 indicates that the neural network based classification provides a better performance than the parametric and the nonparametric methods. It should be noted that these results represent the average statistics. Also, there is a trade-off between the TP and FP rates. For example, the low TP rate of the quadratic classifier for Set-2 features is compensated by a low FP rate. The relatively poor performance by the parametric methods may be explained by not meeting the required assumptions about the statistical nature of the data such as the normal density distribution.

The mammograms used in this analysis were digitized at a relatively coarse resolution of 160 microns/pixel. A finer resolution could possibly lead to the inclusion of additional features or the exclusion of features from the current optimal sets of features. It should also be noted that a database of more than 18,000 mammograms (developed by Myron Moskowitz, M.D.) was carefully scanned to select about 100 cases of "difficult-to-diagnose" mammographic microcalcifications used in this study. Because of the greater extent of difficulty, the results obtained using the presented approach can be interpreted as significant.

4. CONCLUSIONS

We have presented a gray-level based feature extraction and classification approach for the analysis of mammographic microcalcifications. The gray-level features are computed as second-order histogram statistics of the microcalcification cluster subimage. The backpropagation artificial neural network was used for classification. We compared the performance of neural network based classification with those of parametric and nonparametric statistical classifiers. We In spite of a limited number of cases used in this study, the results of the image structure features based classification are encouraging. To study the impact of such a computerized analysis on the TP and FP rates, a larger set of cases must be examined. A trade-off in performance between the TP and FP rates was observed. The neural network based classifier can be developed for a five class classification indicating the varying degree of the potential of malignancy. The Receiving Operating Characteristics (ROC) can then be analyzed to study the impact of the computerized mammographic microcalcification analysis on TP and FP rates. We are currently pursuing such an evaluation study. For the limited number of cases examined in this paper, it appears that the image structure features are robust and have significant discrimination power for neural network based classification of mammographic microcalcifications.

ACKNOWLEDGMENT

This work was partially funded by a grant from the National Cancer Institute CA 49976, and the Research Challenge Grant from the University of Cincinnati. The authors are very grateful to Dr. Eric Gruenstein for his valuable comments and discussions.

REFERENCES

[1] D. B. Kopans, J.E. Meyer & N. Sadowsky, Medical progress: Breast imaging, *The New England J. of Medicine* **310**, 960-967, 1984.

[2] G.D. Dodd, Mammography: State-of-the-art, *Cancer* **53**, 652-657, 1984.

[3] M. Moskowitz, Mammography to screen asymptomatic woman for breast cancer, *Amer. J. Roentgenol.* **143**, 457-459, 1984.

[4] E.A. Sickles, Mammographic features of early breast cancer, *Amer. J. Roentgenol.* **143**, 461-464, 1984.

[5] M. Moskowitz, The predictive values of certain mammographic signs in screening for breast cancer, *Cancer* **51**, pp. 1007-1012, 1983.

[6] J.A. Swets, and R.P. Pickett, in *Evaluations of Diagnostic Systems: Methods from Signal Detection Theory*, Academic Press, 1982.

[7] R. Gordon & R.M. Rangayyan, Feature enhancement of film mammograms using fixed and adaptive neighborhoods, *Applied Optics* **23(4)**, 560-564, 1984. "Correction", Appl. Opt. 23(13), 1984.

[8] M.B. McSweeney, P. Sprawls & R.L. Egan, Enhanced image mammography, *Amer. J. Roentg.*.**140**, 9-14, 1983.

[9] M.B. McSweeney, P. Sprawls & R.L. Egan, Enhanced image mammography, in *Recent Results in Cancer Research,* 90, 79-89, Springer-Verlag Berlin - Heidelberg, 1984.

[10] R.A. Kilgore, E.C. Gregg & P.S. Rao, Transfer function for xeroradiographs and electronic image enhancement systems, *Optical Engineering* **13(2)**, 130-133, 1974.

[11] A.P. Dhawan, G. Buelloni, & R. Gordon, Enhancement of mammographic features by optimal neighborhood image processing, *IEEE Trans. on Medical Imaging*, **vol. MI-5(1)**, pp. 8-15, Corrections in MI-5(2), pp. 128, 1986.

[12] A.P. Dhawan, and E. Le Royer, Mammographic feature enhancement by computerized image processing, *Computer Methods and Programs in Biomedicine*, **vol. 27,** pp. 23-35, 1988.

[13] H. Chan, K. Doi, S. Galhotra, C. Vyborny, H. Macmahon, and P. M. Jokich, Image feature analysis and computer-aided diagnosis in digital radiography: Automated detection of microcalcification in mammography, *Med. Phys.* **vol. 14(4)**, pp. 538-548, Jul/Aug 1987.

[14] S. M. Lai, X. Li, and W. BischoF, On techniques of detecting circumscribed masses in mammograms, *IEEE Trans. Med. Imaging,* **vol. 4(4)**, pp. 377-386, 1989.

[15] L.V. Ackerman, and E. Gose, Breast lesion classification by computer and xeroradiography, *Cancer,* pp. 1025-1032, 1972.

[16] F. Winsberg et al., Detection of radiographic abnormalities in mammograms by means of optical scanning and computer analysis, *Radiology*, **vol. 89**, pp. 211-215, 1967.

[17] W. Hand, J.L. Semmlow, and L.V. Ackerman, Computer screening of xeromammograms: A technique for defining suspicious areas of the breast, *Comput. Biomed. Research*, **vol. 12**, pp. 445-460, 1979.

[18] U. M. Pujare, Computer analysis of mammographic classification clusters for breast cancer detection, Masters thesis, Elect & Comp. Eng., Univ. of Cincinnati, 1980.

[19] W.G. Wee, M. Moskowitz, N. Chang, Y. Ting, and S. Pemmerju, Evaluation of mammographic calcification using a computer program, *Radiol.* **vol. 116(3)**, pp. 717-720, 1975.

[20] E. Patrick, M. Moskowitz, E. Gruenstein, V.T. Mansukhani, An Outcome Advisor expert system network for diagnosis of breast cancer, Univ. of Cincin Tech Report: 110/10/87, 1987.

[21] E. Patrick, J.M. Fattu, *Artificial Intelligence and Statistical Pattern Recognition*, Prentice Hall, NJ, 1986.

[22] P. Franklin, and N. Angerman, Consult-I : Breast cancer susbsystem, *Proc. Am Assoc. Med. Systems Info (AAMSI) Cong.* pp. 245-247, 1983.

[23] S.H. Fox, M. Moskowitz, et al., Computer analysis of mammographic calcification, Manuscript, 1981.

[24] S. Morio, S. Kawahara, et al., Expert system for early detection of cancer of the breast, *Comp. in Biol. and Med.,* **vol. 19(5)**, pp. 295-305, 1989.

[25] I.E.Magnin, F.Cluzeau, C.L.Odet Mammographic Texture Analysis: An Evaluation of Risk for Developing Breast Cancer, *Optical Engineering* , **Vol.25 No.6** (1986), 780-784

[26] K.Woods, J.Solka, C.Priebe, C.Doss, K.Bowyer, L P.Clarke Comparative evaluation of pattern recognition techniques for detection of microcalcifications IS&T/SPIE's Symposium on Electronic Imaging:Science & Technology, January 31 - February 4, 1993 San Jose, California, USA

[27] L.Shen, R.M.Rangayyan, J.E.L.Desautels An Automatic Detection and Classification System for Calcifications in Mammograms IS&T/SPIE's Symposium on Electronic Imaging: Science & Technology, January 31 - February 4, 1993 San Jose, California, USA

[28] R.M.Nishikawa et al. Computer-aided detection and diagnosis of masses and clustered microcalcifications from digital mammograms IS&T/SPIE's Symposium on Electronic Imaging: Science & Technology, January 31 - February 4, 1993 San Jose, California, USA

[29] M. Lanyi, *Diagnosis and Differential Diagnosis of Breast Calcifications*, Springer-Verlag, 1986.

[30] M. D. Levine, *Vision in Man and Machine*, McGraw Hill, 1985.

[31] A. Rosenfeld & A.C. Kak, *Digital Picture Processing*, Vol.1 and Vol.2, Academic Press, New York, 1982.

[32] R.O. Duda, and P.E. Hart, *Pattern Classification and Scene Analysis*, Wiley, New York, 1973.

[33] T.W. Anderson, *An Introduction to Multivariate Statistical Analysis*, 2nd Ed., John Wiley, NY, 1984.

[34] R.A. Johnson, D.W. Wichern, *Applied Multivariate Statistical Analysis*, Prentice Hall, NJ, 1992.

[35] B. Widrow, R. Winter, and R. Baxter, Layered neural nets for pattern recognition, *IEEE Trans. Accou. Speech and Sig. Process.*, **vol. 36(7)**, pp. 1109-1118, 1988.

[36] D.E. Rumelhart, G.E. Hinton, and R.J. Williams, Learning internal representation by error propagation, in D.E. Rumelhart and J.L. McClelland (Eds.): *Parallel Distributed Processing: Exploration in Microstructure Cognition*, Vol.1: Foundations, MIT Press, pp.318-362, 1986.

[37] R. Lippmann, An introduction to computing with neural nets, *IEEE ASSP Magazine*, 1987.

Detection and Classification of Mammographic Calcifications

Liang Shen[†], Rangaraj M. Rangayyan[†], J.E.Leo Desautels[‡]
[†]Department of Electrical and Computer Engineering
The University of Calgary
[‡]Department of Radiological Sciences and Diagnostic Imaging
Foothills Hospital
Calgary, Alberta, Canada T2N 1N4

ABSTRACT

We propose a detection and classification system for the analysis of mammographic calcifications. First, a new multi-tolerance region growing method is proposed for the detection of potential calcification regions and extraction of their contours. The method employs a distance metric computed on feature sets including measures of shape, centre of gravity, and size obtained for various growth tolerance values in order to determine the most suitable parameters. Then, shape features from moments, Fourier descriptors, and compactness are computed based upon the contours of the regions. Finally, a two-layer perceptron is utilized for the purpose of classification of calcifications with the shape features. A new leave-one-out algorithm-based parameter determination procedure is included in the neural network training step. In our preliminary study, detection rates were 81% and 85 ± 3%, and correct classification rates were 94% and 87% with a test set of 58 benign calcifications and 241 ± 10 malignant calcifications, respectively. The proposed system should provide considerable help to radiologists in the diagnosis of breast cancer.

Keywords: contour extraction, shape analysis, classification, two-layer perceptron, neural networks, pattern recognition, calcification analysis, mammographic analysis, breast cancer.

1. INTRODUCTION

There is increased concern now about the epidemic of breast cancer. Recent statistics show that approximately one in ten Canadian women will develop breast cancer in their lifetime [1], and that breast cancer will be the most common cancer among Canadian women in 1992 [1]. Although curable, especially when detected at early stages, breast cancer is expected to account for 28% of incident cancer cases and 20% of cancer deaths in women [1]. A similar situation exists in the U.S. and other Western countries. For these reasons, a considerable number of research projects have been directed towards the development of more efficient methods for detecting and treating breast cancer. Although the cause of breast cancer has not yet been fully understood, early detection and removal of the primary tumor is an essential and effective method to reduce mortality, since at such a point in time only a few of the cells that depart a primary tumor succeed in forming a secondary tumor [2]. Currently, mammography is the only reliable procedure for detecting nonpalpable cancers and for detecting many minimal breast cancers when they appear to be curable [3].

The major problem presented with a mammographic screening program would involve the interpretation of the large volume of mammograms, most of which may have no anomalous features. Because of low contrast and the small size of malignant features, mammograms are among the most difficult of radiological images to interpret. Further, only about 20% − 30% of breast biopsy cases recommended by radiologists prove to be cancerous [4]. The price of this imprecision is enormous in terms of emotional and physical trauma for the women and their families, as well as in terms of fiscal costs. This situation could possibly be improved through the use of digital image processing techniques in mammography.

Digital image enhancement techniques have been used in digital radiography for more than 10 years. In 1982, Ram [5] stated that images considered unsatisfactory for medical analysis may be rendered usable through various enhancement techniques. Further, she indicated that application of these techniques in a clinical situation may reduce the radiation dose by about 50%. Chan et al. [6] investigated unsharp-mask filtering for digital mammography. According to their receiver operating characteristic (ROC) studies, the simple unsharp masking procedure could improve the detectability of calcifications on digital mammograms, although this method also increased image noise and resulted in the enhancement of artifacts. Algorithms based on adaptive neighborhood image processing to enhance the contrast of features of mammograms have been reported by Gordon and Rangayyan [7], Morrow et al. [8], and Dhawan and Royer [9]. While the adaptive neighborhood enhancement techniques have been successful in enhancing the diagnostic information in mammograms, enhanced noise continues to be a problem.

Calcifications are the most important and sometimes the only mammographic sign in early, curable breast cancer [10, 11]. Due to their subtlety, detection and classification (as benign or malignant) are two major problems. Wee et al. [12], developed a procedure to evaluate calcifications in mammograms based upon a set of features including area, mean gray level, contrast, gray level deviation, horizontal length, vertical length, shape quantity, and hollow area. Spiesberger [13] proposed a similar procedure for inspection of calcifications based on a feature set including the local maximum gray level, the difference of foreground and background brightness, and compactness. Since 1987, Chan et al. [14, 15, 16] have published a series of papers on a calcification detection system based upon a difference-image technique. Davies and Dance [17] investigated a method to detect clustered calcifications in digital mammograms. Recently, Patrick et al. [18] proposed an expert learning system for the diagnosis of breast calcifications. While most of the researchers focused on the detection of calcifications, only the groups of Wee et al. [12] and Patrick et al. [18] included a classification procedure. We recently reported on the use of three shape factors based on moments, Fourier descriptors, and compactness for the analysis of calcifications [19, 20]. However, the calcifications were manually chosen for analysis in that work. The system proposed in the present paper is designed as an aid to detect and classify mammographic calcifications based upon a multi-tolerance region growing procedure, shape analysis, and neural networks [21].

2. METHODS

2.1. Image data acqusition

We acquire our digital images by digitizing standard x-ray films. Since some significant calcifications may have a size of only $0.1mm$ and the grey level dynamic range in mammogram films can exceed $60dB$, digitization to 10-12 bits/pixel at submillimetre pixel size on the order of $0.1mm$ is essential. Mammograms of biopsy-proven cases chosen from the Radiology Teaching Library of the Foothills Hospital were digitized with high resolution of up to 2560×4096 pixels (12 bits per pixel) using an Eikonix 1412 scanner (Eikonix Inc., Bedford, MA) and a Plannar 1417 light box (Gordon Instruments, Orchard Park, NY). Our digitization procedure includes corrections for nonuniformities in the scanner and the light box.

2.2. Detection of calcifications

After digitization of mammograms, the first step is the detection of potential regions of calcifications. We had initially developed a fixed-tolerance region growing method to extract boundaries of calcifications with manually-selected seed pixels [20]. In this method, the algorithm starts with a selected pixel, called the seed pixel, as the first region pixel. Then, the pixel value $p(i,j)$ of every 4-connected neighbor of pixels belonging to the region is checked for the following condition:

$$(1+\tau)(F_{max}+F_{min})/2 \geq p(i,j) \geq (1-\tau)(F_{max}+F_{min})/2 \qquad (1)$$

where F_{max} and F_{min} are the current maximum and minimum pixel values of the region being grown, and τ is the growth tolerance ($0 \leq \tau \leq 1$). If the condition is satisfied, the pixel is included in the region. This recursive procedure is continued until no connected pixel meets the above condition. The outermost layer of connected pixels of the region grown is then treated as the contour of the region. However, the major difficulty with this method was in determining the value of the tolerance for each calcification. The modified region growing approach proposed in the present paper, which is a multi-resolution procedure, tries to find an appropriate tolerance value τ for each object region.

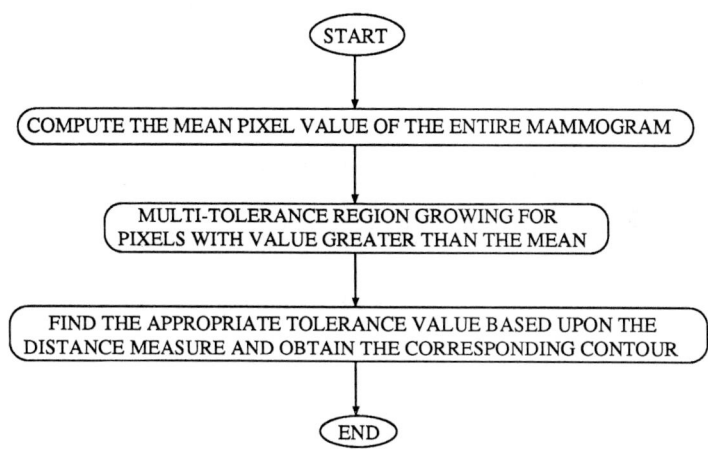

Figure 1: Flow chart of the calcification detection procedure

The complete calcification detection procedure is illustrated in Fig. 1. First, the mean pixel value is computed for the entire mammogram, including the area outside the breast boundary. Every pixel with value greater than the mean (by selecting the highest intensity pixel remaining in raster scan order) is used as a seed pixel for the multi-tolerance region growing algorithm, as long it has not been included in any of the regions already labelled as calcifications. The fractional tolerance value τ for region growing is increased from 0.01 to 0.40 with a step size (SS) determined by the seed pixel (SP) value as SS = 1/SP. A feature set including shape compactness (see Section 2.3), centre of gravity (x-y coordinates), and size (number of pixels), is calculated for the region obtained at each tolerance level. The normalized distance of this feature set between the successive tolerance levels is computed, and the feature set with the minimum distance is selected as the final set. The corresponding region is treated as a calcification region only if the size (S) in pixels and contrast (C) of the region at the final level meet the following conditions:

$$5 < S < 2500 \qquad (2)$$

and

$$C > 0.20 \qquad (3)$$

where

$$C = \frac{f-b}{f+b}, \quad (4)$$

and f and b are mean values of the region (foreground) and a background formed using pixels circumscribing the region contour to a thickness of 3 pixels, respectively.

Two examples are demonstrated in Figs 2 and 3. Fig. 2(a) and Fig. 3(a) show two sections of mammograms (512 × 512 pixels) with benign calcifications and malignant calcifications, respectively, while Fig. 2(b) and Fig. 3(b) show the same mammogram sections but with contours of calcification regions extracted by the algorithm as described above.

2.3. Shape features of calcifications

As Feig et al. [22] and Sickles [4] indicated, one of the major criteria for distinguishing malignant calcifications from benign calcifications is their shape. We have developed a set of shape factors to measure the roughness of objects, which consists of three features m, f, and c from moments, Fourier descriptors, and compactness, respectively, defined as [19, 20]:

$$m = \frac{[\frac{1}{N}\sum_{i=1}^{N}(z_i - m_1)^4]^{1/4} - [\frac{1}{N}\sum_{i=1}^{N}(z_i - m_1)^2]^{1/2}}{m_1} \quad (5)$$

where z_i, $i = 1, 2, \ldots, N$, are the Euclidean distances between the ordered set of contour pixels and its centroid, and m_1 is the mean value of this distance array;

$$f = 1 - \frac{\sum_{k=-N/2+1}^{N/2} \frac{\|NFD(k)\|}{|k|}}{\sum_{k=-N/2+1}^{N/2} \|NFD(k)\|} \quad (6)$$

where

$$NFD(k) = \begin{cases} 0; & k = 0 \\ A(k)/A(1); & k = 1, 2, \ldots, N/2 \\ A(k+N)/A(1); & k = -1, -2, \ldots, -N/2+1 \end{cases}, \quad (7)$$

$$A(n) = \frac{1}{N}\sum_{i=0}^{N-1} Z_i \exp[-j2\pi ni/N]; \quad n = 0, 1, \ldots, N-1, \quad (8)$$

and Z_i is a complex sequence, which is composed of the x-y coordinates of each point in the contour, represented as $Z_i = x_i + jy_i$, $i = 0, 1, \ldots, N-1$; and

$$c = 1 - \frac{4\pi a}{p^2} \quad (9)$$

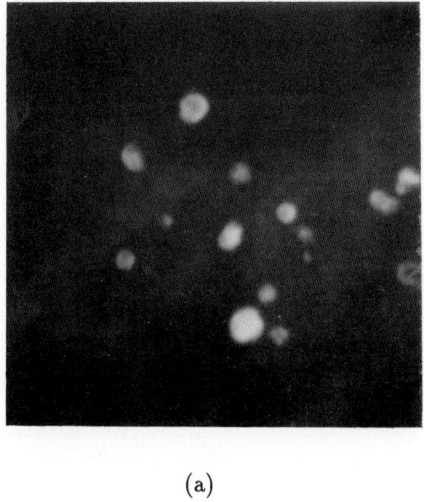

(a)

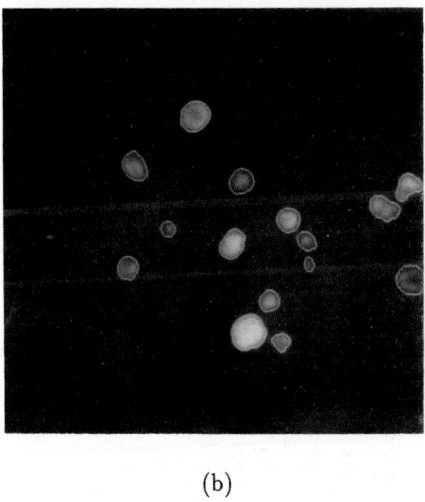

(b)

Figure 2: Mammogram section with benign calcifications. (a) original; (b) with extracted contours of detected calcification regions. The sections shown are of size 512 × 512 pixels, out of the full matrix of 1536 × 4096 pixels of the complete mammogram.

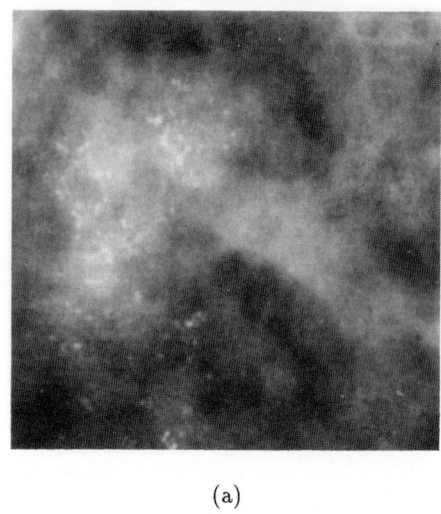

(a)

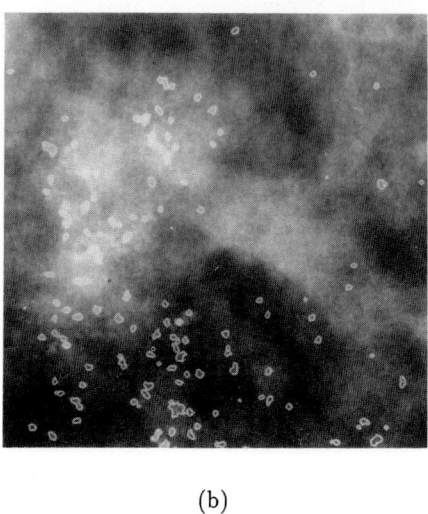

(b)

Figure 3: Mammogram section with malignant calcifications. (a) original; (b) with extracted contours of detected calcification regions. The sections shown are of size 512 × 512 pixels, out of the full matrix of 1792 × 4096 pixels of the complete mammogram.

where p is the perimeter of the region and a is its area.

The three shape features measure shape roughness from different aspects. However, one common characteristic among them is that the rougher the shape, the larger are their values. We have shown [19, 20] that the above shape factors are very effective in characterizing mammographic calcifications, and that using a combination of the three shape factors is better than using any one or two of them. Therefore, the shape factor set as above was computed based on the contours of calcification regions obtained from the detection procedure.

2.4. Classification of calcifications

Since we have no knowledge of the a priori probabilities of calcifications as being malignant or benign, no general classification rules exist for calcifications, and clinical knowledge is unable to create symbolic knowledge bases comprehensive enough to cope with the diverse exceptions that occur in practice, conventional parametric pattern recognition methods seem not well-suited for classification of calcifications. However, Artificial Neural Networks (ANN), with the properties of experience-based learning, fault tolerance, and signal enhancement should be effective in solving such a classification problem. We are developing a two-layer perceptron with one hidden layer and one output layer for classification of calcifications (see Fig. 4). The network learns the similarities among patterns directly from their instances in the training set. That is, it infers classification rules from the training data without prior knowledge of the pattern distributions in the data. Training of the neural network classifier is accomplished by the *back-propagation* algorithm [23, 24]. The actual output Y_k is calculated as

$$Y_k = f(\sum_{j=1}^{J} W'_{jk} X'_j - \theta'_k), \qquad k = 1, 2, \ldots, K \tag{10}$$

where

$$X'_j = f(\sum_{i=1}^{I} W_{ij} X_i - \theta_j), \qquad j = 1, 2, \ldots, J \tag{11}$$

and

$$f(\beta) = \frac{1}{1 + \exp(-\beta)}. \tag{12}$$

In the above equations, θ_j and θ'_k are node offsets, W_{ij}'s and W'_{jk}'s are node weights, X_i's are the input parameters of calcifications, and I, J, and K are the numbers of nodes in the input, hidden, and output layers, respectively. The weights and offsets are updated by

$$W'_{jk}(t+1) = W'_{jk}(t) + \eta[Y_k(1-Y_k)(O_k-Y_k)]X'_j + \alpha[W'_{jk}(t) - W'_{jk}(t-1)] \tag{13}$$

$$\theta'_k(t+1) = \theta'_k(t) + \eta[Y_k(1-Y_k)(O_k-Y_k)](-1) + \alpha[\theta'_k(t) - \theta'_k(t-1)] \tag{14}$$

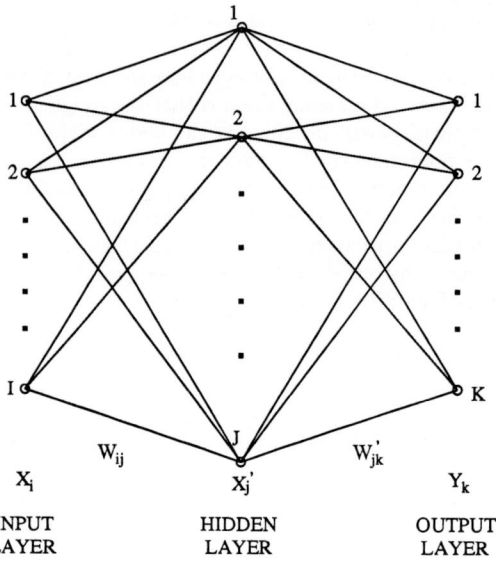

Figure 4: Two-layer perceptron architecture

$$W_{ij}(t+1) = W_{ij}(t)+\eta[X'_j(1-X'_j)\sum_{k=1}^{K}(Y_k(1-Y_k)(O_k-Y_k)W'_{jk})]X_i+\alpha[W_{ij}(t)-W_{ij}(t-1)] \quad (15)$$

$$\theta_j(t+1) = \theta_j+\eta[X'_j(1-X'_j)\sum_{k=1}^{K}(Y_k(1-Y_k)(O_k-Y_k)W'_{jk})](-1)+\alpha[\theta_j(t)-\theta_j(t-1)] \quad (16)$$

where O_k's are the desired ouputs, α is a momentum term, and η is a gain term. The classifier training algorithm is repeated until the errors between the desired outputs and actual outputs for the training data are smaller than a predetermined threshold value (0.1 in our study).

3. RESULTS AND DISCUSSION

3.1. Classifier training

In this study, the shape features (m, f, c) discussed above are employed as inputs $(X_i, i = 1, 2, 3)$, and we classify calcifications into two groups: benign and malignant. Therefore, the numbers of input (I) and output (K) nodes are 3 and 2, respectively. Feature sets of 143 calcifications (64 benign and 79 malignant) obtained from 18 typical mammograms of biopsy-proven cases (chosen from the Radiology Teaching Library of the Foothills Hospital by a radiologist) by manual selection of seed pixels and their growth tolerances [20] were used for training. Fig. 5 provides a three-dimensional plot of the feature vectors for the 143 calcifications which were used as the training data. Three parameters (the number of hidden nodes J, the gain term η, and the momentum term α) need to be determined before training the two-layer perceptron. Unfortunately, there is no general rule available for the selection of these parameters. One of the most common methods is trial-and-error by choosing the set of parameters with which the fastest training speed (the smallest number of iterations) is achieved. However, the major disadvantage of this method is that classification effectiveness (after training) is not considered. To use the training data set more efficiently and to overcome the above-mentioned shortcoming of the trial-and-error method, we propose to include the leave-one-out algorithm [25, 26] in the procedure for determining the three parameters (J, η, and α), as described below.

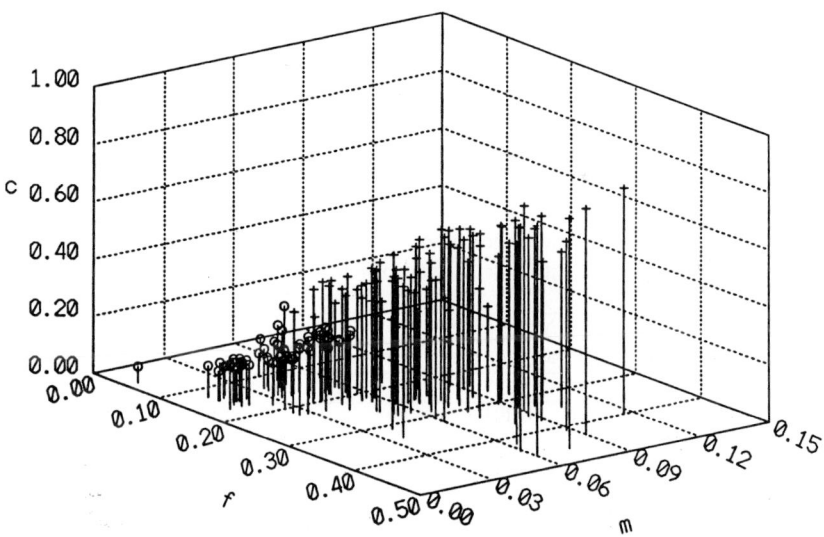

Figure 5: A three-dimensional plot of the shape factors of 143 calcifications, used as the training data set. The +'s represent 79 malignant calcifications, and the o's represent 64 benign calcifications.

First, we fix η and α to determine the optimal number of hidden nodes J. Table 1 and Table 2 list the results (the average number of iterations and the number of erroneous classifications) of the leave-one-out training and parameter determination method in two circumstances: $\eta = 1.0, \alpha = 0.7$ and $\eta = 2.0, \alpha = 0.7$ respectively. Based upon Tables 1 and 2, we find $J = 10$ is an optimal number as it achieved the fewest number of classification errors in a reasonable number of iterations.

Table 1: Results of the leave-one-out training and parameter determination algorithm with $\eta = 1.0$ and $\alpha = 0.7$.

Number of hidden nodes	Number of iterations (mean)	Number of erroneous classifications out of 143 samples
1	1810	4
3	1809	4
5	1774	4
7	1729	4
9	1697	4
10	1697	3
15	1676	3
20	1675	3
30	1676	3

Table 2: Results of the leave-one-out training and parameter determination algorithm with $\eta = 2.0$ and $\alpha = 0.7$.

Number of hidden nodes	Number of iterations (mean)	Number of erroneous classifications out of 143 samples
5	1448	3
10	1391	3
12	1380	4
15	1387	3
20	1401	4

After determining an optimal value for J, we determine a value for η by fixing $J = 10$ and $\alpha = 0.7$. The corresponding results are listed in Table 3. We notice that $\eta = 2.0$ is the best value.

Finally, we determine a value for α with $J = 10$ and $\eta = 2.0$. Table 4 provides the results of various trials. It is clear that the best value for α is 0.7.

Table 3: Results of the leave-one-out training and parameter determination algorithm with $J = 10$ and $\alpha = 0.7$.

Gain η	Number of iterations (mean)	Number of erroneous classifications out of 143 samples
0.3	4088	4
0.7	2145	4
1.0	1697	3
1.5	1431	4
2.0	1391	3
2.3	1430	3
3.0	2691	5

After obtaining the optimal values for the parameter set, we trained the perceptron again by using all the training data (instead of the leave-one-out algorithm), setting $J = 10$, $\eta = 2.0$, and $\alpha = 0.7$. All of the 143 calcifications in the training set were correctly classified in 1268 iterations. The weight set obtained by this procedure was utilized for the classification of calcifications in the test set.

3.2. Detection and classification test

Because of memory limitations of our computer, sections (1024×768, 768×512, 512×768, and 512×768 pixels) of four typical mammograms from complete images of up to 2560×4096 pixels) with biopsy-proven calcifications were utilized for this preliminary study, among which two had a total of 58 benign calcifications while the other two contained 241 ± 10 malignant calcifications. Based upon visual inspection by a radiologist, detection rates of our multi-tolerance region growing algorithm were 81% with 0 false calcifications and $85 \pm 3\%$ with 29 false calcifications for the benign and malignant sections, respectively. After the detection procedure, the detected calcifications were classified by our neural network classifier. The correct classification rate for the detected benign calcifications was 94%, while the correct classification rate for the correctly detected malignant calcifications was 87%.

Table 4: Results of the leave-one-out training and parameter determination algorithm with $J = 10$ and $\eta = 2.0$.

Momentum α	Number of iterations (mean)	Number of erroneous classifications out of 143 samples
0.5	2426	4
0.7	1391	3
0.9	4152	7

3.3. Discussion and future work

Classification errors for benign calcifications arose mainly from overlapping calcifications. One possible solution to this problem is two-view analysis [27]. A likely reason for erroneous classification of malignant calcifications is that not all calcifications within a malignant calcification cluster may possess rough contours, which makes it necessary to include a cluster analysis procedure in the classification algorithm. Further work is in progress with more mammograms of biopsy-proven cases to test our detection and classification approaches and along the directions described above.

4. ACKNOWLEDGMENTS

This work is supported by grants from the Natural Sciences and Engineering Research Council of Canada.

REFERENCES

[1] *Canadian Cancer Statistics (1992)*. National Cancer Institute of Canada, Toronto, Canada, 1992. pp. 8-9.

[2] Spratt JS and Spratt JA. Growth rates. In Donegan WL and Spratt JS, editors, *Cancer of the Breast*, chapter 10, pages 270–302. W. B. Saunders Company, Philadelphia, PA, 3rd edition, 1988.

[3] McLelland R. Screening for breast cancer: Opportunities, status and challenges. In Brünner S and Langfeldt B, editors, *Recent Results in Cancer Research*, volume 119, pages 29–38. Springer-Verlag, Berlin Heidelberg, 1990.

[4] Sickles EA. Breast calcifications: Mammographic evaluation. *Radiology*, 160:289–293, 1986.

[5] Ram G. Optimization of ionizing radiation usage in medical imaging by means of image enhancement techniques. *Med. Phys.*, 9(5):733–737, 1982.

[6] Chan HP, Vyborny CJ, MacMahon H, Metz CE, Doi K, and Sickles EA. ROC studies of the effects of pixel size and unsharp-mask filtering on the detection of subtle microcalcifications. *Investigative Radiology*, 22:581–589, 1987.

[7] Gordon R and Rangayyan RM. Feature enhancement of film mammograms using fixed and adaptive neighborhoods. *Applied Optics*, 23(4):560–564, 1984.

[8] Morrow WM, Paranjape RB, Rangayyan RM, and Desautels JEL. Region-based contrast enhancement of mammograms. *IEEE Transactions of Medical Image Processing*, 11(3):392–406, 1992.

[9] Dhawan AP and Royer EL. Mammographic feature enhancement by computerized image processing. *Computer Methods and Programs in Biomedicine*, 27:23–35, 1988.

[10] Sickles EA. Mammographic features of malignancy found during screening. In Brünner S and Langfeldt B, editors, *Recent Results in Cancer Research*, volume 119, pages 88–93. Springer-Verlag, Berlin Heidelberg, 1990.

[11] Basset LW and Gold RH, editors. *Breast cancer detection: Mammography and other methods in breast imaging.* Grune & Stratton, Inc., Florida, 2nd edition, 1987.

[12] Wee WG, Moskowitz M, Chang NC, Ting YC, and Pemmeraju S. Evaluation of mammographic calcifications using a computer program. *Radiology*, 116:717–720, 1975.

[13] Spiesberger W. Mammogram inspection by computer. *IEEE Transactions on Biomedical Engineering*, BME-26(4):213–219, 1979.

[14] Chan HP, Doi K, Galhotra S, Vyborny CJ, MacMahon H, and Jokich PM. Image feature analysis and computer-aided diagnosis in digital radiography: I. Automated detection of microcalcifications in mammography. *Med. Phys.*, 14(4):538–548, 1987.

[15] Chan HP, Doi K, Vyborny CJ, Lam KL, and Schmidt RA. Computer-aided detection of microcalcifications in mammograms: Methodology and preliminary clinical study. *Investigative Radiology*, 23(9):664–671, 1988.

[16] Chan HP, Doi K, Vyborny CJ, Schmidt RA, Metz CE, Lam KL, Ogura T, Wu YZ, and MacMahon H. Improvement in radiologists' detection of clustered microcalcifications on mammograms: The potential of computer-aided diagnosis. *Investigative Radiology*, 25(10):1102–1110, 1990.

[17] Davies DH and Dance DR. Automatic computer detection of clustered calcifications in digital mammograms. *Phys. Med. Biol.*, 35(8):1111–1118, 1990.

[18] Patrick EA, Moskowitz M, Mansukhani VT, and Gruenstein EI. Expert learning system network for diagnosis of breast calcifications. *Investigative Radiology*, 26(6):534–539, 1991.

[19] Shen L, Rangayyan RM, and Desautels JEL. Shape analysis of mammographic calcifications. In *Proceedings of the Fifth Annual IEEE Symposium on Computer-Based Medical Systems*, pages 123–128, Durham, North Carolina, June 1992.

[20] Shen L, Rangayyan RM, and Desautels JEL. Application of shape analysis to mammographic calcifications. *IEEE Transactions on Medical Imaging*, 1992. submitted.

[21] Shen L, Rangayyan RM, and Desautels JEL. An automatic detection and classification system for calcifications in mammograms. In *Proceedings of the 1993 SPIE/SPSE Symposium on Electronic Imaging*, San Jose, California, February 1993. In Press.

[22] Feig SA, Galkin BM, and Muir HD. Evaluation of breast microcalcifications by means of optically magnified tissue specimen radiographs. In Brünner S and Langfeldt B, editors, *Recent Results in Cancer Research*, volume 105, pages 111–123. Springer-Verlag, Berlin Heidelberg, 1987.

[23] Pao YH. *Adaptive Pattern Recognition and Neural Networks*. Addison-Wesley Publishing Company, Inc., Reading, Massachusetts, 1989.

[24] Lippmann RP. An introduction to computing with neural nets. *IEEE ASSP Magazine*, pages 4–22, April 1987.

[25] Fukunaga K. *Introduction to Statistical Pattern Recognition*. Academic Press, Inc., San Diego, CA, 2nd edition, 1990.

[26] Devijver PA and Kittler J. *Pattern Recognition: A Statistical Approach*. Prentice-Hall, London, 1982.

[27] Shen L, Rangayyan RM, and Desautels JEL. A knowledge-based position matching technique for mammographic calcifications. In *Proceedings of the 14th Annual International Conference of the IEEE Engineering in Medicine and Biology Society*, pages 1936–1937, Paris, France, October 1992.

Comparative Evaluation of Pattern Recognition Techniques for Detection of Microcalcifications in Mammography

Kevin S. Woods[1], Jeffrey L. Solka[2], Carey E. Priebe[2], and W. Philip Kegelmeyer, Jr.[3], Christopher C. Doss[1], Kevin W. Bowyer[1]

1. Computer Science & Engineering, ENG 118,
Univ. of South Florida, Tampa, FL 33620
2. Systems Research & Technology Dept, B10,
Naval Surface Warfare Center, Dahlgren, VA 22448-5000
3. Sandia National Laboratories, PO Box 969, ORG 8117, Livermore, CA 94551

Abstract

Computer-assisted detection of microcalcifications in mammographic images will likely require a multi-stage algorithm that includes segmentation of possible microcalcifications, pattern recognition techniques to classify the segmented objects, a method to determine if a cluster of calcifications exists, and possibly a method to determine the probability of malignancy. This paper focuses on the first three of these stages, and especially on the classification of segmented local bright spots as either calcification or noncalcification. Seven classifiers (linear and quadratic classifiers, binary decision trees, a standard backpropagation network, 2 dynamic neural networks, and a K-nearest neighbor) are compared. In addition, a post-processing step is performed on objects identified as calcifications by the classifiers to determine if any clusters of microcalcifications exist. A database of digitized film mammograms is used for training and testing. Detection accuracy of individual and clustered microcalcifications is compared across the seven methods using area under the ROC curve as a figure of merit.

1. Introduction

Radiologists look for certain signs and characteristics indicative of cancer when evaluating a mammogram. Among these signs is the presence of clustered microcalcifications. A microcalcification is a tiny calcium deposit that has accumulated in tissue in the breast, and it appears as a small bright spot on the mammogram. A cluster is typically defined to be at least 3 microcalcifications within a 1cm^2 region. Between 30% and 50% of breast cancers demonstrate clustered microcalcifications, and in approximately 36% of these cases the clusters are the only sign of malignancy[2]. The calcifications that may be of potential interest as an indication of malignancy vary in size from .1mm to 1.0mm, and a radiologist must carefully examine the mammogram with a magnifier to locate calcifications which may be embedded in dense parenchymal tissue[4]. Due to their size and subtlety, individual microcalcifications can easily be overlooked in the normal manual examination of the mammograms.

This paper compares seven classification techniques for use in automatic microcalcification detection in digitized mammograms. Two Bayesian classifiers are examined. They are the linear classifier (LC), and the quadratic classifier (QC). A binary decision tree (BDT) classifier is examined. Three artificial neural networks (ANN) are examined. They are a standard feed-forward network using backpropagation training (BP), Cascade Correlation (CC) ANN, and Divide and Conquer (DCN) ANN. The CC and DCN are dynamic, or self-organizing, ANNs. A self-organizing ANN is one which automatically determines its topology (architecture) during training. The seventh method of pattern classification is the k-nearest neighbors algorithm (KNN). Common sets of training data and test data are used to evaluate and compare the methods. Therefore, the principal purpose of this paper is to determine which, if any, of the classifiers produces superior results. The classifiers are trained to detect *individual* microcalcifications. Since clusters of microcalcifications are a sign of a possible malignancy, the results of the individual microcalcification detection (for some of the classifiers) are further processed to indicate the presence of clusters.

2. Related Work

Previous research on the detection of clustered microcalcifications (benign and/or malignant) has not yet produced clinically acceptable results[1,2,3,4,5,6,7,8,9,10,11]. Many different pattern recognition methods have been used for microcalcification detection, including k-nearest neighbors[4], thresholds on each computed feature[1,5,6,8,11], binary decision trees[4], and Bayesian classifiers[10]. Most of these algorithms involve a segmentation process followed by a classification process. The two apparently most successful methods are reported by Chan and Doi[1] and Davies and Dance[8]. Davies and Dance used 25 training images and 50 test images, half of which contained clusters of microcalcifications. They report successfully detecting 47 of 49 clusters with a total of 9 false positive clusters detected. Chan and Doi tested their algorithm using simulated microcalcifications superimposed on normal mammograms, and on 20 hand selected clinical images. For the simulated microcalcifications, they report 80% TP cluster detection rate with one FP cluster per image. For the clinical study, they report an 82% TP cluster detection rate with one FP cluster per image. We have not found any paper which has reported results for an automated screening environment, simulated or otherwise.

3. Pattern Classification Techniques

Pattern recognition (PR) techniques can be used to assign objects to one of a fixed number of classes by means of some measured properties or features. The features are usually organized into a feature vector of real values which have been normalized so that all features are weighted equally. The feature vectors can be plotted in a d-dimensional feature space, where d is the number of elements (features) in the feature vector. The classification of an unknown pattern can be determined by its location in feature space. One method is to divide the feature space into regions, where each region corresponds to a different class. The regions are divided by decision boundaries, and it is the job of the classifier to determine where these boundaries should be located in order to provide the highest possible classification accuracy.

A complete pattern recognition system requires data acquisition, data representation, and classification. The data acquisition and representation stages are kept the same for the seven classifiers being compared. In a paper by Jain[12], classifiers are grouped according to the following dichotomies: finite or infinite number of training samples, labelled or unlabelled samples, and known or unknown form of the class-conditional density functions. For the classification problem at hand, we have a finite number of labelled training samples for which the density functions are unknown. At this point, we can either estimate the density functions or use methods which avoid a direct density function estimation. We have chosen to examine both parametric density estimation approaches and also techniques which do not directly estimate the density functions. The former case includes the linear and quadratic classifiers, while the later includes the KNN, the BDT, and the ANNs. The following subsections give thumbnail sketches of the different classifiers.

3.1 Linear and Quadratic Classifiers

The linear and quadratic classifiers are special cases of the general Bayesian classifier. The classifier type is determined by the model which is used to build the conditional density functions, $p(x|c_i)$. In many applications, a feature vector is well modeled by a Gaussian distribution $N(x,m,\Sigma)$ given by

$$N(x,\mu,\Sigma) = \frac{1}{(2\pi)^{n/2}|\Sigma|^{1/2}} \exp(-\frac{1}{2}(x-\mu)^t \Sigma^{-1}(x-\mu))$$

where x is an n-component column vector, μ is the n-component mean vector, Σ is the n-by-n covariance matrix, $(x-\mu)^t$ is the transpose of $x-\mu$, Σ^{-1} is the inverse of Σ, and $|\Sigma|$ is the determinant of Σ.

In the simplest case, the mean of each class is estimated separately and the covariance matrix is computed in a pooled manner, i.e. by averaging the covariance matrices of the two classes. In this case, it can be shown that the classifier boundary that separates the two classes is a hyperplane[18], and hence the classifier is referred to as a linear classifier or linear machine. If each distribution is allowed to have its own covariance matrix, then the decision surfaces are hyperquadrics and the classifier is referred to as a quadratic classifier[18].

3.2 Binary Decision Trees

Binary decision tree[19] (BDT) classification methods provide a means of approximating the optimal Bayesian classification rule for a given situation. A BDT is simply an ordered list of binary threshold operations on the feature vectors, organized as a tree. At each node, one of the features in a vector is compared to a threshold, which moves the vector down the appropriate branch of the tree. This continues until it arrives at a terminal node which assigns a classification.

Practical trees can often contain hundreds of nodes. This is not daunting, however, as they are grown automatically from the training data by recursive reduction of impurity. The control parameters at each node are chosen by simply determining the feature and threshold which best separates the current data, where the quality of the separation is determined by some impurity measure. This process is repeated, recursively partitioning the remaining training samples, until some stopping criteria is met[20]. This recursive selection of the best possible partition enables automatic feature selection and data reduction, both of which are important advantages of the BDT approach. Another advantage of BDTs is that they have a compact representation and are computationally efficient when used for classification, operating at essentially a constant speed, independent of the number of training vectors.

3.3 Neural Networks in General

In general, neural networks are characterized by (a) large numbers of simple processing nodes, (b) larger numbers of weighted connections between nodes in which knowledge is encoded, (c) highly parallel, distributed control, and (d) an ability to learn the internal representation (i.e. values for interconnection weights) automatically[13]. The processing nodes perform a weighted sum of their inputs, for which a single output value is computed using some nonlinear activation function. The node is said to "fire" if the activation value is greater than some threshold associated with the node. Network topology refers to the way that the processing node interconnections are made. The knowledge of a network is encoded in the interconnection weights, and it is the learning algorithm which specifies the initial values of the weights and how they are updated to improve performance. ANNs can be described by their node characteristics, network topology, and the learning algorithm used to train the network.

The ANNs described in this paper are feed-forward networks. In a fully connected network, each node in one layer is connected to every node in the next layer. The input nodes serve only to distribute the input values to other nodes in the network. When the network is used for pattern classification, there is one input node for each element of the feature vector. There may be one or more layers of hidden nodes which perform the weighted summing of inputs and pass an activation value as an output. The hidden nodes are so-called because their outputs are not directly observable, and are used as inputs to other nodes. Finally, there is a layer of output nodes, and it is the activation values of these nodes which are taken to be the output of the network. There is usually one output node for each possible class to which a pattern may be assigned. For a 2-class problem, such as the one examined here, one output node is generally used to represent a target class, and it is thresholded to make a classification. In feed-forward ANNs, the inputs are presented at the input nodes and the activations of the nodes flow through the network towards the output nodes.

The hidden nodes enable internal representations of the input data to be developed by the network during learning. These hidden nodes act as high order "feature detectors" which "fire" (pass a relatively high activation value) in the presence of a particular feature and, conversely, pass an inhibitory signal (a relatively low activation value) if the feature is absent. The term "high order feature" refers to one which is inferred by the ANN from the input data, and is not to be confused with the features that are computed by a user and specified as input to the ANN. An additional weighted input associated with each hidden or output node, referred to as an offset, may be implemented as a bias input value fixed at 1.0 and an adjustable weight. This way the offset is represented as a separate weighted connection, and can be learned during training as if it were any other weight. When an unknown pattern is presented to a trained network, a set of hidden nodes will fire and excite one of the output nodes. The connections from other hidden nodes will pass inhibitory signals to the other outputs, and the pattern is assigned to the class which is represented by the output node that fires. More than one output node may fire, and in this case the node with the maximum activation value is selected.

Neural networks, when applied to pattern classification, define decision regions by the interconnection weights in the network. Programming the weights by hand to specify decision regions is impossible, so they must be learned from a set of training examples which are a set of input values with corresponding desired (target) output values. The basic approach to training a feed-forward ANN is to present the training sample inputs to the network, allow the activations to flow to the output nodes, compare the network outputs with a desired (target) output to compute an error measure, and then somehow adjust the weights so that the error will be reduced. This procedure is repeated until the network converges on a solution. The most common estimate for the error of a network is the sum of squared errors (observed value - target value) over all outputs. Depending on the learning algorithm the error estimate may be computed for individual training samples or for the entire training set. An epoch is defined as one pass of all training samples through the network. Different learning algorithms specify if the network weights are to be updated after each training sample (for which the error estimate is computed for the training sample just presented), or after each epoch (in which case the error estimate is computed over the entire training set), and how they are to be updated. As described here, ANNs used in PR are simply a particular method of implementing a general non-parametric classifier.

3.4 Simple Backpropagation Neural Networks

The first type of ANN considered is a fully connected backpropagation network (BP) with two hidden layers. Each node has a bias input of 1 with an adjustable weight. The activation function for hidden and output nodes is a sigmoid function which produces a real value between 0 and 1 based on the weighted sum of inputs. The term backpropagation stems from the fact that the errors are propagated backwards from the output nodes through the network to adjust the weights in the previous layers. For a more complete description of the BP training algorithm, see [13].

A major drawback of BP networks is the long training times that may be required. Many epochs of the training set may be required for the network to converge on a good solution. There are a number of reasons that BP learning is so slow. One reason is the difficulty of determining the step size by which the weights are changed during training. Too small a step size and the network takes too long to converge on a solution, too large a step size and the network may jump over the solution and possibly oscillate instead of converging. Another reason is that all the weights in the BP network are updated at the same time after each training sample, and this may cause all the weights to adjust to reduce the error for one sample and then adjust differently to reduce the error for the next sample, and so on. This type of training may take a while for the network to settle into a good solution for all the training samples. Another problem associated with these networks is determining a good topology. The number of input and output nodes are defined by the problem at hand, but there are no precise rules which state now many hidden layers or hidden nodes in a layer should be selected to achieve good results. There are a few rules of thumb, but for the most part the network topology is determined by trial and error.

3.5 The Cascade Correlation Neural Network

The cascade correlation (CC) ANN attempts to overcome some of the problems associated with standard BP networks. The CC network is self-organizing, so there is no guessing involved in setting up the network topology. The network begins with input and output nodes only, and hidden nodes are added as needed during the training phase. The CC learning algorithm adds hidden nodes to the network one at a time in such a way that the error estimates can be made for each node directly, and therefore error estimates do not need to be propagated backward through the network. The weights are adjusted using the quickprop algorithm[15] which computes for each weight independently the slope of the error surface for the current training cycle and the previous training cycle, and the change that was made in the weight during the last training cycle. The two slopes and the step between them are used to define a parabola which estimates the error surface, and a jump is made to the minimum value of the parabola. The quickprop algorithm reduces the problem of choosing a step size. The CC algorithm allows only a single hidden unit to evolve at a time, and the weights are updated after a single error estimate is made for the entire training set. This strategy lets each hidden unit move directly towards reducing a specific error. The hidden nodes are not all changing at the same time, and this in turn leads to faster learning.

The CC ANN demonstrates a number of desirable characteristics. The training times (number of epochs) are shorter compared to BP networks. When running the networks on a serial machine, even greater speedup is observed because (1) error estimates do not have to be propagated backwards through the network, and (2) since the network is built dynamically during training, many epochs are run when the network is smaller than its final size. Another advantage is that the network topology does not have to be determined in advance as with standard BP networks. Since input connections to hidden units are frozen when the unit is added to the network, a CC network can be used for incremental learning in which new information is added to a trained network. For a complete description of the CC network and learning algorithm, see Fahlman's[14] paper.

3.6 The Divide and Conquer Neural Network

The divide and conquer network[17] (DCN), like the CC network, is a self-organizing ANN. The DCN learning algorithm consists of two phases: (1) the divide phase, and (2) the conquer phase, which are executed individually for each output during training. Unlike the CC algorithm which creates single node hidden layers, the DCN algorithm will create multiple hidden nodes in the hidden layers if they are needed. Like the CC algorithm, the DCN algorithm only trains one unit at a time, allowing the new unit to attempt to correctly classify some of the training samples and eliminating the need to propagate an error signal backwards though the network. Since backpropagation is not required, a simple delta rule can be used to update the weights in the network, and a threshold activation function is suitable. Training the outputs separately is similar to training different networks for each different class, and DCN allows cells trained for one output to be used while training another output. This is called "cell-sharing"[17].

The DCN algorithm has some desirable features. Like the CC networks, no specification of the network topology is required, as hidden layers and units are added as needed. Avoiding backpropagation of the error signal allows the use of simple learning rules for updating the connection weights. Unlike CC networks, no correlation measure is computed, and the networks created can have multiple hidden units in the hidden layers. This may lead to a higher degree of parallelism in a hardware implementation.

3.7 The Traditional K-Nearest Neighbors Algorithm

The K-nearest neighbor (KNN) algorithm is a very simple but powerful method of pattern classification. Unknown patterns are classified based on their similarity to known patterns. The KNN algorithm computes the distance from an unknown test pattern to every training pattern and selects the K nearest training samples to base the classification on. We use the Mahalanobis[18] distance in the experiments reported here. The test sample is assigned to the class which has the most samples among the K nearest samples. We are dealing with a two class problem, so the value of K is usually chosen to be odd to ensure that a majority among the two classes can be found.

A variation of the KNN algorithm can be used to bias the decision towards one of the two classes. In this approach, a threshold k less than or equal to K can be used for one of the classes instead of a majority vote among the K nearest neighbors of the test sample. This modified KNN rule now states that an unknown test pattern is assigned to a particular class if at least k of the K nearest neighbors is in that particular class. This type of biased decision may be desirable in an application where the penalty for misclassifying one class is much greater than the penalty associated with the misclassification of another class. In our attempt to screen for a sign of cancer, more specifically microcalcifications, we are more concerned with detecting a high percentage of calcifications and are willing to trade off for a lower recognition rate of other objects. By selecting a k less than K/2 for the calcification class, the KNN rule will be more sensitive to calcification detection, and conversely less sensitive to noncalcifications.

4. Experimental Methods

To obtain the training and test data, a segmentation routine is run on a set of digitized mammograms. The result of the segmentation routine is a template for each image which indicates the locations of possible microcalcifications called candidates. The segmentation routine is designed to locate small, bright spots (a characteristic of microcalcifications) in the raw image. It is important that most individual calcifications and all clusters of calcifications be segmented since the overall cluster detection accuracy can be limited by the results of the segmentation. Since the segmentation routine will detect objects other than microcalcifications, it is the job of the classifiers to label the candidates as either yes (a microcalcification) or no. A set of 7 features is systematically chosen and values are computed for each candidate. The feature values are organized into a feature vector, normalized, and written to a data file. Therefore, the training and test data is 7-dimensional feature vectors which are normalized between 0 and 1 using the *(value-min)/(max-min)* formula, where value is the feature vector element being normalized, and max and min are the maximum and minimum training set values for that feature.

4.1 Images and Data Sets

A set of 24 mammograms, each containing at least one biopsy-proven malignant cluster of microcalcifications, are digitized at 70 micron resolution with a DuPont NDT Scan II, Model 35. The images are then divided into a training set of 9 images and a test set of 15 images. The training and test sets are selected so that each includes images with calcification clusters that are embedded in dense parenchymal tissue and are therefore more difficult to detect. It should be noted here that due to the small number of images, some bias of our split of the data into training and test sets is unavoidable. An alternate approach would be to segment all the images and then randomly select candidates from all images for the training and test sets. We feel this would produce overly optimistic classification rates. Another possibility would be to perform "leave one out" evaluation on a per image basis.

All seven methods of classification (LC,QC,BDT,KNN,CC,DCN, and BP) require a training set. Results are reported for 5 different sizes of training sets: 100, 200 300 400, and 524. An equal number of training samples from each of the two classes are randomly selected from the set of training images, making sure that we get some samples from every image. For example the training set with 300 samples contains 150 samples of microcalcifications and 150 samples of non-microcalcifications. The training set with 524 patterns (262 from each class) includes all the microcalcifications in the training images. In addition, 5 different sets of random samples are collected for each of the different sizes of training sets, for a total of 25 different training sets. Therefore, there are 5 training sets with 100 samples, 5 sets with 200 samples, etc. The reason for keeping the calcification and non-calcification sets equal in size is so that the PR algorithm will not be inherently biased toward one decision.

4.2 Segmentation Routine

A segmentation procedure is used to extract candidate objects from the mammogram images for classification. This routine is able to segment most individual microcalcifications, and all clusters of microcalcifications from the training set images while picking up as few non-microcalcifications as possible. By segmenting candidates from the raw image, the problem becomes one of classification of a hundred or so objects, rather than the classification of millions of individual pixels for which a limited number of useful features can be computed. Thus, the segmentation step serves primarily as an important data reduction stage. (For an example of a by-pixel classification approach, see Kegelmeyer's paper in this volume.)

The segmentation routine used in this work is now described. A local contrast image is computed by subtracting from every pixel the average of a 1.13mm (15 by 15 pixels) square region surrounding it. Depending on the maximum pixel intensity in the square region of the local contrast image, the lowest values are discarded, leaving only those pixels with the greatest contrast. If the maximum value in the local contrast image is greater than 15, then a threshold of 10 is selected, otherwise the threshold is 5. Note that this threshold is computed for each pixel in the local contrast image. The result of this is an image with only the locally bright spots remaining. Next, region growing is performed on the local contrast image to group pixels into objects. In order to reduce the number of candidates segmented, a histogram of the object to background contrast for all objects is created, and only those objects with the highest contrast are retained. This is done by selecting a threshold so that 3% of the total number of segmented objects with the highest contrast (with a minimum of 100) are kept. Also, any single pixel objects are eliminated since the high resolution digitization should ensure that all important microcalcifications are larger than one pixel. Pixels that remain at this stage in the local contrast image are assigned a constant value, and the result is a binary template of candidate objects. The template is overlaid on the original image to extract features for each candidate object from the raw data.

Once the segmentation is done, all objects are manually labelled as either microcalcifications or non-microcalcifications. Thus, we have a 2-class classification problem: (1) microcalcification, or (2) non-microcalcification. Labelling produces training and test sets for which detection accuracy can be computed. An experienced radiologist located the clusters of microcalcifications, and then we were left with the task of labelling the individual microcalcifications.

4.3 Definition of Feature Space

Once the segmentation is done, features can be computed for all candidate objects remaining in the template. Since feature selection can be the most crucial component of a pattern recognition system, a systematic evaluation of features that might be useful is performed to select a subset of "best" features. In order to select the "best" features, the full set of 24 segmented, labelled images is used. A set of 29 features is chosen to begin with, some are from previously published papers and a few are our variations on previously published features. From the set of 29 features, some are eliminated because a similar feature exists that gives better values. Eighteen features are finally selected for testing. The 18 feature values for all the labelled images are computed, and frequency histograms are plotted for each feature for each class (microcalcifications and non-microcalcifications). If the frequency histograms of the two classes are visually well separated, the feature is retained and included in the feature vector. This assures that each feature kept is one which has some merit on its own. (However, this approach would not pick up groups of features which are only useful as a group.)

The full set of 29 features considered is listed in Appendix A. Seven features are eventually selected to form the feature vector, they are:
1) Area of object - number of pixels
2) Average grey level of the object
3) Gradient strength of the object's perimeter pixels
4) Root mean square (rms) noise fluctuation in the object
5) RMS noise fluctuation in the 3.5mm by 3.5mm local background
6) Contrast - average grey level of the object minus the average of a two pixel wide border surrounding the object
7) A low order moment based shape descriptor[16]

Only one paper reviewed so far attempted to select features in a systematic manner. Fox et al[4] examined sixty-nine different features and selected the best five using Fisher's linear discriminant. No other paper discusses why certain features were chosen, though some features are obvious. One group did some testing on some shape features[16], but this was to differentiate between malignant and benign calcifications. A number of groups appear to have determined upper and lower bounds for a feature value associated with microcalcifications. This approach is useful for determining thresholds but does not indicate how well the feature will separate microcalcifications from other objects that may be detected in earlier stages of the algorithms. This could explain why some of the previously mentioned (see section 2) attempts at automatic microcalcification detection have only been moderately successful.

4.4 Cluster Detection

A simple post-processing routine is used to check the classifier results for the existence of clusters of microcalcifications. All objects that are labelled as calcifications by a classifier are checked to determine if at least three exist within a 1 cm^2 window. If a cluster is detected, then any other detected objects that are within 1 cm of the cluster are added to the cluster. This process is repeated iteratively until no more objects can be added to the cluster, and then the centroid of the cluster is computed. If the computed cluster centroid is with 1 cm of a known cluster, then a true positive detection is the result, otherwise the cluster is a false positive.

4.5 Method of Comparing Classifiers

The diagnostic accuracy of a classifier can be completely characterized in its operating environment by its receiver operating characteristic (ROC) curve. The ROC is the single analytical technique known to provide both a desired accuracy index, and the desired basis for a description of utility in terms of cost and benefit[21]. The advantages of ROC analysis over alternative methods of analysis have been clearly established[22,23].

The ROC curve is a plot of the classifier's true positive detection rate versus its false alarm rate. The false alarm (FA), or false positive, rate is the probability of incorrectly classifying a nontarget object (eg. a normal tissue region) as a target object (eg. a tumor region). Similarly, the true positive (TP) detection rate is the probability of correctly classifying a target object as being a target object. The TP and FA rates both are specified in the interval from 0.0 to 1.0, inclusive. In medical imaging, the TP rate is referred to as sensitivity, and (1 - FA rate) is called specificity. Statistical classifiers have parameters that can be varied to alter the FA and TP rates. Using these parameters, an ROC curve can be generated which shows the TP/FA trade-off associated with the different values that the parameter(s) may assume. It would then be possible to trade a lower (higher) FA rate for a higher (lower) TP detection rate by choosing appropriate value(s) for the parameter(s) in question.

The area under the ROC curve (AUC) is an accepted way of comparing the performance of two or more classifiers[21,22]. Obviously, the greater the AUC, the better the classifier's performance. A perfect classifier would have a TP rate of 1 (or 100%) and a FA rate of 0, and therefore would have an AUC of 1.0. When a benefit or cost can be associated with the decisions made by the classifier, it is very desirable for a user to be able to adjust the sensitivity of a classification system. "Profits" can be maximized for decisions that are based on this type of gain/loss scenario by selecting appropriate TP and FA rates, which are given as points on the ROC curve. This requires that the parameters that affect the FA and TP rates for the classifier be easily manipulated to facilitate selection of the classifier's operating point[24].

The AUCs are estimated by using the trapezoid rule for the discrete operating points. The AUC can also be computed by fitting a continuous binormal curve to the operating points, requiring an assumption to be made about the functional form of the ROC curve[22]. This type of curve fitting is generally done for medical imaging studies when operating points are obtained by presenting a reader with normal and abnormal images in random order, and the reader is asked to rank each image on a discrete ordinal scale of 5 or 6 categories ranging from definitely normal to definitely abnormal[21,22,25,26]. This is known as a confidence rating. The ROC points are obtained by successively considering broader and broader categories of abnormal. In other words a threshold is applied to the confidence rating scale, and any images rated above the threshold are labeled abnormal, while any images rated below the threshold are labeled normal.

The methods used to obtain ROC points in this paper, and in statistical pattern recognition in general, can be considered as applying a threshold to a confidence rating scale that is continuous. Some parameter is varied over a range of values, and the resulting TP and FA rates are noted. The range of the parameter is the continuous confidence rating scale, and the value of the parameter corresponds to a threshold applied at some point on the scale. Thus, potentially many operating points can be used to estimate the ROC curve and the AUC. Only a limited number of operating points (maybe 5 or 6) can be obtained using the discrete ordinal confidence rating scale mentioned above, and an area computed using the trapezoidal rule will be underestimated. For ROC curves estimated from the continuous confidence rating scale, the area under the curve estimated by the trapezoidal rule will be virtually identical to any area underneath a fitted, smoothed curve[25]. Therefore, complex curve fitting is not necessary. In addition, when the continuous rating scale is used and an infinite number of samples are assumed, the AUC is equal to the probability of a correct decision[25].

4.6 Method of Obtaining ROC Points

For the ANN classifiers, the weights are initialized to random values using 4 different seeds for the random number generator for each of the 25 training sets. This means each of the ANN classifiers is trained 20 different times for each size of training set. Both dynamic ANNs add new hidden nodes during training. The BP network requires a fixed topology to be specified from the beginning. Therefore, the BP network is trained and tested with various numbers of nodes (5 to 20) in the hidden layers, and various numbers of hidden layers (1 to 3). The best detection rates are found for 10 hidden nodes in each of the 2 hidden layers, and these are the results reported. The dynamic ANNs are designed to build a topology with enough hidden nodes and layers such that a complete solution (100% correct classification) for the training set can be found. The BP network must search for a solution without changing its configuration, and therefore it may not be possible to get 100% classification rates on the training set. The BP network is trained for 3000 epochs and the error over all training patterns after each epoch is computed, and the network configuration which produces the lowest overall error is saved to be used for the classification results. In order to obtain ROC points for the ANNs, the bias unit value is varied over a range (recall the bias unit value is usually fixed at 1.0), and the corresponding TP and FA rates of the networks are observed. It is beyond the scope of this paper to explain how adjusting the bias unit value affects ANN classifier performance, but we have shown that statistically significantly better ROC curves can be generated for ANNs using this method rather than applying a threshold to the output node[27]. The bias unit value is varied over a range in 0.01 increments such that TP detection rates from 0% to 100%, and the corresponding FA rates, are obtained.

The KNN algorithm we described has two parameters that can be varied, (1) K the number of nearest neighbors to base the decision on, and (2) the threshold k which determines the minimum number of the K-nearest neighbors that must be microcalcifications before an unknown pattern is classified as a microcalcification. ROC points for a specific value of K are obtained by varying k from 1 to K and observing the resulting TP and FA rates. We run the KNN classifier with values of K running from 5 to 19 for each training set for a total of 9 different trials for each of the 25 training sets. By ensuring that K is at least 5, we are able to obtain a sufficient number of ROC points. KNN classifiers show a general dependency of accuracy of classification on the value of K used. As K is increased starting from values which are "too small", accuracy will increase. Then, as K is increased beyond some range of appropriate values, accuracy will begin to fall off. Therefore it is important to vary K over a large enough range during classifier design such that this basic behavior is observed. Otherwise it is problematic whether the "right" value of K has been chosen. By increasing K up to 19, we are able to observe this increase and subsequent decrease of the classifier accuracy. This large range for K ensures that we find the best value of K for each training set.

The LC and QC classifiers are evaluated by first training on each of the 25 training sets. This training consists of computing the parameters (mean vector and covariance matrices) of the models from the training set. Once trained, the models are used to estimate the class-conditional probabilities, $p(x|c_i)$, of an unknown sample for both classes. We base our decision on the ratio of the likelihood for the two classes $p(x|c_0)/p(x|c_1)$. We set a decision threshold, T, such that if the ratio is greater than T, the unknown sample is classified as a microcalcification, otherwise it is labelled a non-microcalcification. To obtain ROC points, threshold T on the likelihood ratios is varied from 0 to 15 in small increments (0.01), and the resulting TP and FA rates are noted. The BDT ROC points are obtained by simply varying a threshold over some range on the terminal nodes of the tree.

5. Results

The maximum AUC found for each classifier for individual microcalcification detection, along with the number of ROC points generated by each classifier for its corresponding ROC curve, is shown in Table 1. For example, the ANNs were each trained and tested 100 times, and the AUC of all 100 resulting ROC curves for each ANN were computed. The maximum AUC found over the 100 trials is used for comparison. The linear classifier and the backprop ANN produce the best results with AUCs of approximately 0.935, which corresponds to a 93.5% probability that a segmented object is correctly classified. The KNN classifier has a maximum AUC of 0.929. The quadratic classifier and the CC ANN have the same maximum AUC, which is 0.918. The BDT and DCN ANN have maximum AUCs of 0.900, and 0.887, respectively. (It should be noted that for our data set a KNN classifier utilizing the Euclidean distance produces inferior results compared to using the Mahalanobis KNN.)

Table 1. Number of ROC points and AUC of seven classifiers for individual calcification detection.

Classifier	Number of ROC points	Area Under ROC Curve
Linear Classifier	60	0.936
Backprop ANN	75	0.935
K-Nearest Neighbor	17	0.929
Quadratic Classifier	42	0.918
CasCor ANN	70	0.918
Binary Decision Tree	6	0.900
Divide & Conquer ANN	57	0.887

The classification results of the five classifiers with the best AUCs, namely the LC, BP, KNN, QC, and CC classifiers, are run through the cluster detection routine. The result is to derive an ROC curve representing cluster-level detection from the results of calcification-level detection. The number of operating points on the ROC curves for cluster-level detection is limited to, at most, the number of points on the corresponding ROC curve for calcification-level detection. In practice the number of ROC points is always reduced, and we are able to obtain approximately 5 or 6 points for the cluster-level detection results of each classifier. The ROC curves for cluster detection are shown in figure 1. Once again, the linear classifier has the maximum AUC of 0.964. The other four classifiers in descending order of AUC values are: the CC ANN with an AUC of 0.935, the quadratic classifier with an AUC of 0.926, the BP ANN with an AUC of 0.907, and finally the KNN classifier with an AUC of 0.857.

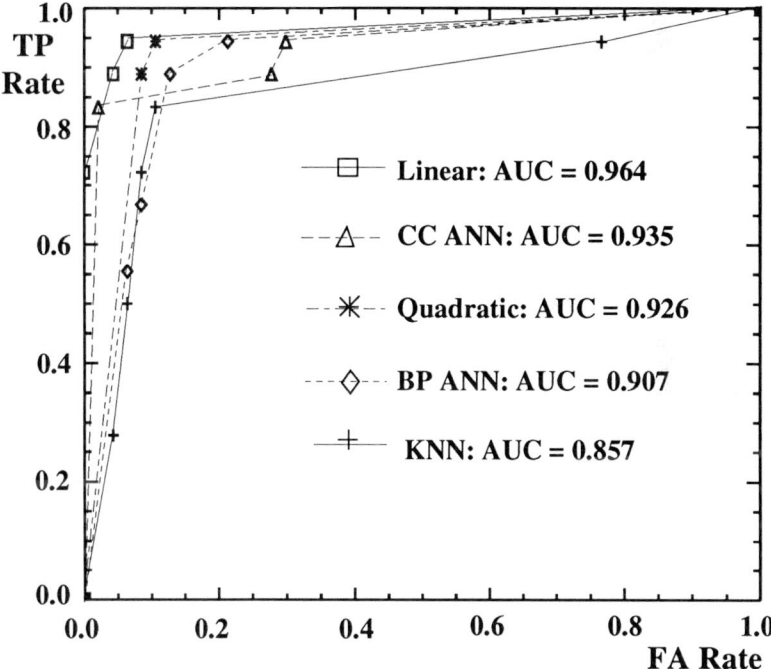

Figure 1. ROC curves for microcalcification cluster detection.

One of the best operating points found is for the linear classifier in which 17 of 18 clusters are detected with 3 FP cluster detected. This operating point for cluster detection is obtained when the LC classifier operating point is chosen such that the individual calcification TP rate is around 73% with about 3.5% FPs. Also for the LC classifier, 16 of 18 clusters are detected with only 2 FP clusters when the LC operating point for individual calcification is about 68% TP rate and 2.5% FP rate. For the CC ANN classifier, 15 of 18 clusters are detected with only a single FP cluster when operating points are selected which correspond to 50% TP rate and 2.4% FP rate for detection of individual calcifications. Finally, for the LC classifier operating at 49% TP rate and 0.8% FP rate for individual calcification detection, 12 of 18 clusters are detected with 0 FP clusters. These results are summarized in Table 2.

Detection rates at the image level are even better than those at the cluster level because 2 of the FP clusters detected (for the LC classifier in rows 1 and 2 of table 2) are on the same image. With regards to the LC classifier (row 1, table 2), 12 of the 15 test images are classified completely correct. That is, all calcification clusters are detected with no FP clusters. The two images for which a FP cluster is detected also contain at least one TP cluster, and therefore classifying these images as abnormal is correct. Only a single test image is incorrectly classified as normal (i.e a cluster was not detected).

Table 2. Best cluster level detection rates. Operating point is for individual calcification detection.

Classifier	Operating Point (TP rate, FA rate)	# TP Clusters (18 possible)	# FP Clusters
Linear Classifier	(73%, 3.5%)	17	3
Linear Classifier	(68%, 2.5%)	16	2
CasCor ANN	(50%, 2.4%)	15	1
Linear Classifier	(49%, 0.8%)	12	0

6. Discussion

The objective of this study is to determine which method or methods of pattern classification is best-suited for automatic detection of clusters of calcifications. A complete automated detection system would be composed of several building blocks. It is difficult to determine the best set of blocks all at once. A more practical approach is to work on optimizing each stage of the algorithm separately. From our experiments, we note that the simple Bayesian linear classifier performed best at not only individual calcification detection, but also cluster detection. This may at first glance seem surprising, since the linear classifier might be considered in some sense "less sophisticated" than the other classifiers examined. However, the PR problem is perhaps better viewed as an attempt to match level of sophistication of technique to level of complexity in distribution of feature data. That is, if the feature data for each class is reasonably well described by a Gaussian distribution, then a "more sophisticated" technique (one allowing more complex distributions) may well produce poorer results due to over-adapting itself to random fluctuations in the training data.

The detection rates reported here, although on a limited number of images, are very promising. Comparison to other published works is not possible without a common database, however the results reported here certainly seem competitive. Testing on a much larger data base is planned in the near future to help determine the clinical value of the automated detection scheme outlined in this paper. The ability to easily control a classifier's sensitivity via selection of an operating point is very desirable. The Bayesian techniques and the ANNs were able to produce many ROC points, and this is an indication of the inherent flexibility of these classifiers. This type of "dial-in" control will almost certainly be required in a clinical situation.

One interesting point illustrated by these results is that detection of individual calcifications which is moderately good (say 75% TP rate) can result in very high cluster detection rates (approaching 95%). Another point illustrated here is that a relative ranking of classifiers based on accuracy of individual calcification detection does not necessarily hold for cluster detection. This can be true due to different spatial groupings of the individually detected calcifications by the different classifiers.

Acknowledgements

The mammography studies used in this work were selected by Robert A. Clark, M.D., of the Department of Radiology, H. Lee Moffitt Cancer Center and Research Institute, at the University of South Florida. The authors would like to express sincere appreciation for his help in this project. Part of this work was performed while the first author was with the Department of Radiology at USF under the administrative direction of Laurence P. Clarke. We would also like to thank Robert Velthuizen and Maria Kallergi for help in data acquisition. Finally, we would like to thank Larry O. Hall for help in using his DCN neural network system.

Appendix A: Features for Microcalcification Detection

Type of Feature [Reference]	Method of Computing Feature
Moments about Centroid [16]	Low order moments computed using Euclidean distance between centroid and ordered set of perimeter pixels.
Fourier Descriptors [16]	Boundary as a complex sequence $Z_i = x_i + jy_i$
Compactness [16]	$C = p^2 / a$ where p is perimeter and a is area.
Area [2]	Number of pixels in object
Average Grey Level [2]	Absolute values of calcification pixels are averaged
Smoothness [2]	Root-mean-Square (RMS) of grey level fluctuation in the calcification
Shape [2]	RMS of the Euclidean distance from centroid to ordered set of perimeter pixels.
Dimensions of Calcification [2]	Horizontal and vertical length
Holes in Calcification [2]	Hollow area in center of calcification.
Contrast [4]	Binary decision tree, calcification must contain a local maximum.
Contrast[4]	Difference between 3 by 3 central area and mean of the operator boundary pixels.
Compactness [4]	Ratio: number of object-background transitions to total number of object pixels.
Area Descriptor [3]	Standard deviation of calcification area divided by the mean calcification area.
Cluster size [3]	Number of calcifications in cluster.
Dimensions [3]	Mean of individual calcification aspect ratio.
Dimensions [3]	Standard deviation of individual calcification aspect ratio.
Local Background [1]	RMS noise fluctuation of local background in an N by N window.
Local Background [1]	Mean of local background grey level.
Contrast [1]	Maximum intensity in calcification minus mean of local background intensity.
Contrast [6]	Ratio of calcification average grey level to the local background average.
Contrast [6]	Difference between calc. average grey level and average local background.
Shape [8]	Ratio of the calcification area to the square of the maximum linear dimension.
Shape [8]	$P / 4\pi A$ where P is perimeter and A is area.
Edge Strength [8]	Mean value of Robert's gradient for each perimeter pixel.
Shape [10]	Magnitude and direction of the gradient are used to calculate a shape parameter.

Appendix A Continued: Features for Microcalcification Detection

Type of Feature [Reference]	Method of Computing Feature
Smoothness [USF]	Center pixel intensity minus the average of the perimeter pixel intensity, all divided by the RMS noise fluctuation in the object.
Shape [USF]	Calcification aspect ratio defined as Rmax divided by Rmin, where Rmax is the maximum radius and Rmin is minimum radius.
Contrast [USF]	Average grey level of calcification minus the average of 2 pixel width surround.
Edge Strength [USF]	Average of 3 by 3 gradient for perimeter pixels.

A [USF] reference is for a feature not encountered in any digital mammography literature we found, and was either developed by our group or taken from an image processing text.

7. References

1. H.P. Chan, K. Doi, C.J. Vyborny, K.L. Lam, and R.A. Schmidt. "Computer-aided detection of microcalcifications in mammograms, methodology and preliminary clinical study". Investigative Radiology, 23(9): pp. 664-671, Sep 1988.
2. W.G. Wee, M. Moskowitz, N.C. Chang, Y.C. Ting, and S. Pemmeraju. "Evaluation of Mammographic Calcifications Using a Computer Program". Radiology, 116: pp. 717-720, Sep. 1975
3. S.H. Fox, U.M. Pujare, W.G. Wee, M. Moskowitz, and R.V.P. Hutter. "A Computer Analysis of Mammographic Microcalcifications: Global Approach". In Proceedings of IEEE Pattern Recognition Conference, pp. 624-631, 1980.
4. W. Spiesberger. "Mammogram Inspection by Computer". IEEE Transactions on Biomedical Engineering, **BME-26(4)**: pp. 213-219, Apr. 1979.
5. H.P. Chan, K. Doi, S. Galhotra, C.J. Vyborny, H. MacMahon, and P.M. Jokich. "Image Feature Analysis and Computer-aided Diagnosis in Digital Radiography. 1. Automated Detection of Microcalcifications in Mammography". Medical Physics, **14(4)**: pp. 538-548, Jul./Aug. 1987.
6. B.W. Fam, S.L. Olson, P.F. Winter, and F.J. Scholz. "Algorithm for the Detection of Fine Clustered Calcifications on Film Mammograms". Radiology, **169**: pp. 333-337, 1988.
7. S.L. Olson, B.W. Fam, P.F. Winter, F.J. Scholz, A.K. Lee, and S.E. Gordon. "Breast Calcifications: Analysis of Imaging Properties". Radiology, **169(2)**: pp. 329-332, Nov. 1988.
8. D.H. Davies and D.R. Dance. "Automatic Computer Detection of Clustered Calcifications in Digital Mammograms". Physics in Medicine and Biology, **35(8)**: pp. 1111-1118, 1990.
9. J. Dengler, S. Behrens, and J.F. Desaga. "Segmentation of Microcalcifications in Mammograms". Mustererkennung 1991, Informatik Fachberichte, **290**: pp. 380-385, 1991.
10. N. Karssemeijer. "A Stochastic Model for Automated Detection of Calcifications in Digital Mammograms". In Information Processing in Medical Imaging, 12th International Conference, IPMI'91 Proceedings, pp. 227-238, 1991.
11. I.N. Bankman, W.A. Christens-Barry, I.N. Weinberg, D.W. Kim, R.D. Semmel, and W.R. Brody. "An Algorithm for Early Breast Cancer Detection in Mammograms". In Fifth Anual IEEE Symposium on Computer-based Medical Systems, pp. 362-369, 1992.
12. A.K. Jain, "Pattern Recognition". In International Encyclopedia of Robotics Applications and Automation, pp. 1052-1063, edited by Dorf, John Wiley and Sons, Inc., 1988.
13. K. Knight, "Connectionist Ideas and Algorithms". Communications of the ACM, **33(11)**: pp. 59-74, Nov. 1990.
14. S.E. Fahlman and C. Lebiere, "The Cascade Correlation Learning Architecture". Neural Information Processing Systems 2, pp. 524-532, (Ed. D. Touretzky), Morgan-Kaufmann, San Mateo, CA.
15. S.E. Fahlman, "Faster-learning variations on back-propagation: An empirical study". In Proceedings of the 1988 Connectionist Models Summer School, Morgan-Kaufmann Publishers, San Mateo, CA. pp. 38-51, 1988.
16. I. Shen, R.M. Rangayan, and J.E. Desautels, "Shape Analysis of Mammographic Calcifications". In Proceedings of the Fifth IEEE Symposium on Computer-Based Medical Systems, June 1992.

17. S.G. Romaniuk and L.O. Hall, "Divide and Conquer Neural Networks", Accepted for publication in the Journal of Neural Networks, to appear in 1993.
18. R.O. Duda and P.E. Hart, *Pattern Classification and Scene Analysis*, John Wiley and Sons, 1973.
19. L. Breiman, J.H. Friedman, R.A. Olshen, and C.J. Stone, *Classification and Regression Trees*, Wadsworth International Group, Belmont, CA, 1984.
20. S.B. Gelfand, C.S. Ravishankar, and E.J. Delp, "An Iterative Growing and Pruning Algorithm for Classification Tree Design", IEEE Transactions on Pattern Analysis and Machine Intelligence **13(2)**, pp. 163-174, Feb. 1991.
21. J.A. Swets, "ROC Analysis Applied to the Evaluation of Medical Imaging Techniques",Investigative Radiology, **14**: pp. 109-121, 1979.
22. C.E. Metz, "ROC Methodology in Radiologic Imaging", Investigative Radiology 1986;21:720-733
23. C.E. Metz, "Some Practical Issues of Experimental Design and Data Analysis in Radiological ROC studies", Investigative Radiology, **24**: pp. 234-245, 1989.
24. R.M. Haralick, and L.G. Shapiro, *Computer and Robot Vision: Volume 1*, Addison-Wesley Publishing, 1992.
25. J.A. Hanley, and B.J. McNeil, "The Meaning and Use of the Area Under a Receiver Operating Characteristic (ROC) Curve", Radiology, **143**: pp. 29-36, 1982.
26. J.A. Hanley, and B.J. McNeil, "A Method of Comparing the Areas Under Receiver Operating Characteristic Curves Derived from the Same Cases", Radiology, **148**: pp. 839-843, 1983.
27. K.S. Woods, and K.W. Bowyer, "Generating ROC Curves for Artificial Neural Networks", Department of Computer Science and Engineering Technical Report #93-03, University of South Florida.

Digital mammography: Image analysis and automatic classification of calcifications in ductal carcinoma in situ

J Parker, D R Dance and D H Davies

Joint Department of Physics,
Institute of Cancer Research and Royal Marsden Hospital, London, U.K.

L J Yeoman[*], M J Michell[*] and S Humphreys[+]

Departments of Radiology[*] and Pathology[+], King's College Hospital, London, U.K.

1. Introduction

Ductal carcinoma in situ (DCIS) is a disease characterised by tumour development within the ducts of the breast. In many cases mammographic abnormality is the only sign of this disease. With the advent of screening programmes the number of cases of DCIS diagnosed has risen. Cases of DCIS account for about 20% of cancers detected by screening[1].

DCIS is widely believed to be a precursor of invasive cancer[2] and is therefore treated as a malignancy. Using radical mastectomy as the standard treatment, a cure rate approaching 100% has been achieved[3], but at the expense of a disfigurement and trauma for the patient. However, there is evidence that some DCIS tumours may have a low risk of progressing to invasive disease[4,5]. Attempts are now being made to identify the sub-set of patients with low risk DCIS for whom breast-conserving therapy may be the most appropriate treatment[6].

DCIS can be categorised according to cell-type and growth pattern into the following tumour types: comedo, cribiform, micropapillary, papillary and solid[4]. The disease may be multicentric and contain several categories of tumour within the same breast. Retrospective studies have suggested that comedo tumours are more aggressive, i.e. they are more likely to become microinvasive even at an early stage of development[4]. It is therefore important to be able to detect a comedo component in a DCIS lesion.

An estimated 70-80% of mammographically detected DCIS cases have calcifications on the mammogram[1,4,6]. These appear as clusters of small bright spots on the mammogram. Many authors have reported that comedo tumours produce calcifications which are more elongated in shape than other types of DCIS. The underlying causes of this phenomenon are illustrated in Figure 1.

Key:
- calcification
- necrotic material
- tumour cell

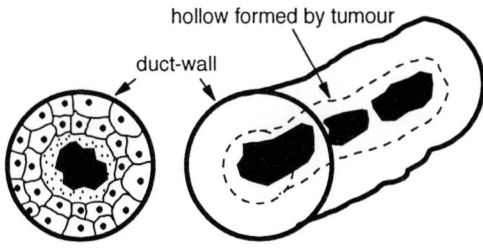

(a) Growth pattern for comedo DCIS

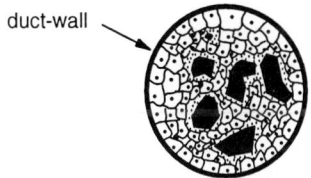

(b) Growth pattern for non-comedo DCIS
(cribiform)

Figure 1. DCIS tumour architecture and formation of calcifications

The growth pattern of the comedo tumours often leads to a solid tumour which entirely fills and enlarges the duct, causing a region of necrosis to appear along the axis. Calcifications forming in this region are cast into elongated shapes. Elongation may be increased when objects in the same duct coalesce as the disease progresses.

Non-comedo tumours generally have less necrosis and a different growth pattern. Calcifications forming in recesses in the sponge-like tumour structure are cast into more compact shapes.

Attempts to distinguish between comedo and non-comedo cases from the mammographic appearance have used visual estimates of basic shape features. Holland et al^6 report a significant difference between the shape distributions in predominantly comedo cases and those with little or no comedo component. In this work we applied digital image analysis techniques to objectively study the imaging features of the DCIS calcifications. The aim was to use image features to develop an automatic classifier for detection of cases with a significant comedo component from the appearance of the calcifications on the mammogram.

2. Data Acquisition

Cases of DCIS containing calcifications were taken from the United Kingdom Breast Screening Programme. The original pathology slides were reassessed to check which categories of tumour were present in each case. A data-set of 32 cases was obtained comprising 23 comedo and 9 non-comedo cases. No cases of mixed category were used in the study.

A mammographic film taken using the magnification technique (magnification = 1.5) was obtained for each case. An area of each film containing all significant calcifications was digitised using a Joyce-Loebl SCANDIG III scanning microdensitometer. The scanning aperture was 25 microns with 8-bit resolution of optical densities in the range 0 to 3. In this way a pixel size of approximately 17 microns square was obtained. Visual comparison showed the magnified views were noisier than standard view films, thus reducing the contrast of the calcifications. However, we felt the high resolution was necessary to measure objects of minimum dimension 50 microns.

Before receiving the true pathology data, as many calcifications as possible were manually labelled. Examples of these segmentations are shown in Figure 2. This procedure was facilitated using in-house computer graphics software enabling windowing, magnification and linear enhancement of contrast. Calcifications which were obviously due to a benign process were not marked. The marking of all calcifications was checked by a radiologist experienced in breast screening.

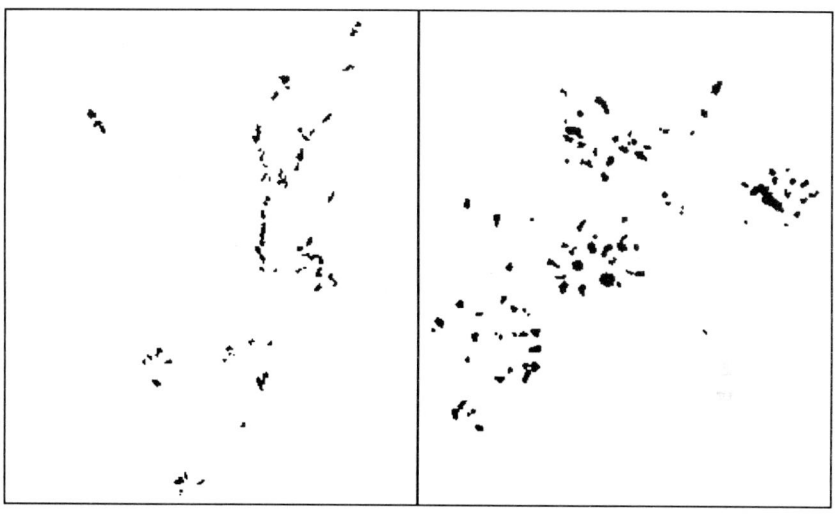

a) typical comedo (cluster width 23 mm)   b) typical non-comedo (cluster width 22 mm)

c) atypical comedo (cluster width 28 mm)   d) typical comedo (cluster width 9 mm)

Figure 2. Binary representations of manually segmented calcifications
(scale indicated by actual cluster width)

3. Automatic Classification

The development of the classifier fell into the two stages: feature extraction and classification. The objective of the feature extraction stage was to develop a set of measures to be calculated from the digitised images which would reflect the imaging properties of the individual calcifications. In the classification stage an algorithm was developed, trained and optimised to automatically partition cases of DCIS based upon a combination of these measures.

3.1. Feature extraction

A wide variety of features was calculated for each calcification including second-order statistics which are difficult to assess by eye. A list of the features is given in Table I. Full definitions are given in the Appendix.

The features Φ_1 and Φ_2 are combinations of regular moments which remain invariant to shift, scale and rotation. These are the first two of seven moment invariants described by Hu[7]. The other five invariants were close to zero for all calcifications and had no discriminatory potential.

Eccentricity$_1$ is calculated from the length r_{min} of the vector joining the centre of mass to the nearest boundary pixel. Therefore as the centre of mass approaches the boundary of the object the feature value increases sharply for little change in eccentricity. The length r_{min} was given a lower limit of one pixel to prevent an infinite value for *eccentricity$_1$*. *Eccentricity$_2$* and *eccentricity$_3$* are moment based and have more stable behaviour.

Radius of gyration is normalised to the length r_{max} of the vector joining the centre of mass to the farthest boundary pixel. This compensates for the variation in size between objects.

The *pair* feature is a measure of the combined directionality of the calcification with its nearest neighbour on the mammogram. The magnitude of *pair* falls off rapidly when the distance to the nearest neighbour is greater than 10 pixels. This makes the feature sensitive to pairs of elongated calcifications which are very close together. These are likely to be adjacent comedo calcifications on the point of coalition.

In order to eliminate features which contained closely similar information the product-moment correlation coefficient (r where $|r| \leq 1$) between pairs of features was evaluated. Two pairs of features were highly correlated: *foreground* and *background* (r=0.99) and *contrast* and *difference* (r=0.98). The features *foreground* and *contrast* were therefore excluded from further consideration leaving 17 features available for classification.

Table I. Feature descriptions

feature name	description	measure of:
area	number of pixels in the object	contrast
foreground	mean greylevel of pixels of object	contrast
background	mean greylevel of pixels 8-connected to object boundary	contrast
difference	foreground - background	contrast
contrast	difference / (foreground + background)	contrast
shape	compares perimeter to disk of same area	shape
entropy	entropy of greylevels of object pixels	texture
$eccentricity_1$	ratio of r_{max} to r_{min} vectors	shape
edge-strength	mean gradient in greylevel at object boundary	contrast
variance	variance of greylevel of object pixels	texture
directionality	ratio of sides of bounding rectangle	shape
fullness	ratio of object area to bounding rectangle area	shape
$eccentricity_2$	ratio of axes of best-fit ellipse	shape
$eccentricity_3$	ratio of moments of inertia of best-fit ellipse	shape
radius of gyration	about centre of mass	texture
Φ_1	moment invariant	shape
Φ_2	moment invariant	shape
pair	directionality of object combined with nearest neighbour	shape
comio	binary feature: whether centre of mass lies inside or outside the object	shape

3.2. Classification

The k-nearest neighbours method[8,9] (kNN) was chosen for the classifier. This non-parametric statistical method was preferred as it can operate with a sparse data-set. Being supervised, it made full use of all the prior information which was available in the form of the true pathology. The method imposed no constraints on the shape and number of decision boundaries, these being determined by the data.

The 32 cases of the data-set were divided into two sub-sets, one formed the basis of the classifier and the other was used to optimise classifier performance. The first set consisted of three comedo and three non-comedo cases which were specified to be of typical appearance by an expert radiologist. The objects from these cases formed the feature-space required by the kNN classifier. The second set consisted of the remaining 26 cases (6 non-comedo and 20 comedo). These cases were used to assess classifier performance.

Classification of each case was in two steps. Firstly, each object was classified as having comedo or non-comedo appearance using the kNN classifier. The Euclidean distance in feature space was used as the similarity measure. Objects having equivocal appearance were not classified. Secondly, the case itself was classified as being comedo or non-comedo according to the fraction of objects having comedo appearance by applying a threshold T in the range 0 to 1.

3.3. Classifier optimisation

There were three parameters which controlled the operation of the kNN classifier:

k   the number of nearest neighbours
M_0 the minimum majority required for class 0 (comedo)
M_1 the minimum majority required for class 1 (non-comedo)

The value of k was set to five, a small value being preferred given the sparse data-set. As there were considerably more comedo objects than non-comedo objects, we took two measures to prevent the feature space being swamped. Firstly, the 20 largest objects only from each case were used. Secondly, the values of M_0 and M_1 were set to 5 and 1 respectively so that only objects of distinctly comedo appearance would be classified as comedo.

A receiver operating characteristic (ROC)[10] curve was produced for the classifier by varying the threshold T in 100 steps between 0 and 1. The area under this curve was taken as a measure of the performance of a classifier having a particular combination of features. The ROC curve axes were defined as true positive fraction (tpf) versus false positive fraction (fpf).

These were defined as follow:

$$tpf = tp / total\_p$$

$$fpf = fp / total\_n$$

and where:

tp = number of true positives ie comedo cases correctly classified
fp = number of false positives ie non-comedo cases classified as comedo
total_p = total number of positive (comedo) cases
total_n = total number of negative (non-comedo) cases

This produced a number of points which were joined by straight lines to form a rough curve. The smoothness of the curve depends on the number of test-cases. The area under the curve was taken as a measure of the performance of the classifier for a given set of features. The classifier was optimised by calculating this area for all possible combinations of one to five of the features (a total of 9401 cases).

4. Results

Table II gives an indication of the variability of number and subtlety of the calcifications.

Table II. Variation in number, size and contrast of calcifications.

	minimum	maximum	mean	standard deviation
number per case	14	412	68	73
area [pixels]	10	9920	352	457
contrast [greylevels]	3	22	5	3

Table III gives details of the distribution of each feature. Most features showed a wide variability especially *area* and *shape*.

Table III Statistical parameters for measured features for all data

feature name	minimum	maximum	mean	standard deviation
area	10	9920	352	457
foreground	117.9	235.7	200.3	19.4
background	112.3	233.4	195.5	20.5
difference	3.0	21.8	4.7	2.6
contrast	0.001	0.065	0.012	0.007
shape	1.49	8.27	2.59	0.85
entropy	1.60	5.43	3.54	0.66
eccentricity$_1$	1.18	158.95	4.14	6.84
edge-strength	1.30	14.86	5.77	2.16
variance	0.55	127.45	14.17	13.76
directionality	1.00	8.63	1.63	0.54
fullness	0.30	1.25	0.73	0.11
eccentricity$_2$	0.79	1.22	1.00	0.05
eccentricity$_3$	0.02	25.56	1.40	1.54
radius of gyration	0.42	0.74	0.57	0.05
Φ_1	7.08×10^{-4}	5.42×10^{-3}	1.05×10^{-3}	3.34×10^{-4}
Φ_2	8.20×10^{-12}	2.85×10^{-5}	4.36×10^{-7}	1.15×10^{-6}
pair	0.00	14.17	1.06	1.16
comio	0	1	0.009	0.093

Table IV shows the top five performing classifiers found by systematic trial of all combinations of one to five features. The ROC curve for the best performing classifier is shown in Figure 3. This has area 0.80 and uses the five features *difference, entropy, eccentricity$_1$, eccentricity$_2$* and Φ_1.

Table IV. Results of systematic feature selection

Area under ROC curve	combination of features
0.80	*difference, entropy, eccentricity$_1$, eccentricity$_2$*, Φ_1
0.80	*entropy, eccentricity$_1$, eccentricity$_2$*, Φ_1, Φ_2
0.79	*entropy, variance, eccentricity$_2$*, Φ_1
0.79	*entropy, eccentricity$_1$, variance, eccentricity$_2$*, Φ_1
0.78	*eccentricity$_2$, eccentricity$_3$*, Φ_2, *pair, comio*

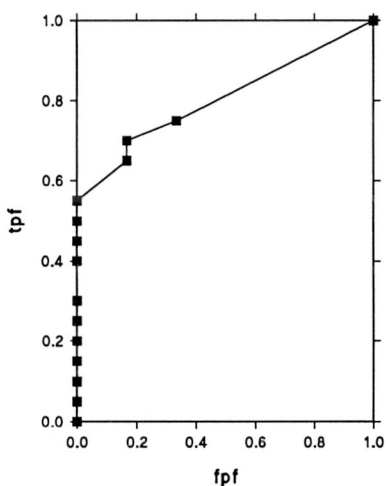

Figure 3. ROC curve for best classifier with five features

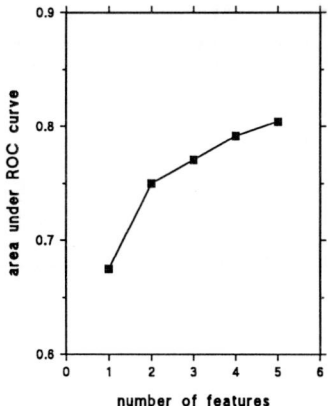

Figure 4. Area under ROC curve for best combinations of 1 to 5 features

5. Discussion

We have measured performance levels for automatic classification of DCIS from the appearance of the individual calcifications. Using the kNN classifier we have achieved an area under the ROC curve of 0.80 using five features. The performance levels of a typical radiologist in performing the same recognition task are not currently known, so a comparison with the performance of the radiologist cannot currently be made.

The cohort of 32 cases is small compared to the large number of DCIS cases detected by screening. Therefore assessment of the performance of the classifier was limited to a number of cases which may not be representative of the full range of appearances. Also, the ROC curves were not very smooth due to the small number of test-cases. The use of automatic calcification detection algorithms[11] should allow an increase in the size of the data-set and hence improve statistical precision.

The results of our systematic search showed that several of the best classifiers can have similar performance whilst containing different features. It is possible that better performance would be obtained by sub-dividing each class and developing separate classifiers for each sub-class.

In general, increasing the number of features improved the performance of the classifier. Figure 4 shows that increasing the number of features beyond three gave marginal improvement in classifier performance. The trend shown in Figure 4 appeared to reach a plateau at a ROC area of approximately 0.81.

We have investigated the application of an object oriented classifier to the problem of identifying high-risk cases of DCIS from associated calcifications. We are encouraged by the performance of the automatic classifier developed, given the wide variability and overlap in appearance of the different types of calcifications.

6. References

1. J. F. Wilson, J. M. Destouet, D. P. Winchester, R. R. Kuske, V. G. Vogel, "1991 RSNA Special Focus Session: Current Controversies in the Management of Ductal Carcinoma in Situ of the Breast", *Radiology* **185** (1992) 77-81.

2. J. A. Andersen, M. Nielsen and J. Jensen, in *Early Breast Cancer*, ed. J. Zander and J. Baltzer (Springer-Verlag, Berlin, 1985).

3. J. A. Sunshine, H. S. Moseley, W. S. Fletcher and W. W. Krippaehne, "Breast carcinoma in situ: a retrospective review of 112 cases with a minimum 10 year follow-up", *Am. J. Surg.* **150** (1985) 44-51.

4. A. S. Patchefsky, G. F. Schwartz, S. D. Finkelstein, A. Prestipino, S. E. Sohn, J. S. Singer and S. A. Feig, "Heterogeneity of intraductal carcinoma of the breast", *Cancer* **63** (1989) 731-41.

5. P. C. Stomper, J. L. Connolly, J. E. Meyer and J. R. Harris, "Clinically occult ductal carcinoma in situ detected with mammography: analysis of 100 cases with radiologic-pathologic correlation", *Radiology* **172** (1989) 235-41.

6. R. Holland, J. H. C. L. Hendriks, A. L. M. Verbeek, M. Mravunac and J. H. Schuurmans Stekhoven, "Extent, distribution, and mammographic/histological correlations of breast ductal carcinoma in situ", *Lancet* **335** (1990) 519-22.

7. M. K. Hu, "Pattern recognition by moment invariants", *Proc. IRE* **49** (1961) 1428.

8. R. O. Duda and P. E. Hart, *Pattern classification and scene analysis* (John Wiley & Sons, New York, 1973) 103-5.

9. P. A. Devijver and J. Kittler, *Pattern Recognition: A Statistical Approach* (Prentice/Hall International,London,1982) Ch.3.

10. C. E. Metz, "ROC methodology in radiologic imaging", *Invest Radiol* **21** (1986) 720-33.

11. D. H. Davies and D. R. Dance, "Automatic computer detection of clustered calcifications in digital mammograms", *Phy. Med. Biol.* **35** (1990) 1111-8.

7. Appendix: definition of features

For an image set I (containing all image pixels), foreground object set F (a subset of I containing all pixels which make up the calcification object) and a background set B (a subset of I containing pixels 8-connected to calcification boundary pixels but not in set B), the following features were defined:

$area = $ size of set F

$$foreground = \frac{1}{area} \sum_{gl_i \in F} gl_i \quad (gl_i = greylevel\ of\ pixel\ i)$$

$$background = \frac{1}{N} \sum_{gl_i \in B} gl_i \quad (N = size\ of\ set\ B)$$

$difference = foreground - background$

$$contrast = \frac{difference}{foreground + background}$$

$$shape = \frac{P^2}{4\pi . area} \quad (P = perimeter\ length\ [pixel])$$

$$entropy = -\sum_{i=1}^{i_{max}} p_i . \log_2(p_i) \quad (p_i = frequency\ of\ i'th\ greylevel \neq 0)$$

$$eccentricity_1 = \frac{r_{max}}{r_{min}} \quad (r_{max}, r_{min}\ defined\ in\ text)$$

$$edge\ strength = \frac{1}{P} \sum_{L_i \in B} \overline{\delta g} \quad (L_i = 2x2\ mask\ containing\ boundary\ pixel\ i$$
and at least one background pixel
$\overline{\delta g} = mean\ gradient\ of\ diagonals\ of\ L_i$)

$$\text{variance} = \frac{1}{\text{area}} \sum_{gl_i \in F} (gl_i - \text{foreground})^2$$

$$\text{directionality} = \frac{\max(a,b)}{\min(a,b)} \qquad (a,b \text{ dimensions of bounding rectangle})$$

$$\text{fullness} = \frac{\text{area}}{a.b}$$

$$\text{eccentricity}_2 = \frac{A}{B} \qquad (A,B \text{ semi-axes of best-fit ellipse})$$

$$\text{eccentricity}_3 = \frac{I_{\max}}{I_{\min}} \qquad (I_{\min}, I_{\max} \text{ moments of inertia about } A,B)$$

$$\text{radius of gyration} = \left(\frac{I}{M}\right)^{\frac{1}{2}} \cdot \frac{1}{r_{\max}} \qquad (I = \text{moment of inertia about centre of mass}$$
$$M = \text{foreground} \times \text{area})$$

$$\phi_1 = \mu_{2,0} + \mu_{0,2}$$
$$\text{where: } \mu_{p,q} = \frac{v_{p,q}}{v_{0,0}^{1+(p+q)/2}}$$
$$v_{p,q} = \text{central moment of order } p+q$$

$$\phi_2 = (\mu_{2,0} - \mu_{0,2})^2 + 4\mu_{1,1}^2$$

$$pair = diry_1.diry_2.e^{-\left(\frac{d_{min}}{10}\right)}$$ ($diry_1, diry_2$ *directionalities of neighbouring objects*
d_{min} = *distance of closest approach*)

$$comio = \begin{cases} 0 & \text{if centre of mass inside object} \\ 1 & \text{if centre of mass outside object} \end{cases}$$

AUTOMATED DETECTION OF BREAST ASYMMETRY USING ANATOMICAL FEATURES

Peter Miller and Sue Astley

Department of Medical Biophysics, University of Manchester, Stopford Building, Oxford Road, Manchester M13 9PT, England, pim@wiau.mb.man.ac.uk

Breast asymmetry is an important radiological sign of cancer. This paper describes the first approach aiming to detect *all* types of asymmetry; previous asymmetry-based research has been focussed on the detection of mass lesions. The conventional approach is to search for brightness or texture differences between corresponding locations on left and right breast images. Due to the difficulty in accurately identifying corresponding locations, asymmetry cues generated in this way are insufficiently specific to be used as prompts for small and subtle abnormalities in a computer-aided diagnosis system. We have undertaken studies to discover more about the visual cues utilized by radiologists. As a result, we propose a new automatic method for detecting asymmetry based on the comparison of corresponding anatomical structures, identified by an automatic segmentation of breast tissue types. We describe methods for comparing the shape and brightness distribution of these regions, and we present promising results obtained by combining evidence for asymmetry.

1. Introduction

Breast screening programmes have been introduced in many countries, with the aim of detecting cancer at an early stage in asymptomatic women. In Britain, for example, it is estimated that 1 in 12 women will be affected by breast cancer at some point in their lives. Screening generates a large number of mammograms requiring interpretation, and a variety of computer-based aids have been proposed to improve the performance of radiologists searching for small, subtle and infrequent abnormalities. One viable application of current image processing technology would be a system for prompting radiologists by indicating to them any suspicious regions.

There is a wide variation in the appearance of mammograms from different women, but normal left and right mammograms from the same woman are generally symmetric; radiologists consider asymmetry an important sign of abnormality. Masses are the most common asymmetric sign of cancer, and appear brighter than surrounding tissue, often with discernible margins. When a mass is obscured by other structures, it will usually be seen as a focal, though poorly defined, asymmetric density. A disturbance in the normally symmetrical flow of structures towards the nipple may also be indicative of cancer, which can have the effect of pulling structures in towards a point. This sign is particularly important in screening of asymptomatic women, when masses may be very small or barely visible.

2. Automated detection of asymmetry

2.1. Previous approaches

Several investigators have used asymmetry in computerized schemes for the detection of mammographic masses. More subtle types of asymmetry – focal density and architectural distortion – have not previously been tackled using automated methods. Firstly, digitised left and right mammograms are registered by matching the breast boundaries extracted from each image. This creates a mapping between the two images, which enables features from corresponding locations in the left and right breast to be compared. The resulting map of local asymmetries is processed to remove spurious responses and to determine the most suspicious regions.

The methods differ mostly in their choice of image features for the measurement of local asymmetry. Yin et al [1] used brightness; Kimme et al [2] and Lau and Bischof [3] used brightness and texture; and Hand et al [4] used brightness, texture and shape. Several tests are commonly used to determine which asymmetric locations should be regarded as suspicious: *magnitude*: only high asymmetry values are considered; *size*: the asymmetric locations must form a cluster above a certain size; *shape*: the cluster should be circular or star–like. If only a few regions on each mammogram satisfy these criteria, they could then be indicated to a radiologist for final diagnosis.

2.2. General problems

Conventional methods are based upon the assumption that breast asymmetry is adequately represented by image asymmetry, once the left and right breast images have been registered. Unfortunately, there are many factors contributing to image asymmetry which have no radiological importance. Although the anatomy of normal left and right breasts is largely symmetric, several asymmetric factors are inherent in the process of mammographic examination. For instance, the amount and angle of compression applied to each breast will determine the position, size, density and brightness of structures on the mammogram [5]. Other spurious asymmetries can be introduced when registering the left and right breasts. For example, if one breast image is warped [3] to match the other in shape and size, the resulting magnification and distortion of internal structures may cause further false cues.

Moreover, these false asymmetries often outweigh and outnumber any true abnormalities which may be present on the mammogram. This explains the need for the supplementary tests mentioned above, as the true abnormalities must be differentiated from the many false cues. Any improvement in specificity is likely to degrade sensitivity, leaving small, subtle cancers undetected. We therefore believe that conventional methods are limited to the detection of conspicuous mass lesions, a task which radiologists are themselves capable of performing to an acceptable standard. A successful prompting system for breast screening must also recognize small masses and architectural distortion, which may be the only asymmetric signs of early cancer, and are difficult for radiologists to detect.

The fundamental difficulty in detecting breast asymmetry – for image analysis systems and radiologists alike – is that asymmetry cannot be precisely defined. There is no minimum or maximum size or brightness, or typical shape; indeed secondary signs of cancer such as increased vascularity and skin thickening may affect the whole mammogram. In this light the approach adopted by other researchers is a practical one: to detect the subset of asymmetries which *can* be defined unambiguously. However, our approach is to gain greater insight into the processes used by a radiologist in labelling certain subtle asymmetries as suspicious, and hence develop a more comprehensive automatic system suitable for breast screening.

3. How do radiologists detect asymmetry?

Our basic understanding of the nature and mammographic appearance of breast asymmetry has been gained from the literature and in detailed discussions with experienced breast radiologists. It is apparent that several levels of symmetry are considered in mammographic interpretation. Firstly, an impression of overall symmetry of the whole breast and gland tissue is gained by viewing the images at a distance. Then each quadrant of the two breasts is compared, looking for architectural disturbance and localized increases in density [6]. Some experts suggest moving masks slowly across both mammograms, to ensure that no asymmetries are missed [7]. Many additional techniques are used to evaluate any suspicious asymmetries in detail.

It is also noticeable that much of radiologists' reasoning is performed on a regional basis. As well as the four quadrants already mentioned, the region containing all of the gland tissue, called the *gland disc*, is an important feature in the comparison. This is because cancers which attack mainly fatty tissue or supporting structures, form bright, isolated foreground regions, and are relatively easy to detect on the darker background. The majority of cancers attack gland tissue, and can be obscured by other bright structures in the gland disc, so radiologists must also compare the shape and density of the gland discs to detect any underlying disease.

In summary, we believe that radiologists compare anatomically similar regions, independently of their precise location on the mammograms. This is in contrast with conventional automated methods, which are dependent on similar structures lying in corresponding locations. To test our hypothesis, and to discover which visual cues are used in the comparison of regions, we have employed a series of experiments to test radiologists; these are described below.

3.1. Materials and methods

Two consultant breast radiologists selected 30 screening mammogram pairs (D_1 in table 1). Twelve of these cases contained abnormalities, which were visible as varying degrees of asymmetry. Several of the normal cases also exhibited some degree of asymmetry. Both radiologists delineated the non–fat regions of each mammogram on registered transparent overlays. On most mammograms the gland disc was the only non–fat region (excluding the pectoral muscle), though two of the abnormal cases contained isolated mass lesions.

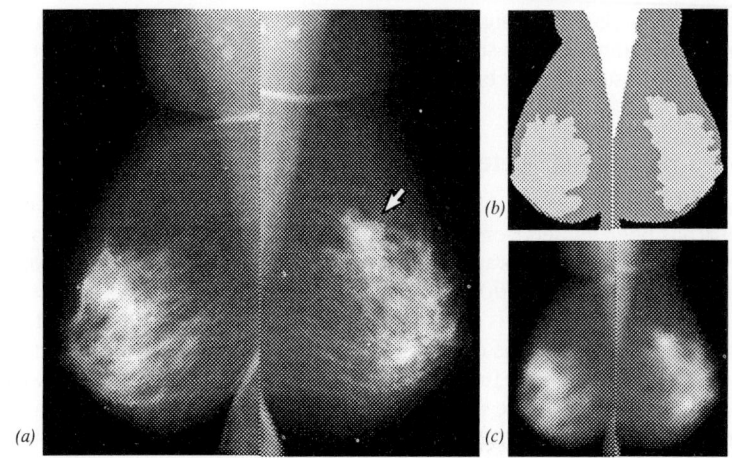

Figure 1. Example mammogram (a) with abnormality marked by arrow (b) in shape study (c) in density study

Table 1. Information on mammogram data sets used in this paper
(ML = Medio-lateral, MLO = Medio-lateral oblique)

Data set	Cases	Pairs	View	Normals	Abnormals	Pixel size (mm)	Depth (bits)
D_1	30	Yes	MLO	18	12	0.20	8
D_2	74	Yes	MLO or ML	29	45	0.15	8
D_3	40	No	MLO	40	0	0.40	6

The mammograms in our first experiment were processed to remove all brightness information, by superimposing the radiologists' annotations of non-fat regions onto silhouettes of each breast. These data were designed to test if asymmetry could be detected using just shape and size cues from the non-fat regions. Both sets of annotations were used in random order to extend the data set to 60 pairs. In the second experiment the mammograms were blurred to remove structural details and texture, leaving only density and brightness information. Figure 1 shows an abnormal mammogram pair, together with processed versions for the shape and density experiments. The style of presentation was kept as familiar as possible, by positioning the mammograms back-to-back on a dark background.

We have conducted a pilot experiment with three experienced breast radiologists. The processed mammograms were reduced to one-sixth of their digitised resolution, and printed on paper four to a page, each mammogram pair occupying an 80 x 70 mm area. Participants were asked to rate the suspiciousness of each case on a scale from 1 (definitely normal) to 6 (definitely abnormal), and also to mark the suspicious regions on the mammogram.

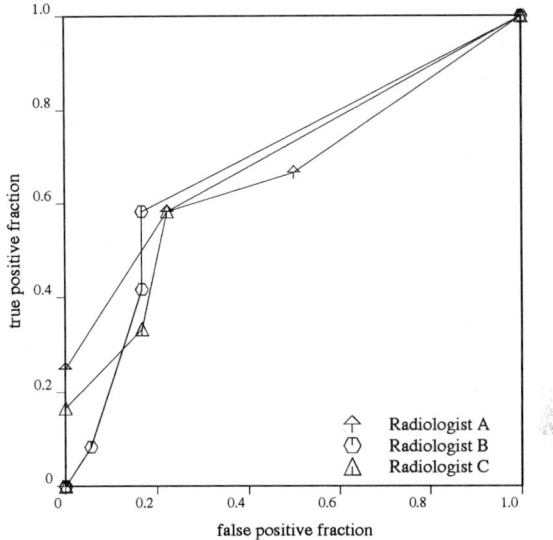

Figure 2. ROC analysis of shape experiment, with radiologists classifying mammograms on the basis of silhouettes of non–fat regions

3.2. Results

The six–point scale was used to construct a receiver operating characteristic (ROC) curve for each participant (figure 2). This shows that diagnosis based purely on shape comparison of anatomical regions can detect up to 60% of abnormal cases, while misclassifying 20% of normal cases. This corresponds to an overall accuracy of approximately 70% on the whole data set (table 2).

Table 2. Accuracy of shape experiment participants

Radiologist	Accuracy %
A	70.0
B	73.3
C	70.0

3.3. Discussion

These results provide initial evidence for our assertion that asymmetry is detected using a comparison of regions. Further examination of the results has revealed that normal mammograms misclassified as abnormal frequently exhibit significant differences in the amount of glandular tissue in each breast; thus these cases are arguably suspicious. Further and more extensive analysis and experimentation will allow us to measure and compare the radiological importance of each type of visual cue. The shape and density experiments have now been distributed to 30 breast radiologists around the country, and analysis of these results is in progress. The protocol for the

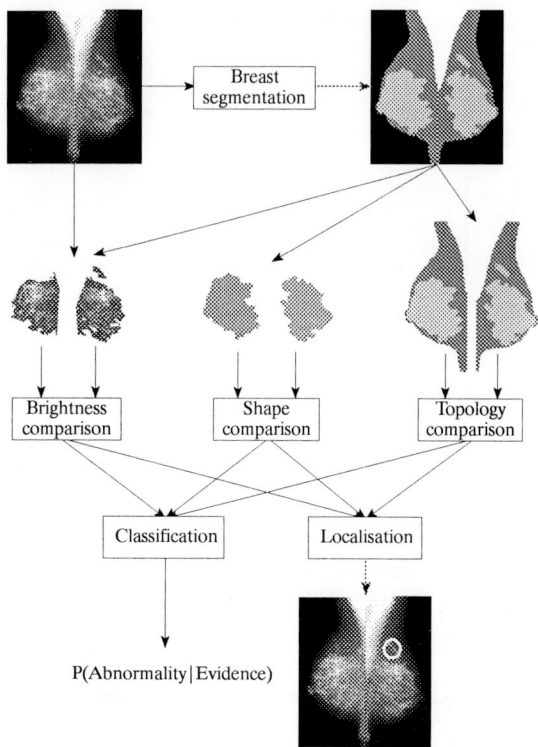

Figure 3. Schematic diagram of automated system for detecting asymmetry using anatomical features

density experiment is the same as for the shape experiment, but as the density mammograms contain more detail they are only reduced to quarter resolution, and printed three to a page, each pair occupying an 110 x 90 mm area. Participants are instructed to complete the shape experiment first, because the same mammograms are used for the density experiment, providing additional information on each case.

4. A new automated approach

In our discussion of radiologists' technique, we made the assertion that asymmetry is detected by comparing anatomically similar regions of the left and right breast. We propose that a successful automated system can be developed using the same principle. The system is explained with the aid of the diagram in figure 3. Firstly, tissue types in the digitised mammogram are segmented to form anatomically homogeneous fat or non–fat regions. Asymmetry is then detected by comparing various features of non–fat regions in the left and right mammogram. Finally, the evidence from these comparisons is combined, in order to classify the case as normal or abnormal, and to locate any suspicious regions. The main advantage of this approach over conventional methods is that the non–fat regions are extracted from the mammogram and compared directly, so asymmetry measurements are likely to be more robust than those obtained using problematic breast alignment procedures. It is also possible to compare the *shape* of the regions, and thus recognize certain signs of architectural distortion which were not available to previous methods.

The following sections describe the development of the major components of our system in detail: breast segmentation, asymmetry measurement, and classification. The system is designed to be completely automated, though we have found it necessary to separate the development of the segmentation and asymmetry components, temporarily using ideal segmentations for asymmetry measurement.

5. Breast segmentation

The objective of this work is the automatic segmentation of mammograms into anatomically distinct regions.

5.1. Materials and methods

Two consultant breast radiologists selected a representative data set of 40 normal screening mammograms (D_3 in table 1). To establish a standard against which the methods could be tested, both radiologists delineated the non–fat regions on transparent overlays. The overlays were also digitised, and combined to produce a consensus annotation for each mammogram; regions in which the two opinions differed were excluded from subsequent analysis.

A semi–automated procedure was used to find the breast area on each mammogram, and to remove the pectoral muscle region. Feature images were generated using Laws' texture energy method [8], morphological granulometry techniques [9], and the original image grey levels. A threshold for each feature was determined using leave–one–out training across the data set. This threshold was used to segment each breast into fat and non–fat regions, which were compared with the consensus annotation to calculate the segmentation accuracy.

5.2. Results

The discriminating power of the best texture and grey–level features is compared using ROC curves in figure 4. The best texture energy feature (R5R5) measures the spottiness of the texture. The granulometry coarseness feature calculates the most prominent size of structure in the texture. The corresponding segmentation accuracies achieved using trained thresholds are listed in table 3, and an example mammogram successfully segmented using texture energy is shown in figure 5. We define segmentation accuracy as the percentage of correctly classified pixels in the breast region, and calculate the mean value for the 40 mammograms.

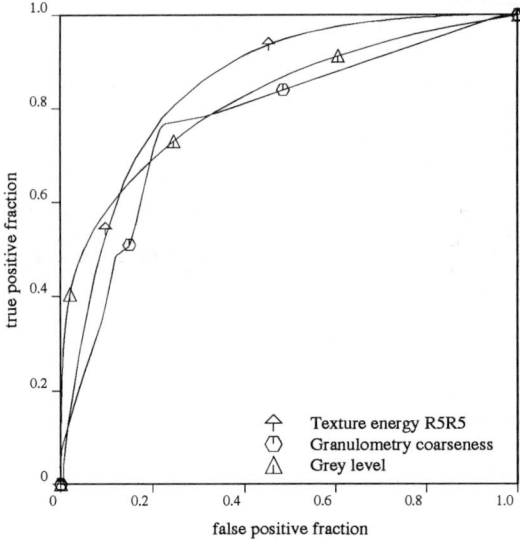

Figure 4. ROC comparison of feature performance for breast segmentation

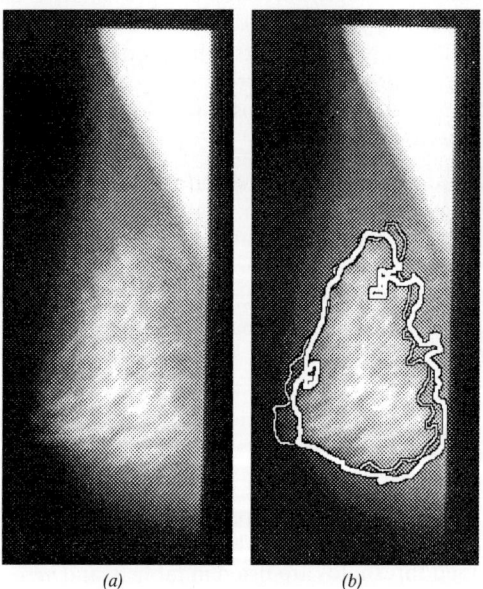

Figure 5. (a) Example mammogram (b) Comparison of radiologist's delineation (thin line) with automatic segmentation (thick line)

Table 3. Mean segmentation accuracy obtained using trained thresholds

Feature	Accuracy %
Texture energy R5R5	80.3
Granulometry coarseness	75.7
Grey level	71.0

5.3. Discussion

Our results show that texture energy was the most successful segmentation method tested, though still some way short of the 91% agreement between radiologists [10]. Initial results suggest that similar accuracies can be achieved using the higher resolution D_1 and D_2 mammograms. The majority of misclassifications were of dense glandular regions which appear relatively uniform, and were classified as fat. By combining evidence from grey–level and texture features we should be able to achieve more reliable tissue classification. A further problem occurs in mammograms with diffuse glandular tissue over much of the breast, as confusion arises as to whether the whole area or just concentrated regions should be classified as non–fat. Further improvements could be made using a region–based segmentation approach, rather than thresholding. Until the accuracy of automated breast segmentation has been improved, we have elected to use the radiologists' annotations as the basis of asymmetry measurements.

6. Asymmetry cues

The aim of these experiments is to identify successful methods for the detection of asymmetry between non–fat regions of the left and right breast.

6.1. Materials and methods

Two types of region features can be used in the comparison of non–fat regions: *global features*, which use a single value to describe some property of the whole region; and *local features*, which describe each location in the region individually. To compare global features of regions, it is only necessary to measure the difference between two values. To compare local features, an alignment process must first be performed, so that the locations in each region correspond. The difficulty in creating such a correspondence between whole breasts was discussed previously, but it is likely that the problems in aligning smaller regions would not be as severe. We have initially concentrated on global features.

Data sets D_1 and D_2 were used for these experiments. Of the 104 pairs, there were 47 normals, 28 asymmetric densities, 16 architectural distortions and 13 masses. The radiologists' non–fat annotations were used as a temporary replacement for the automated breast segmentation method, to exclude the effects of segmentation errors from our analysis of comparison methods.

6.1.1. Shape

Cancer is known to distort the shape of anatomical structures, in some cases even before a mass is detectable [11]. By comparing the shape of gland discs from left and right mammograms, we may be able to detect both this architectural distortion, and any masses affecting the disc boundaries. Shape features can only be calculated from single closed regions, so for these experiments we assumed that the largest non–fat region in each breast was the gland disc, and discarded all smaller regions. An alternative approach would be to use the convex hull of non–fat regions. We calculated a shape feature of left and right gland discs, and used the difference as a measure of asymmetry. No registration of the gland discs was required.

After exploring a number of shape measurement techniques [eg 12,13], we found that compactness, circularity, eccentricity, and fourier features all achieved some degree of discrimination between normal and abnormal cases. We did not consider model-based shape descriptors, as they rely on the identification of reliable landmark points and minimal (or predictable) variation. The definition of the shape features used are as follows:

$$compactness = \frac{p^2}{a}$$

$$circularity = \frac{\bar{r}}{\sigma_r}$$

$$eccentricity = \frac{max\,chord}{max\,\perp chord}$$

$$elongation = \frac{|C_1| + |C_{N-1}|}{|C_1| - |C_{N-1}|}$$

$$roughness = \frac{\sum_{i \in HF} |C_i|}{\sum_{i \in LF} |C_i|}$$

$$deviation = \frac{\sum_{i \in HF} |C_i|^2}{\sum_{i \in LF} |C_i|^2}$$

$$contour\,energy = \sum_{i=1}^{N-1} |C_i|^2$$

where p, a, r are perimeter, area and radius, C_i ($0 \leq i \leq N-1$) are the first N fourier coefficients of the contour, and HF, LF are the high and low frequency coefficients.

The fourier transform was calculated by treating the coordinates of the gland disc contour as a one–dimensional complex function, always starting and ending at the pixel closest to the nipple. The fourier features were calculated using a subset containing the most significant coefficients ($N=20$). Fourier features are sensitive to shape rotation, enabling similarly shaped regions at different orientations to be correctly rated as asymmetric.

6.1.2. Brightness distribution

A limitation of shape features is their inability to detect masses which are not near the border of the gland disc. This section describes two techniques for comparing the distribution of brightness within non–fat regions: *moments* and *transportation*. Moments are defined as follows:

$$moment_{u,v} = \sum_{(x,y) \in S} f(x,y)(x - \bar{x})^u (y - \bar{y})^v$$

where S is the set of non–fat coordinates, and f is the image function. Asymmetry features are calculated as the difference in moment values for the left and right breast. The second and third order moments have analogies with the mechanics of bodies

[14], and can be interpreted as the following features:

$moment_{11}$ ≡ diagonality
$moment_{20}, moment_{02}$ ≡ horizontal, vertical centralness
$moment_{12}, moment_{21}$ ≡ horizontal, vertical divergence
$moment_{30}, moment_{03}$ ≡ horizontal, vertical imbalance

In operations research, the *transportation problem* is that of minimizing the cost of transporting goods from many warehouses to many shops, each having different availabilities or requirements. There is a cost associated with each route, so the optimal solution must fulfil shop requirements using local warehouses where possible. We decided to use this analogy to calculate the minimal cost of matching regions from left and right mammograms. This cost could then be considered a measure of asymmetry between the regions. Transportation can be formulated as a linear programming problem [15]:

$$\text{minimise} \quad t = \sum_{s,d} c_{sd}\, q_{sd}$$

$$\text{subject to} \quad \sum_{d} q_{sd} = A_s \quad \text{for all } s$$

$$\sum_{s} q_{sd} = R_d \quad \text{for all } d$$

$$q_{sd} \geq 0 \quad \text{for all } s, d$$

$$\sum_{s} A_s = \sum_{d} R_d$$

where t is the total transportation cost, q_{sd} is the quantity transported from source s to destination d, c_{sd} is the cost per unit transportation from source s to destination d, A_s is the availability at source s, and R_d is the requirement at destination d. If the total availability and requirement are unequal, then a dummy site is added to satisfy the final constraint.

In our model, the domain of source sites is represented by non–fat pixels in the left breast, and destination sites by non–fat pixels in the right breast. Pixel values represent the availability or requirement at each site. The cost of transportation between sites should be a measure of distance, so as to minimize the warping required for a match. As the source and destination sites are on different mammograms, the domains are aligned (with respect to nipple locations) to allow distances to be calculated. We found that by reducing the size of the images (eg 4 mm/pixel), the transportation problem could be solved rapidly [16], with only a minor effect on results.

6.1.3. Topology

Further diagnostic information can be extracted from the topology of non–fat regions within the breast. For instance, a small region isolated from the gland disc is suspicious, especially if it is in an unusual location, such as between the gland disc and the pectoral muscle. So far the only topology features we have considered are area and binary moments, which compare the distribution of non–fat tissue in left and right mammograms. The method is the same as for brightness moments, except that the image function $f(x,y) = 1$ for non-fat coordinates. A rule-based expert system would be appropriate for providing further asymmetry evidence from topology.

6.2. Results

For each asymmetry feature described above, observations were generated from the data set of mammogram pairs. The *variance–ratio test* (or *F–test*) was used to find the best features for discriminating between normal and abnormal groups. This test measures the degree of separation of two group means, as the ratio of between–group to within–group variances; good features give ratios above one. The different asymmetry types were considered both together and separately, each time with the same set of normal cases. Six features were found to be effective discriminators (table 4).

Table 4. Variance–ratio test for measuring the discriminating power of asymmetry features

Feature	All asymmetries	Type of asymmetry		
		Density	Distortion	Mass
Contour	3.8	5.8	1.0	0.2
Deviation	3.8	7.8	0.0	0.9
Roughness	1.3	2.6	0.0	0.7
Circularity	0.3	0.0	5.6	0.0
Transportation	6.7	6.6	4.3	4.6
Area	4.6	0.1	7.4	6.3

6.3. Discussion

The strongest shape features are derived from the fourier transform, which is a powerful method for describing the significant deviations of the gland disc contour. The best brightness feature is transportation, and non–fat area was a useful topology feature. It can be seen that different features are successful in discriminating the distinct types of asymmetry from normal cases. This suggests that asymmetry should be detected using separate classification schemes for each asymmetry type.

We are currently investigating texture as a further global feature, to aid recognition of architectural disturbance. Brightness, density and texture will also be considered for the local comparison of non–fat regions. Another question being considered is whether the left and right breasts should be corrected for size and shape differences before the non–fat regions are compared. Although this might eliminate differences due to breast compression, warping could introduce unnatural distortion of internal structures, especially if the breasts are actually different in size. Further analysis of the transportation solution and moment values should allow positional information for asymmetries to be generated.

7. Classification

The purpose of this work is to classify mammogram pairs into normal and abnormal categories, based on their degree of symmetry.

7.1. Materials and methods

Our approach relies on many automated measurements, each providing evidence on the presence of asymmetry. As the signs of asymmetry are subtle, the evidence supplied by any single feature is likely to be too weak for classification purposes. However, combination of evidence may improve discrimination considerably. This technique was used successfully by Astley and Taylor [17] for the detection of microcalcifications.

We tested three classifiers for the combination of asymmetry evidence: linear discriminant, quadratic discriminant and k–nearest–neighbour (kNN) [18]. We found that the linear classifier gave the best performance for this application. Discriminant classifiers create decision boundaries in feature space for classifying observations into groups. Optimal decision boundaries are calculated from the means and covariances of training observations of each group. These classifiers assume normal distributions for the features, though they are robust to minor violations.

Three data sets were derived from the 104 mammogram pairs, each containing examples of only one asymmetry type, and all of the normal cases. In this way we were able to develop and test separate classification schemes for densities, distortions and masses. Each classifier used the six features described above, and was trained and tested on a leave–one–out basis. No attempt has yet been made to optimise the classifier by adjusting the prior group probabilities, which are currently assumed to be equal.

Table 5 presents the classification performance obtained when considering asymmetry types separately and together. The final column indicates the performance of the separate-type classifiers on the whole data set.

Table 5. Classification results using linear discriminant classifier, with equal prior probabilities and leave-one-out training

%	Asymmetries together	Type of asymmetry			Asymmetries separately
		Density	Distortion	Mass	
Hit rate	53	68	56	77	67
False alarm rate	23	19	19	14	17
Accuracy	64	76	75	84	74

7.2. Discussion

Use of the three separate classification schemes in combination is clearly more effective than the original scheme in which all types of asymmetry were considered together. Although the combined hit rate is as yet only moderately high, we believe that further optimisation of our methods will improve the results to a clinically acceptable extent. We now have evidence that prompting may still be effective at lower hit rates provided that the false alarm rate is kept low [19]. In this light, our results are very encouraging.

8. Conclusions

The detection of breast asymmetry is a difficult problem, even for experienced radiologists. The ill–defined, variable and subjective nature of asymmetric visual cues makes the problem even harder to define in terms of computer vision techniques. Nevertheless, we must focus our effort toward such challenging problems if computers are to provide useful assistance to radiologists. We have developed a new automated approach to the detection of breast asymmetry, modelled on the regional comparison identified in radiologists' technique. Digitised mammograms are segmented into regions of fat and non–fat tissue; non–fat regions in the left and right breast are compared using shape, brightness and topology features. Shape is used to detect architectural distortion of the gland disc; brightness distribution detects masses and focal densities; and topological rules specify other suspicious asymmetries. As breast registration is not required by this approach, we believe that it will eventually be possible to detect smaller and more subtle abnormalities than those detected by conventional methods.

We have described a texture analysis method for segmenting the breast image into anatomical regions, on average classifying 80% of the breast area correctly. We need to combine several texture and brightness features to improve this accuracy, and enforce spatial constraints on the segmentation to produce contiguous regions suitable for asymmetry analysis. Non–fat regions of the left and right breast are compared using shape and brightness features from the literature. We adopted a divide–and–conquer strategy: separate data sets for each distinct type of asymmetry were assembled, so that the best features for each type could be identified and combined to improve the overall detection of asymmetry.

The asymmetry evidence from different features has been combined to achieve 74% correct classification of a data set of 104 very subtle mammographic cases. We are now exploring methods for improving the detection of asymmetry, and for generating locations of potential abnormalities, with the aim of producing a technique suitable for prompting radiologists in a computer–aided diagnosis system for breast screening.

9. Acknowledgements

This research is funded by SERC and IBM UK Scientific Centre. The authors would particularly like to thank Drs Caroline Boggis and Mary Wilson, consultant radiologists at The Nightingale Centre, Withington Hospital, for their invaluable participation in discussions and experiments.

10. References

1. Yin F-F, Giger ML, Doi M, Metz CE, Vyborny CJ, Schmidt RA. Computerized detection of masses in digital mammograms: analysis of bilateral subtraction images. *Medical Physics* 18:955–963, 1991.
2. Kimme C, O'Loughlin BJ, Sklansky J. Automatic detection of suspicious abnormalities in breast radiographs. *Data Structures, Computer Graphics and Pattern Recognition*, Academic Press, New York, 1975.
3. Lau T-K, Bischof WF. Automated detection of breast tumours using the asymmetry approach. *Computers and Biomedical Research* 24:273–295, 1991.
4. Hand W, Semmlow JL, Ackerman LV, Alcorn FS. Computer screening of Xeromammograms: a technique for defining suspicious areas of the breast. *Computers and Biomedical Research* 12:445–460, 1979.
5. Egan RL. *Breast imaging – diagnosis and morphology of breast diseases*. WB Saunders, London, 1988.
6. Boggis CRM, Hufton AP, Asbury DL et al. *Manchester breast screening manual*. Withington Hospital, 1990.
7. Tabar L, Dean PB. *Teaching atlas of mammography*. Thieme, New York, 1985.
8. Laws KI. *Textured image segmentation*. Report 940, Image Processing Institute, University of Southern California, Los Angeles, 1980.
9. Serra J. *Image analysis and mathematical morphology*. Academic Press, New York, 1982.
10. Miller PI, Astley SM. Classification of breast tissue by texture analysis. *Image and Vision Computing* 10:277–282, 1992.
11. Kopans DB. *Breast imaging*. Lippincott, Philadelphia, 1989.
12. Marshall S. Review of shape coding techniques. *Image and Vision Computing* 7:281–294, 1989.
13. Veillon F. Study and comparison of certain shape measures. *Signal Processing* 11:81–91, 1986.
14. Giuliano VE. Automatic pattern recognition by a Gestalt method. *Information and Control*, 1961.
15. Hartley R. *Linear and nonlinear programming*. Ellis Horwood, Chichester, 1985.
16. Numerical Algorithms Group. *The NAG Fortran library manual*, Mark 14, 1990.
17. Astley SM, Taylor CJ. Combining cues for mammographic abnormalities. *Proceedings of the British Machine Vision Conference*, pp. 253–258, 1990.
18. Therrien CW. *Decision, estimation, and classification: an introduction to pattern recognition and related topics*. John Wiley, New York, 1989.
19. Astley S, Hutt I, Adamson S, Miller P, Rose P, Boggis C, Taylor C, Valentine T, Davies J, Janette Armstrong. Automation in mammography: computer vision and human perception. In this publication.

Evaluation of Stellate Lesion Detection in a Standard Mammogram Data Set

W. Philip Kegelmeyer, Jr.
Sandia National Laboratories
P.O. Box 969, ORG 8117
Livermore, CA, 94551

Abstract

We have previously reported on a method for the automatic detection of stellate lesions in digitized mammograms, and on our tests of that method on image data with known diagnoses. This earlier investigation was based on a limited set of 10 test images, each with a stellate lesion. As our approach is one of supervised training, half of the data was used as a training set, and so the performance results were necessarily coarse.

Accordingly there is value in testing these algorithms on a larger data set that will not only provide more lesions but also truly undiseased tissue. A new mammogram data set addresses both of these concerns, as it contains examples of twelve stellate lesions, as well as fifty examples of entirely normal mammograms. Further, as this data set has been made widely available to all interested researchers, performance results for specific algorithms on this data set are of particular value, as they can be directly compared to the performance of other algorithms similarly applied.

Thus the main contribution of the current paper is to exhaustively evaluate the performance of this stellate lesion detection algorithm on the new mammogram data set. A secondary aim is to present a revision of the spatial integration step which generates the final report of a lesion's existence, one that facilitates the extraction of ROC performance statistics.

1 Introduction

Breast cancer is a leading cause of cancer deaths among women, currently exceeded only by lung cancer. It is a disease that will eventually affect one in nine women in the United States[1]. Early detection is the most effective means of preventing death from breast cancer, and mammographic screening is currently the only effective method of early detection[2]. There has accordingly been a fair amount of investigation into automated image analysis systems designed to make the radiologist's screening efforts more efficient or accurate.

The eventual aim of the current investigation is to allow the computer to operate as a second reader, to draw the attention of the radiologist to suspicious areas she might have missed on her own. Accordingly, here the focus is on detection and general localization of the lesions, and not on their detailed segmentation.

The visual signs for which radiologists search during mammographic screening have been codified into three basic categories[3], each of which have received study in the automated mammographic analysis literature; circumscribed lesions, calcifications, and stellate lesions. Of these, stellate lesions are arguably the most important, due to the fact that most breast carcinomas are first indicated by stellate lesions and that they are so often malignant that there is only one rare case where they do not immediately require biopsy[3]. As stellate lesions are also the most subtle and varied in appearance of the three classes, they are quite difficult to detect. Accordingly, much of the computer analysis of stellate lesions has involved the characterization of a lesion, detected by some other process, as circumscribed or stellate[4, 5, 6]. Algorithms for detection proper have often hinged on asymmetry between the left and right views, with pioneering work on xeromammograms[7] and more recent efforts on film-screen mammograms[8, 9]. This approach has the merit that it can detect more suspicious conditions than just stellate lesions, but it will be challenged by lesions embedded in dense, glandular regions present in both breasts. Thus a single-view stellate lesion method is of value, both on its own and as an integrated complement to multi-view methods.

2 A Review and Criticism Of Previous Work

2.1 *An Algorithm Review*

2.1.1 *A Summary*

In previous work[10] we have reported on a method for the automatic detection of stellate lesions in digitized mammograms. The technique is to extract image features from the neighborhoods of every pixel in the known images, so that each pixel becomes associated with a vector of features. These feature vectors are used to grow a binary decision tree (BDT), and that tree used to label each pixel of a new mammogram with its probability of being located on an abnormality. After each pixel is independently labeled, a crude spatial filtering step is applied to force a local consensus on the presence or absence of a lesion.

The effect, then, as suggested in Figure 1, is to expand each mammogram into a stack of feature images which is then compressed back into a single "probability of suspiciousness" image, with values on $[0, 1]$, by the binary decision tree classifier.

2.1.2 **Analysis of Local Oriented Edges (ALOE)**

The first of the features, ALOE, was designed specifically for the detection of stellate lesions. The basic idea is to key on the architectural distortion induced by a stellate lesion. A normal mammogram has a duct structure which radiates from the nipple to the chest wall. The veins and superposition of parenchyma can complicate this tendency, but the primary effect is of a roughly radial pattern, particularly at low resolution. A stellate lesion changes

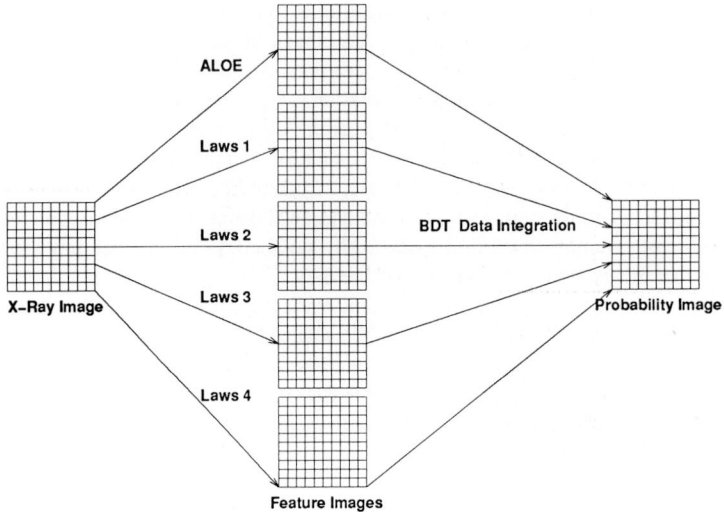

Figure 1: Densities Expanded to Features and Compressed to Probabilities

this pattern, and creates *another* center from which rays radiate; the basic idea is illustrated schematically in Figure 2.

To detect such behavior, one can begin by noting that a primary difference between normal areas and those with stellate lesions is that the suspicious areas will have edges which exist in many different orientations, whereas the normal areas will have edge orientations which are all rather similar. A summary of how ALOE detects this difference is as follows:

- Center a window around each pixel. (See Section 4.1 for comments on the selection of window size and other parameters.)

- Compute edge orientation values in that window.

- Extract a histogram of edge orientations across the window.

- Measure the flatness of the histogram by computing the standard deviation of the bin height.

- The standard deviation is the ALOE feature for that pixel.

In a window on a normal section of a mammogram tissue, most edges will be oriented in the same direction, and so a histogram of those orientations will show a clustered hump. If the window is located on or near a stellate lesion, the edges go in all directions, and so the histogram will be flatter. Both such behaviors are illustrated in Figure 3. Measuring the standard deviation of the height of the histogram bins will thus capture the "stellateness" of the area, and it is this standard deviation which serves as the ALOE feature.

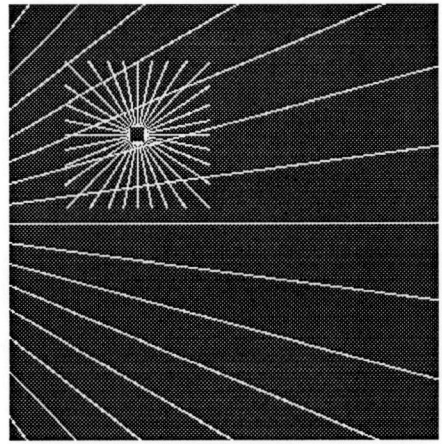

Figure 2: A Schematic Representation of a Stellate Lesion

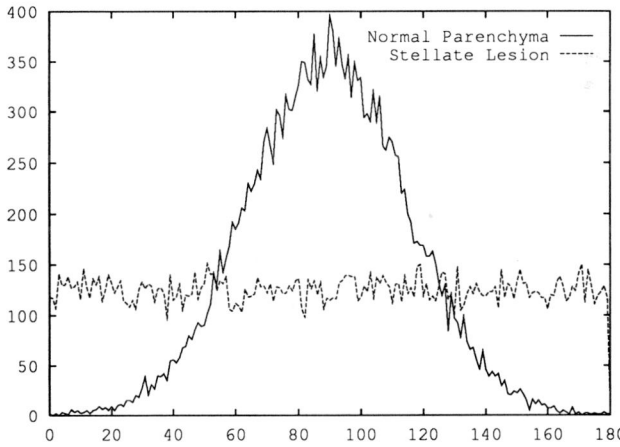

Figure 3: Sample ALOE Histograms, With and Without a Lesion

2.1.3 Laws Texture Features

The ALOE feature was the first developed, and while it proved to be quite sensitive in its detection of stellate lesions, it was not very discriminating, and when acting on its own would generate multiple false alarms per image. To counteract this tendency a feature responsive to normal tissue was desired, one that could be used by the BDT to provide a counterbalance to ALOE's sensitivity, and thus reduce the number of false alarms. The range of possible manifestations of normal tissue is vast, and so it was clear that a general texture measure was desired, one that could represent a wide range of appearances.

Accordingly, attention was turned to the Laws texture energy measures[11]. These texture features are based on the application of a small set of convolution kernels to the image (each kernel designed to respond to a different local behavior), followed by the measurement of various statistics on the convolution images. These kernels and statistics have been refined to the point that the use of four particular convolution kernels, all followed by the computation of the local sum of absolute values[12], has been shown to "work as well, or better, as most other approaches in texture classification problems"[13]. (Interestingly, the Laws texture features have also recently been independently selected for the discrimination of glandular and fatty regions in mammograms[14].)

In the notation of Pietikainen et. al.[12], the convolution kernels which have been shown to be most efficacious and which are used in this study are L5*E5, E5*S5, L5*S5, and R5*R5. The size of the window for the computation of the sum of absolute values texture energy measure was 15 by 15 pixels, as suggested by Laws[11].

2.1.4 Binary Decision Trees (BDTs)

Bayesian hypothesis testing is the optimal way to do pattern recognition from features, but Bayesian approaches require extensive knowledge about the probability distribution functions of the features. This is usually unavailable in practical problems, and is certainly so in the case of mammographic screening. Binary decision tree classification methods, however, provide a formal, rigorous means of approximating the optimal Bayesian classification rule for a given situation[15].

Practical trees for stellate lesion detection can often contain hundreds of nodes. This is not daunting, however, as they are grown automatically from the training data, by recursive reduction of impurity. The control parameters at each node are chosen by determining the feature and threshold which best separates the current data, where the quality of the separation is determined by some impurity measure. This process is repeated, recursively partitioning the remaining training samples, until some stopping criterion is met[16]. This recursive selection of the best possible partition is the source of one of the major advantages of the BDT approach, which is its capacity for automatic feature selection and data reduction.

Another advantage of BDTs is that they have a compact representation and are computationally efficient when used for classification, operating at essentially a constant speed, independent of N, the number of training vectors. This is particularly important in the case of mammographic screening, as a single four-view case can contain 12 million pixels, *each* to be classified through being dropped down the tree.

Probability Images. Our use of BDTs in mammographic screening contains two innovations. One is in nature of the classification. With a traditional BDT, after growing the tree each node is associated with a distinct class (whichever class was most prevalent among the training samples which fell into that node), and each new feature vector is thus assigned the class of the terminal node into which it falls. In the current application, this implies that each pixel would be immediately labeled as definitely suspicious or definitely not. This uniform certainty is unwarranted, however, as the various nodes of the tree can vary in the reliability of their classification. One measure of that reliability, resubstitution error rate, can be computed by dropping the training set back into the tree and noting the number of misclassified features which fall into each node.

Since here we have a two class problem ("normal" and "suspicious"), the resubstitution error rate of a node can be easily converted to the probability that a vector which falls into that node is suspicious. It is this "probability of suspiciousness", independently computed for each pixel, which is the final output of the classifier.

Recomputation of Resubstitution Error Rates Only a random sampling of the training set is used to generate feature vectors for the tree-growing process. One reason for this is that spatial correlation tends to make the feature vectors from adjacent pixels redundant for mapping out the feature space. Another issue is that though BDTs are very computationally efficient when used to classify a vector, they can be as slow as $O(N^2)$ to grow. A BDT, then, must be a compromise between the quality of the tree and the amount of time available to grow it.

This compromise can be mitigated here by recomputing the resubstitution error rates for the tree's nodes based on the *entire* training data set, not just the sampled set used for growing. Though *growing* a tree on all of the pixels is prohibitive, pouring them all through the tree is only an $O(N)$ process, and generates a much more sensitive measure of the probability of suspicion associated with each node.

2.2 The Limitations of the Prior Data Set

The earlier investigation was based on a limited set of test images, only 10 cases of four views each, with a stellate lesion in one view of each case. No entirely normal cases were available, and so the undiseased tissue from the opposing breasts was used to determine the false alarm rate. Further, since the approach here is one of supervised training, half of the data had to be used as a training set, and so there were only six true lesions in the test set. Thus the performance results (a sensitivity of 83% and 0.6 false alarms per image) were necessarily coarse.

2.3 The Limitations of the Prior Spatial Consensus Method

When the BDT classifies a feature vector, and so assigns a probability of being on a lesion to a pixel, it does so without direct reference to the pixel's neighbors. Thus noise and other errors can cause neighboring pixels to occasionally have very different probabilities, in contradiction to the fact that lesion pixels are usually adjacent to lesion pixels, and normal pixels adjacent to normal pixels. Since we are concerned with raw detection here, and not the fine details of lesion segmentation, the noise classifications can be simply addressed by spatial smoothing.

In the original investigation, the approach was to first threshold the probability image at 0.5 (so that pixels more likely than not to be on a lesion would be classified as lesion pixels) and then to use median filtering. This filtering choice was suggested by the fact that the primary noise effect in the thresholded probability image was that of small salt-and-pepper inversions, generally much smaller in scale than the true (and false positive) lesion reports.

Median filtering proved effective but inflexible, primarily because of the large window size required, 25 by 25 pixels. In particular, it is slow enough, even on binary images, to discourage exhaustive examination of the probability of detection (P_D) vs. false alarm rate (FAR) trade-offs permitted by examining thresholds other than the intuitive choice of 0.5.

3 Improved Spatial Consensus on Standard Data

Given those earlier constraints on the extraction of performance statistics, there is value in testing this stellate lesion detection technique on a larger data set, one that will not only provide more lesions but also truly undiseased tissue, and to do so with a revised spatial filtering post-processing step that eases determination of the ROC[17] curve for the technique.

3.1 *The USF Public Data Set*

A new mammogram data set[1] was made publicly available in mid-1992 by the University of South Florida. It contains examples of twelve stellate lesions, as well as fifty examples of entirely normal tissue, spanning a wide range of benign appearances, and so will permit a much more accurate examination of the false positive behavior of this stellate lesion detection technique. Further, as this data set has been made widely available to all researchers involved in the computer analysis of mammograms, performance results of specific algorithms on this data set are of particular value, as they can be directly compared to the performance of other algorithms similarly applied.

3.2 *A New Spatial Consensus Method*

The revision of the spatial filtering method is fairly straightforward, simply a reversal of the order of the thresholding and filtering steps. That is, the floating point probability images are first mean filtered to smooth out discontinuities, and *then* thresholded. This change was first inspired by the realization that precise segmentation of the lesion shape is not necessary for simple detection, and that accordingly the edge-preserving properties of the median filter were overkill for this purpose.

It has the further advantage that arranging the thresholding to be the last step in the processing permits the easy extraction of ROC curve extraction, as the both the P_D and the

---

[1]This data set was provided courtesy of the Center for Engineering and Medical Image Analysis and the H. Lee Moffitt Cancer Center and Research Institute at the University of South Florida. Use anonymous ftp to `figment.csee.usf.edu` for access.

FAR of the final images can be incrementally decreased by increasing the applied threshold, which allows fewer and fewer pixels to survive. By way of example, Figure 4 illustrates the effect of increasing the threshold from 0.2 to 0.8 on the smoothed probability image generated from case 63 of the USF data set.

4 Materials and Methods

4.1 *The Algorithm Parameters*

There are four parameters which control various aspects of this detection system. We describe them here, and discuss the design considerations that led to the values used in this study.

ALOE Window Size: Subsequent investigations have shown that the ALOE feature remains sensitive to small stellate lesions even with a large window size, but that it can miss large stellate lesions and architectural distortions if not sufficiently large. Thus it is best to set the window size to the size of the largest expected lesion; here we choose 4 cm, as any lesion larger than this should certainly be spotted by the screening radiologist. Given the pixel size of the USF data set (see section 4.2), this results in an ALOE window of width 174 pixels and height 189 pixels.

Weeding of the Training Images: As mentioned in Section 2.1.4, only a randomly sampled fraction of each training image is used to grow the tree. This is both because the correlation of adjacent pixels makes use of every feature vector unnecessary, and because our BDT implementation requires simultaneous virtual memory access to every training vector. As a result, 3.5 Mbytes of training data is roughly what our system[2] can support, and this works out to about 5000 samples per training image. The use of the resubstitution error rate renormalization discussed earlier insures that this sampling does not unduly affect the discriminatory ability of the final tree.

BDT Node Size: When growing a binary decision tree, it is necessary to set a stopping condition. Classically the desire is to have pure terminal nodes, affording a crisp classification of whatever feature vectors fall into that node. However, growing the tree out to this point generally runs afoul of the need to keep the node sizes large enough so that the node splitting criteria remain statistically significant.

One innovation of the current approach, however, is that crisp classifications are not necessary. A mixed terminal node is perfectly acceptable, as long as it is populous enough to accurately reflect its resubstitution error rate. So the stopping condition here is to require that each terminal node be no smaller than 100 feature vectors. This may on occasion prevent a further sensible split from occurring, but as segmentation is not as important as detection, this should cause no great difficulty.

Mean Filter Size: From the previous work it was learned that the precise size of the smoothing filter was not important, only that it be some small fraction of the ALOE

---

[2]A SPARC-2 with 64 Mbytes of RAM

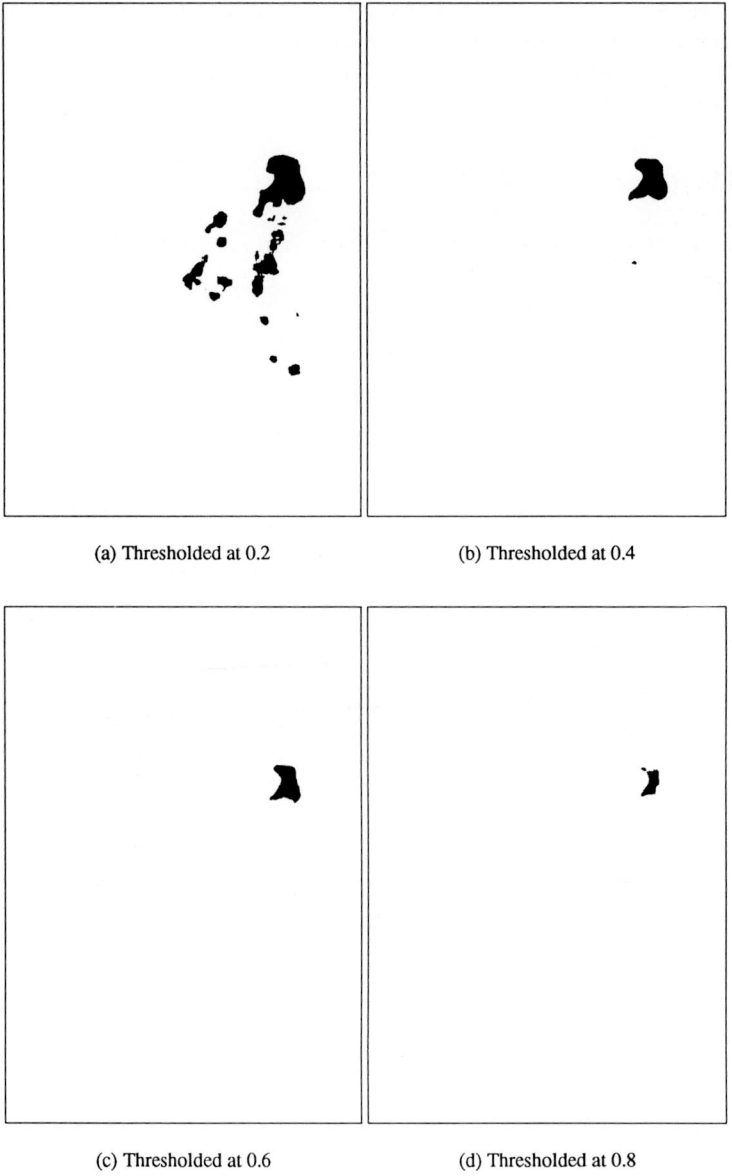

Figure 4: Probability Image For Image 63 at Various Thresholds

window size so as to not smooth over small lesions. Accordingly the window here was set to be 7.5 by 7.5 mm, or 35 by 32 pixels.

4.2 The Data Description

With the algorithm's control parameters described, we now turn to a description of the data to be processed. The USF data set consists of 100 8-bit images with a width of 800 pixels and a height of 1040 pixels, each pixel itself 229 microns in width and 211 microns in height. Each image is a single view from a four-view mammographic screening case, with images 1 through 50 depicting entirely normal tissue and images 51 through 100 depicting various sorts of confirmed malignancies. Table 1 lists the images that were examined in the current study; the "Abnormal" images used were the ones containing at least one stellate lesion.

Table 1: The USF Mammogram Images Used

Normal	Images 1–50
Abnormal	Images 54, 63, 66, 67, 71, 73, 75, 77, 78, 81, 87, 90.

An important characteristic of the USF dataset is that each abnormal image comes with a "truth" image as well, one in which the pixels corresponding to various sorts of abnormalities are flagged. This facilitates both the ready training of the BDT and the eventual scoring of the computer reports.

In order to provide performance results for the *entire* data set, it was randomly separated into two sets, A and B, each with 25 normal and 6 stellate lesion cases; see Table 2. These

Table 2: The Half/Half Separation

Set A	1 2 3 5 8 10 14 15 16 17 18 23 24 26 28 30 31 34 37 42 43 45 46 49 50 54 63 66 71 77 78
Set B	4 6 7 9 11 12 13 19 20 21 22 25 27 29 32 33 35 36 38 39 40 41 44 47 48 67 73 75 81 87 90

data sets were used to conduct a half/half classification test. That is, two separate BDTs were grown from the two separate data sets. Then the tree from set A was used to convert the original images in set B into probability images, and vice versa. Finally, all of these probability images were mean filtered, as discussed above.

4.3 Performance Measurement

To determine the ROC statistics of the smoothed probability images, they were thresholded 100 times, at increments of 0.01, forming binary report images consisting of segmented regions; see again Figure 4 for examples. At each threshold level, each of the 62 report images were compared to their truth images. For the 50 normal images, any report region was counted as a false alarm. For the 12 abnormal images, a report was counted as a correct detection if it overlapped at least 50% of a true lesion, else it was called a false alarm. Any true lesion that was so overlapped was considered have been detected, else missed. The total number of false alarms detected at each threshold level was divided by 62 to generate the rate of false alarms per image, FAR, and the number of correct detections was divided by 12, the total number of lesions, to determine the probability of detection, P_D.

5 Results

The result of primary importance is thus the ROC curve traced out by the changes in FAR and P_D as the threshold varies. Figure 5 presents that curve for both the raw tree and the

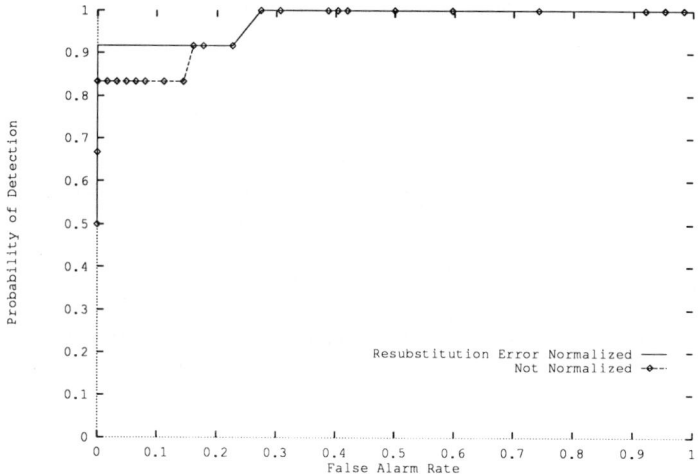

Figure 5: False Alarm Rate for USF Data Set

resubstitution error normalized (REN) tree, and Table 3 lists some of the change points in those curves, along with the thresholds that caused them. Some points to note:

- As expected, the two trees are similar in shape, but the REN tree is more sensitive, and its ROC curve dominates that of the unnormalized tree.

- For both trees, a perfect $P_D = 1.0$ can be achieved at a false alarm rate of 0.27 false alarms per image, or one every 3.7 images. This turns out to be achieved at a threshold of 0.44.

- Similarly, on the REN tree, a perfect FAR= 0 can be achieved with a P_D of 0.92, at a threshold of 0.61.

Table 3: Interesting Points on the ROC Curves

The REN Curve			The Unnormalized Curve		
Threshold	P_D	FAR	Threshold	P_D	FAR
0.01	1.00	13.3	0.01	1.00	13.9
0.44	1.00	0.27	0.44	1.00	0.27
0.45	0.92	0.23	0.45	0.92	0.23
0.50	0.92	0.11	0.47	0.92	0.16
0.61	0.92	0.02	0.48	0.83	0.15
0.62	0.92	0.00	0.61	0.83	0.02
			0.62	0.83	0.00

- At the "intuitive" threshold of 0.5, both curves have a FAR of 0.11, or 1 false alarm in 9 images. The REN tree achieves a P_D of 0.92, and the standard tree a P_D of 0.83.
- The lesion that is lost in both cases when moving from threshold 0.44 to 0.45 is that in image 77, which, upon inspection, is both very small and located at the chest wall, allowing the detectable spiculations to extend in one direction only. The lesion that is lost by the unnormalized tree at threshold 0.48 is that in image 54, which is also small and not highly spiculated, and so both its architectural distortion and its spiculations had only a faint radial impact of the sort to which ALOE is sensitive.

For a more visual rendering of these results, consider Figures 6 through 9, which present two examples, first showing the original image and then a composite image in which the true lesion has been rendered in white and the detection report (generated with a threshold of 0.5) has been indicated by a black border around the detected region.

6 Conclusions

We have demonstrated that this stellate lesion detection works quite well on a standard data set, presenting both objective and visual performance results. In particular, the technique can achieve either perfect detection with a false alarm rate of 0.27, or zero false alarms with a probability of detection of 0.92. These values come from a ROC curve description of the performance results, the determination of which was facilitated by a revision of the spatial integration method previously reported.

Further, as this data set is publicly available and as we have endeavored to be detailed in the description of our study, it is hoped that we have enabled the direct comparison of this technique to others addressing the same problem.

7 Acknowledgments

This research was supported by the United States Department of Energy, Sandia National Laboratories, California. This paper is an expanded treatment of material that was first

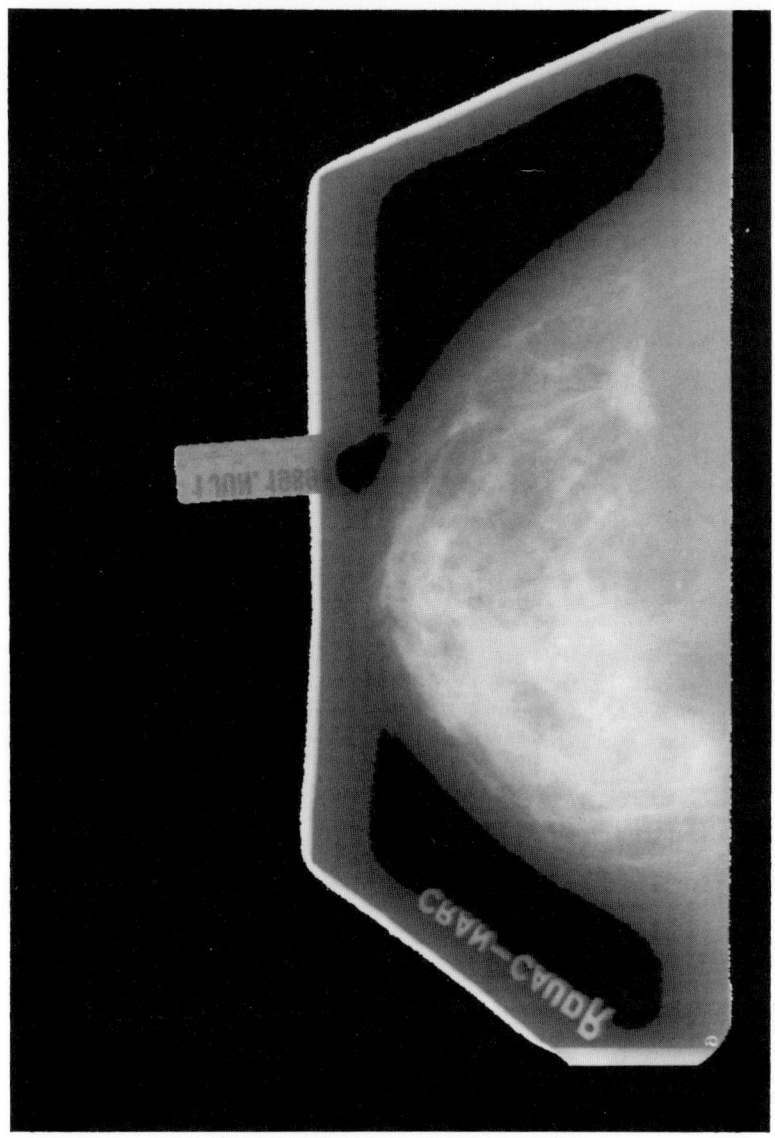

Figure 6: Original Image 63

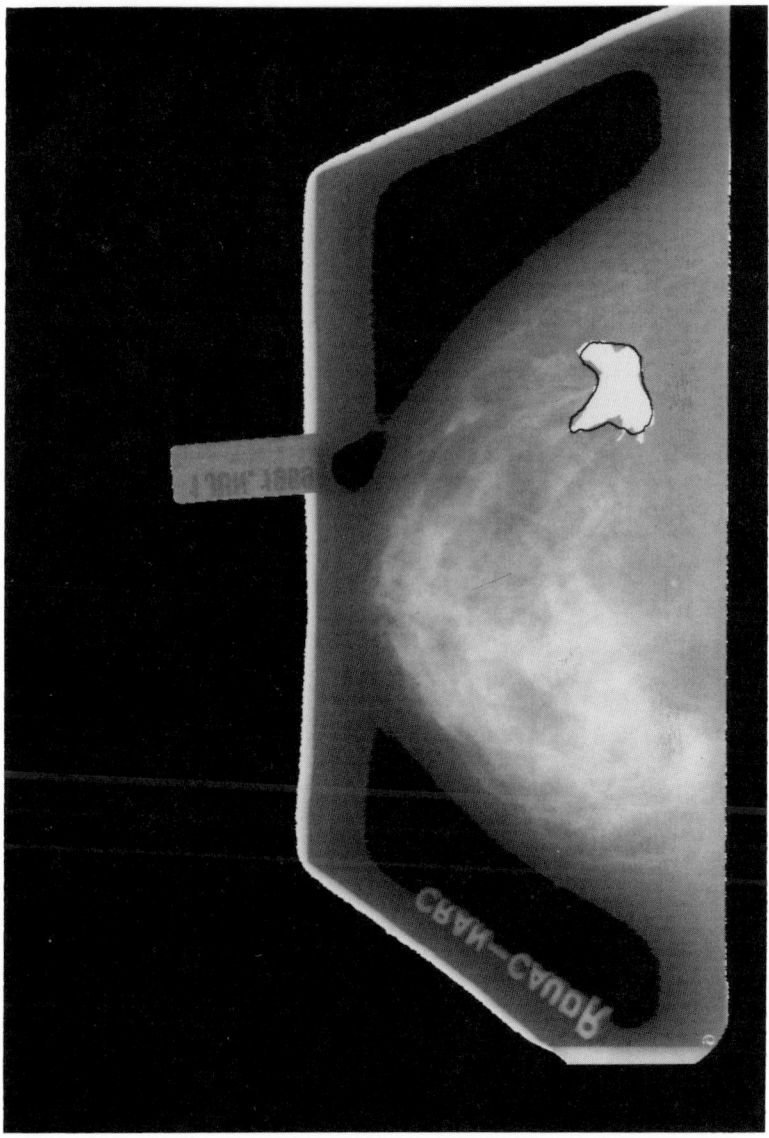

Figure 7: Truth (White) And Detection Output (Black) For Image 63

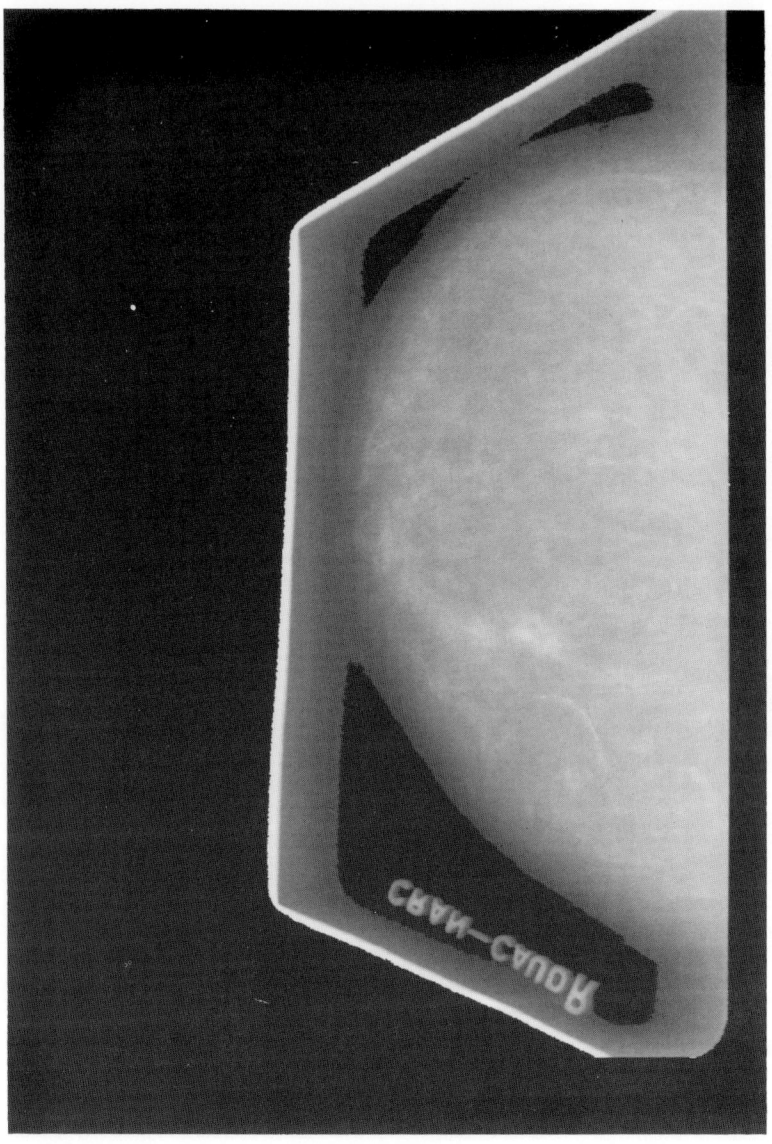

Figure 8: Original Image 71

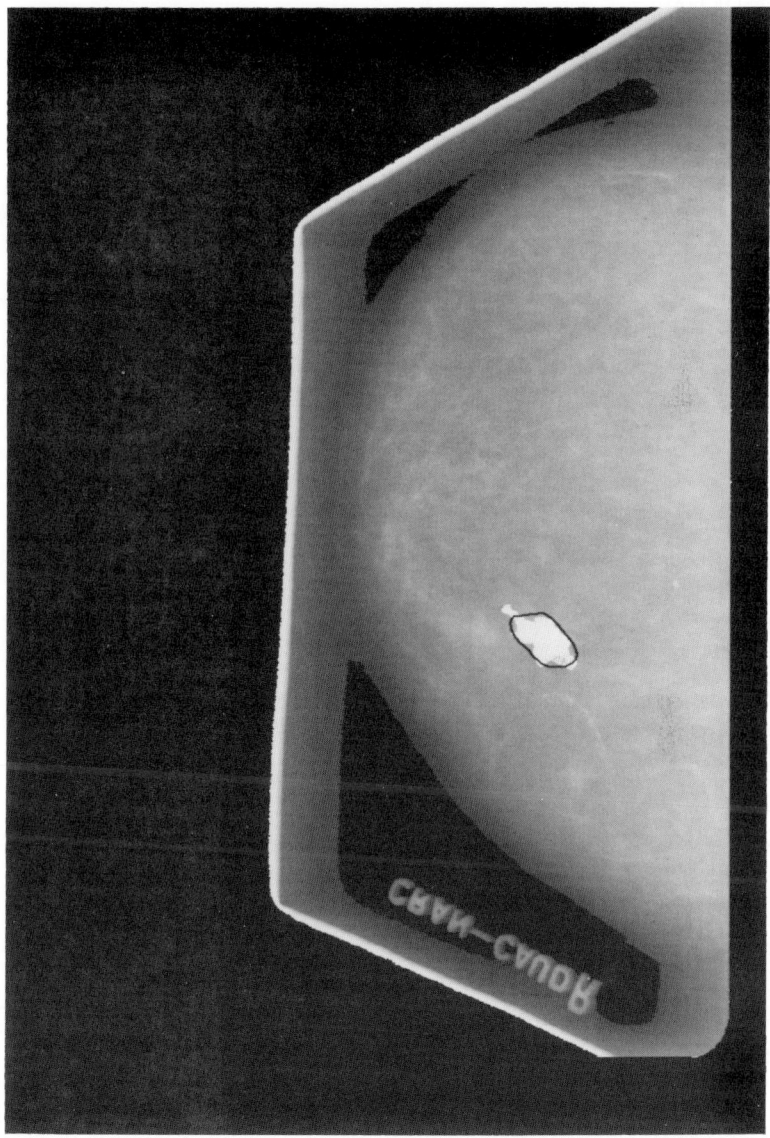

Figure 9: Truth (White) And Detection Output (Black) For Image 71

presented in [18].

References

[1] Cancer facts & figures. Technical report, American Cancer Society, 1991.

[2] H.C. Zuckerman. The role of mammography in the diagnosis of breast cancer. In Irving M. Ariel and Joseph B. Cleary, editors, *Breast Cancer, Diagnosis & Treatement*, chapter 12, pages 152–172. McGraw-Hill, New York, 1987.

[3] Laszlo Taber and Peter B. Dean. *Teaching Atlas of Mammography*. Georg Thieme Verlag, Thieme Inc., Stuttgart, New York, 2nd revised edition, 1985.

[4] Laurens V. Ackerman and Earl E. Gose. Breast lesion classification by computer and xeroradiograph. *Cancer*, 30:1025–1035, 1972.

[5] D. Brzakovic, X.M. Luo, and P. Brzakovic. An approach to automated detection of tumors in mammograms. *IEEE Transactions on Medical Imaging*, 9(3):233–241, September 1990.

[6] Maryellen L. Giger, Fang-Fang Yin, Kunio Doi, Charles E. Metz, Robert A. Schmidt, and Carl J. Vyborny. Investigation of methods for computerized detection and analysis of mammographic masses. In *Proceedings of the SPIE Conference on Medical Imaging IV: Image Processing*, volume 1233, pages 183–184. SPIE, 1990.

[7] Caroyln Kimme, Bernard J. O'Loughin, and Jack Sklansky. Automatic detection of suspicous abnormalities in breast radiographs. In *Proceedings of the Conference on Computer Graphics, Pattern Recognition, and Data Structures*, pages 84–88. IEEE, May 1975.

[8] Tin-Kit Lau and Walter F. Bishof. Automated detection of breast tumors using the asymmetry approach. *Computers and Biomedical Research*, 24:273–295, 1991.

[9] Susan M. Astley and Chistopher J. Taylor. Combining cues for mammographic abnormalities. In *Proceedings of the British Machine Vision Conference 1990*, pages 253–258, 1990.

[10] W. Philip Kegelmeyer, Jr. Computer detection of stellate lesions in mammograms. In *Proc. of the 1992 SPIE Conference on Biomedical Image Processing and 3-D Microscopy*, volume 1660, pages 446–454, February 1992.

[11] K. I. Laws. *Textured Image Segmentation*. PhD thesis, University of Southern California, 1980.

[12] Matti Pietikainen, Azriel Rosenfeld, and Larry S. Davis. Texture classification using averages of local pattern matches. In *Proceedings of the Conference on Computer Vision and Pattern Recognition*, pages 301–303. IEEE, 1982.

[13] J.Y. Hsiao and A.A. Sawchuck. Supervised texture image segmentation using feature smoothing and probablistic relaxation techniques. *IEEE Transactions on Pattern Analysis and Machine Intelligence*, 11(12):1279–1292, December 1989.

[14] Peter Miller and Sue Astley. Classification of breast tissue by texture analysis. *Image and Vision Computing*, 10(5):277–282, June 1992.

[15] Leo Breiman, Jerome H. Friedman, Richard A. Olshen, and Charles J. Stone. *Classification and Regression Trees*. Wadsworth International Group, Belmont, California, 1984.

[16] Saul B. Gelfand, C.S. Ravishankar, and Edward J. Delp. An iterative growing and pruning algorithm for classification tree design. *IEEE Transactions on Pattern Analysis and Machine Intelligence*, 13(2):163–174, February 1991.

[17] Charles E. Metz, Stuart J. Starr, and Lee B. Lusted. Quantitative evaluation of visual detection performance in medicine: ROC analysis and determination of diagnostic benefit. In *Proceedings of the 7th L.H. Gray Conference — Medical Images: Formation, Perception and Measurement*. The Institute of Physics, April 1976.

[18] W. Philip Kegelmeyer, Jr. Evaluation of stellate lesion detection in a standard mammogram data set. In *Proc. of the 1993 SPIE/SPSE Conference on Biomedical Image Processing IV and Biomedical Visualization*, volume 1905-78, February 1993.

Image Processing and Computer Aided Diagnosis in Digital Mammography: A Radiologist's Perspective

by

Etta D. Pisano, M.D.[1]
Chief, Breast Imaging
Assistant Professor of Radiology
University of North Carolina at Chapel Hill

and

Faina Shtern, M.D.
Chief, Diagnostic Imaging Research Branch
Radiation Research Program
National Cancer Institute

1 Introduction

Screening mammography has proven to be an effective test in identifying early breast cancer. Large randomized trials have demonstrated that breast cancer mortality among screened women over 50 years old can be reduced up to 30% when compared with unscreened controls [1] - [3]. The cancers found by mammography tend to be smaller and of less advanced stages than those found by breast physical examination or breast self-examination [4] - [6]. Smaller and lower stage breast cancers tend to have better survival rates over time [7] - [10].

Unfortunately, approximately 10% of clinically obvious breast cancers are not visible with mammography [4]. This occurs most frequently in patients with large amounts of breast glandular tissue [4], [11]. The density of this tissue tends to obscure underlying pathology. Premenopausal women and women undergoing estrogen replacement therapy are more likely to have dense glandular breasts. This may partially explain why some randomized trials of mammography have failed to demonstrate a significant reduction in breast cancer mortality for women under 50 years old [12]. Furthermore, tumor doubling times may be shorter in younger women. With current technology, for women under 50, the average interval between mammographically apparent disease and clinically apparent disease averages only 1.5 to 2 years. For women over 50, this interval averages 3.5 to 4 years [13]. The American College of Radiology (ACR) and the American Cancer Society (ACS), among other organizations,

---

[1] Communications regarding this manuscript should be sent to Dr. E. Pisano

currently advocate screening mammography for women between 40 and 49 years old every one to two years. It is desirable to increase the sensitivity of mammography in these patients so that their cancers are apparent earlier. This earlier detection may result in significantly reduced mortality in this population. In the United States, 24% of breast cancers occur in women under 50 years of age and 24% of deaths from breast cancer occur in women whose diagnoses were made before age 50. This means that 41% of the years of life lost occur in this age group [14].

Another major issue raised by the advent of widely available screening mammography is the frequency of false positive interpretations. In fact, among nonpalpable lesions that are submitted to needle localization and open surgical biopsy, only 10-30% prove to be malignant [1], [15]-[21]. The biopsy yield is higher with very little sacrifice in sensitivity in centers in which six month follow-up mammography is judiciously used in place of biopsy for the majority of probably benign lesions [22]. Generally speaking, the medical morbidity from open biopsies and needle aspirations is minimal [23]. The psychological costs to the patients have not been well explored [24]. The monetary costs are quite high with approximately 32% of the total cost of screening is caused by open biopsy for benign disease [25]. According to Eddy, if screening is performed on women under 50 years old, the total dollars spent for work-up for false positive mammograms in this age group alone will amount to $40,654,00 in 1984 dollars, in the year 2000 [26]. Clearly, this expenditure is a significant drain on a burdened health care system. If a less expensive or more specific technique were available, a large sum of money might be saved.

Mammographic technology has improved dramatically in the last two decades. These improvements include the development of dedicated mammography equipment with appropriate x-ray beam quality, grid capability, adequate breast compression and automatic exposure control. In addition, magnification techniques with very small focal spot size have become widely available. Better film-screen systems and appropriate film processing have also been developed to improve image contrast [27], [28]. Over the same time period, the average glandular radiation dose from mammography has dropped, generally because of the development of faster film-screen combinations [29].

The advent of digitally acquired mammograms offers the possibility of further improvements in early breast cancer detection [30]. Specifically, digital acquisition systems decouple the process of x-ray photon detection from image display by using a primary detector that directly quantifies transmitted photons. This allows digital systems to be more efficient in utilization of radiation dose. Digital systems also allow a wide dynamic range so that a wider range of tissue contrast can be appreciated. Subtle contrast differences can be amplified and the distinction between benign and malignant might be increased. Furthermore, digital systems have the capacity to bring revolutionary advantages to breast cancer detection and management: 1) image processing for increased lesion conspicuity; 2) computer-aided diagnosis for enhanced radiologic interpretation; 3) teleradiology, or image transmission, as a means of bringing world-class expertise to community hospitals and remote areas; 4) improved image access and communication through digital image archiving and transmission; and 5) dynamic, or "real-time" imaging for use during biopsy and localization procedures.

This paper will focus on the current and future clinical utility of image processing and computer-aided diagnosis in breast lesion detection and characterization.

2 Greyscale Image Processing: Summary of Previous Work

Relatively few investigators have directed their attention to manipulation of the contrast and greyscale assignment in the digital environment as applied to mammography. Those researchers who have done so have concentrated mostly on the detection of microcalcifications. McSweeny used an analog technique which improved the image by enhancing small object contrast and edges, but clinical results were not reported [31]. Smathers applied a combination of high and low-band pass filters to digitized images of a breast phantoms and found that they could detect smaller sized specks than with unprocessed images [32]. Chan used matched spatial filtered digitized images combined with signal suppressed (contrast-reversed) images for the purpose of developing computerized detection of microcalcification clusters [33]. His group also did an ROC study to determine the effect of pixel size and unsharp-mask filtering on the detection of subtle microcalcifications. They concluded that processing digital images by unsharp-masking appeared to improve radiologist performance in detection of microcalcifications and that digital systems with lower spatial resolution than that of conventional mammograms might be successful if image processing techniques were applied. They also pointed out that if observers were trained to make diagnoses from processed mammograms and image processing techniques were optimized, even greater improvements might occur [34].

Another study was conducted by Chang where contrast limited adaptive histogram equalization (CLAHE) was applied to digitized mammograms and reprinted on film at array sizes of 2k × 2k, 1k × 1k, and 512 × 512. The ROC analysis showed no statistically significant difference between the original films and the enhanced images at lesser array sizes [35]. This study was criticized because of the small number of cases and insufficient spread of difficulty in detection task. Nevertheless, the study suggests that image enhancement can compensate to some extent for spatial resolution.

Oestmann did a comparison of digitized storage phosphors and conventional mammography in the detection of microcalcifications where a mammography phantom was imaged. The digital images (digitized at 0.1mm × 0.1mm) were presented on film with no enhancement techniques applied. ROC analysis showed equivalence between conventional mammography and the digital system. They also commented that for morphologic analysis of microcalcifications, a higher resolution would be required [36]. Higashida et al. compared the ability of radiologists to detect calcifications using either digitized storage phosphors with unsharp-mask filtering or using standard film-screen mammography. With nine observers and ROC analysis, they concluded that the detectability of subtle microcalcifications was better using the film-screen systems, probably because of the resolution restrictions of the storage phosphors [37]. The consensus from the literature is that detection of microcalcifications requires digitization of at least 100μ pixels and probably 50μ. Image processing appears to improve detection, but it can also increase false positives.

Few authors have addressed what some clinicians believe to be the more exciting issue, that is, how an optimized greyscale assignment might aid in the detection of structural abnormalities such as spiculation and architectural distortion. These mammographic features, in particular, are more frequently pathognomonic of malignancy [38]. Image processing techniques might be useful in optimizing display of these types of structures. Geiger has shown success in quantifying the degree of spiculation in digital mammographic images [39]. Odagiri states that application of edge enhancement and contrast adjustment to digital mammograms showed them to be superior in demonstrating vascular and glandular structures, especially in dense breasts [40]. Yamada reports no significant differences in tumor detection rates for spiculations and calcifications between computed radiographic (CR) and conventional non-screen methods. However, they point out that recognition of the calcifications was "extremely good" because of image processing [41]. Kimme-Smith compared standard display Fuji Computer Radiology (FCR) digital mammograms to those that were processed with a form of enhancement based on the image histogram. While normal mammograms were considered equal by either system, pathology was better perceived when the image was processed in this fashion. They conclude that "for specific types of mammograms, and with carefully designated enhancement procedures, digitized and enhanced images are an acceptable adjunct to conventional mammograms" [42].

3 Computer-Aided Diagnosis: Summary of Previous Work

There have been many attempts over the years to evaluate mammograms using a computer [43] - [50]. The early work in this area was limited in its diagnostic accuracy. Because of recent advances in the technology of film-screen mammography and image digitization, [28, 51] as well as improvements in computer vision [52], more recent studies have demonstrated better results.

As mentioned earlier, Chan developed a method for automatic detection of clustered microcalcifications [33, 53, 54]. Using 60 subtle calcification cases, this technique yielded a sensitivity of 87% with 4 false positives per image. Nishikawa has subsequently improved upon this technique and has reduced the false positive rate [55]. Other laboratories have also had some success with computer-aided microcalcification detection [56] - [59]. In addition, several groups have developed CAD methods for the detection of masses in mammography [60] - [64].

Another approach that has shown some promise is the **ex**traction of features by a human or computer observer in the evaluation of mammographic abnormalities, both masses and calcifications [64] - [67]. The types of features that have been extracted for mass discrimination by the various programs include degree of spiculation, edge distance variation, edge intensity variation, shape and area. For calcification discrimination, shape, center of gravity, breadth, length, orientation, area, perimeter, and convex parameters have been utilized. Human observers have extracted similar feature information in other studies with encouraging improvement in diagnostic accuracy with discriminant analysis to classify lesions [68] - [70], but such techniques are extremely time consuming and expensive.

Most of the studies included in this volume extend upon this work for masses and calcifications with some of the authors broadening the scope of CAD research to include the computer detection of spiculation (or architectural distortion) and asymmetric densities.

4 Greyscale Image Processing and Computer-Aided Diagnosis: Future Work

There should be two major goals in the development of digital mammography: 1) to increase the sensitivity of breast cancer screening in women with dense breasts and, 2) to increase the specificity of breast cancer screening so as to further reduce the number of unnecessary needle and open biopsies. Achieving these goals will require close cooperation between computer scientists, engineers and radiologists who specialize in breast imaging.

The problem of how to determine what is the optimal type of image processing or CAD algorithm for the display or interpretation of a clinical image is a substantial one. There are many available algorithms, each with a number of parameters that can be varied. We do not want to sacrifice specificity for improved sensitivity, and vice versa. Furthermore, the optimal algorithm for increased detection of calcifications will probably differ from the algorithms that yield increased detection of masses, which will probably differ from the algorithms that yield increased detection of spiculations or areas of architectural distortion.

It is therefore important that scientists studying this field follow some general principles in arriving at results that are clinically useful. The prime requirement is of course understanding the clinical problems involved. In most instances this will mean working closely with a radiologist specializing in breast imaging. All algorithms should be tested on real clinical images before they are applied to real patients prospectively. The clinical material to be used should be existent digitized or digital images of pathologically proven cases of benign and malignant lesions, along with known normal mammograms. For the purposes of this type of research, a mammogram should be considered to be a true normal only after at least one year of absence of evidence for malignancy by mammography and physical examination. Three years of normal follow-up would be even better. Images of only the highest quality should be utilized. This will involve discarding clinical images that display poor mammographic positioning, contrast or density, or excessive blur or artifacts. When digitization is used, it should be performed at the best contrast and spatial resolution possible.

Furthermore, impeccable observer studies must be performed before any algorithm should be embraced by the radiologists practicing clinical mammography. This will require radiologist observers who have undergone training in how to interpret images that do not resemble standard film-screen images. Training sets must be developed to accomplish this goal. Both the test and training sets should be constructed to allow for optimal evaluation of both the sensitivity and specificity of the algorithm being evaluated, that is, ROC analysis. This requires not only a range of pathologic abnormalities but a range of difficulty in the detection task. The observer studies must be carefully constructed so that the interpretation task closely mimics that which occurs in the clinical setting with an emphasis on limiting distractions and interruptions. The standard and non-standard presentation must be counterbalanced so as to limit the effects of learning and fatigue on study outcome.

Finally, there must be a sufficient number of observers and observations to assure that the study is powerful enough to find even a small improvement in sensitivity or specificity (e.g. between 5 and 10%). Note the emphasis on the importance of small improvements here. Since breast cancer is a common disease, a small increase in sensitivity might translate into many lives saved. Likewise, given the frequency of breast biopsy for benign diagnoses, a small increase in specificity could save a substantial amount of patient anxiety and money.

Obviously, these types of observer studies cannot be undertaken lightly. The expenditure of time and money required to do the "right" type of research is substantial. Therefore, some cheaper, quicker screening technique to sort through the various algorithms and their associated parameters is required. This might involve the use of phantom images or computer generated test images with an array of unknown hidden test objects. Both types of screening tasks are currently being developed and tested at the University of North Carolina-Chapel Hill [71]. Ideally, since the visual system is the same across all normal observers, the initial selection of potentially useful algorithms and parameters might be performed by non-radiologists.

Furthermore, and finally, we must remember to consider potentially useful algorithms as adjuncts to the "unprocessed" or standard film-screen image display. It is possible at least that these techniques will help us produce the lowest number of false positives only in conjunction with the current or relatively unprocessed method of display. We should begin to consider image processing and CAD as routine components of mammographic examination, similar to the way we use intensity windowing in computed tomography. We would not want to discard either our soft tissue or our bone windows. Both give useful information about different types of structures. Similarly, it is likely that we will eventually find it useful to view mammograms in several ways to bring out different types of features. If this is to occur in a user-friendly manner and with the rapid through-put required by a high volume screening program, it is evident that film display is not suitable. Therefore, the development of a workstation that allows for optimal breast cancer screening with multiple different display parameters should be a high priority.

5 Conclusion:

The development of digital mammography holds forth the possibility of tremendous improvement in the early diagnosis of breast cancer. We scientists and radiologists must work closely together for the optimal utilization of this new modality. With proper clinical scrutiny of the algorithms available to us, we may be able to improve both the sensitivity and specificity of our evaluation of the breast for cancer.

While digital mammography has generated considerable enthusiasm in the academic community, a note of caution should be introduced. The ultimate goal of digital mammography is to surpass diagnostic capabilities currently offered by conventional mammography, and the ultimate test of digital systems will be the improvement in the outcome of breast cancer patients. Perhaps the most frequent concern raised in connection with digital mammography is the potential cost of the proposed technology development, evaluation and implementation versus the gain in patient benefit compared to conventional film-screen systems. It is rather difficult to speculate about the cost-benefit ration and the cost-effectiveness of digital technology. However, the current body of evidence suggests that potential benefits of digital mammography will outweigh potential problems, and it has been predicted that image processing and computer-aided diagnosis may play an important part in improved breast cancer detection and management.

References

[1] Shapiro S., Venet W., Strax P., Venet L., Roeser R.: *Ten to fourteen year effect of screening on breast cancer mortality*, JNCI 69, 349-355, 1982.

[2] Tabar L., Fagerberg G., Duffy S.W., Day N.E.: *The Swedish two county trial of mammographic screening for breast cancer: recent results and calculation of benefit*, J Epid Com Health 43, 107-114, 1989.

[3] Shapiro, S., Venet W., Strax P., Venet L. (eds.): *Periodic screening for breast cancer*, Baltimore, Johns Hopkins Press, 1988.

[4] Baker L.H.: *Breast cancer detection demonstration project: five-year summary report*, CA 32(4), 194-225, 1982.

[5] Saltzstein S.L.: *Potential limits of physical examination and breast self-examination in detecting small cancers of the breast: an unselected population-based study of 1302 cases*, Cancer 54, 1443, 1984.

[6] Fletcher S.W., O'Malley M.S., Bunce L.A.: *Physicians abilities to detect lumps in silicone breast models*, JAMA 251, 1580, 1984.

[7] Fisher B., et al.: *Cancer of the breast: size of neoplasm and prognosis*, Cancer 24, 1071, 1969.

[8] Wanebo H.J., Huvos A.G., Urban J.A.: *Treatment of minimal breast cancer*, Cancer 33:349, 1974.

[9] Gallager H.S., Martin J.E.: *An orientation to the concept of minimal breast cancer*, Cancer 28:1505, 1971.

[10] Frazier T.G., Copeland E.M., Gallager H.S. et. al., *Prognosis and treatment in minimal breast cancer*, Am. J. Surg 133, 697, 1977.

[11] Stomper P.C., Gelman R.S.: *Mammography in symptomatic and asymptomatic patients*, Hem/Onc Clinics NA, 3(4), 611-640, 1989.

[12] Shapiro S., Venet W., Strax P., Venet L.: *Current results of the breast cancer screening randomized trial: the health insurance plan (HIP) of greater New York study*, presented at **UICC workshop on Evaluation of Screening for Breast Cancer**, Helsinki, Finland, April 5-7, 1986.

[13] Moskowitz M.: *Breast cancer: Age-specific growth rates and screening strategies*, Radiology 161, 37-41, 1986.

[14] Smart C.: *The role of mammography in the prevention of mortality from breast cancer*, Cancer Prev., 1-16, June 1990.

[15] Feig S.A.: *Decreased breast cancer mortality through mammographic screening: results of clinical trials*, Radiology 1988, 167:659-665.

[16] Shapiro S.: *Evidence of screening for breast cancer from a randomized trial*, Cancer 1977, 39:2772-2782.

[17] Schwartz G., Feig S., Patchefsky A.: *Significance and staging of nonpalpable carcinoma of the breast*, Surg Gynecol Obstet, 1988, 166:6-10.

[18] Skinner M., Swain M., Simmon R., et. al.: *Nonpalpable breast lesion at biopsy*, Ann Sug. 1988, 208:203-208.

[19] Landerscaper J., Gundersen S., Gunderson A., et al.: *Needle localization and biopsy of nonpalpable lesions of the breast*, Surg Gynecol Obstet, 1982, 164:399-403.

[20] Wright C.: *Breast cancer screening*, Surgery, 1986, 100(4):594-598.

[21] U.S. Preventative Services Task Force: *Guide to clinical preventive services: an assessment of the effectiveness of 169 interventions*, (Baltimore, Md: Williams & Wilkins), Chapter 6, pp. 39-62, 1989.

[22] Sickles E.: *Periodic mammographic follow-up of probably benign lesions: results in 3,184 consecutive cases*, Radiology, 1991; 179(2):463-8.

[23] Helvie M.A., Ikeda D.M., Adler D.D.: *Localization and needle aspiration of breast lesions: complications in 370 cases*, AJR, 1991, 157:711-714.

[24] Hirst P., Whitehead D: *A minor surgical procedure?*, Nursing Times, Sept. 12, 1984;45-46.

[25] Cyrlak D.: *Induced costs of low-cost screening mammography*, Radiology, 1988; 168:661-663.

[26] Eddy D.M., Hasselblad V., McGwney W., Hendee W.R.: *The value of mammography screening in women under age 50 years*, JAMA, 1988; 259:1512-1519.

[27] Kimme-Smith C., Bassett L.W., Gold R.H., Zheutlin J., Grombein J.A.: *New mammography screen/film combinations: imaging characteristics and radiation dose*, AJR 154, 713-719, 1990.

[28] Haus A.G.: *Technologic improvements in screen-film mammography*, Radiology 174(3), 628-637, 1990.

[29] Feig S.A., Ehrlich S.M.: *Estimation of radiation risk from screening mammography: recent trends and comparison with expected benefits*, Radiology 174, 638-647, 1990.

[30] Shtern, F.: *Digital mammography and related technologies: a perspective from the National Cancer Institute*, Radiology 1992, 183:629-630.

[31] McSweeney M.B., Sprawls P., Egan R.L.: *Enhanced image mammography*, AJR 140:9-14, 1983.

[32] Smathers R.L., Bush E., Drace J., Stevens M., Somer F.G., Brown W.B., Karras B.: *Mammographic microcalcifications: detection with xerography, screen-film, and digitized film display*, Radiology, 159, 673-677, 1986.

[33] Chan H.P., Doi K., Galhorta S., Vyborny C.J., MacMahon H., Jokich P.M.: *Image feature analysis and computer-aided diagnosis in digital radiography: I. automated detection of microcalcifications in mammography*, Med Phys, 14(4), 538-547, 1987.

[34] Chan H.P., Vyborny C.J., MacMahon H., Metz C.E., Doi K., Sickles E.A.: *Digital mammography ROC studies of the effects of pixel size and unsharp-mask filtering on the detection of subtle microcalcifications*, Investigative Radiology 22:581-589, 1987.

[35] Chang J.C.H., Martin N.L., Dwyer III S.J.,et. al.: *An adaptive histogram for contrast enhancement of digitized mammographic films:an initial study*, unpublished manuscript, 1987.

[36] Oestmann J.W., Kopans D., Hall D.A., McCarthy K.A., Rubens J.R., Green R.: *A comparison of digitized storage phosphors and conventional mammography in the detection of malignant microcalcifications*, Investigative Radiology, 23:725-728, 1988.

[37] Higashida Y., Maube N., Morita K., Katsuda N., Hatemura M., Takada T., Takayashi M., Yamashita J.: *Detection of subtle microcalcifications: comparison of computed radiography and screen film mammography*, Radiology 1992, 183:483-486.

[38] Moskowitz M.: *The predictive value of certain mammographic signs in screening for breast cancer*, Cancer 51, 1007-1011, 1983.

[39] Geiger M.L., Doi H.K., Yin F., Schmidt R.A., Vyborny C.J.: *Computerized classification of mass lesions in digital mammograms: lesion spiculation in analysis of malignancy*, Radiology 173(P), 394, 1989.

[40] Odagiri K., Ohkoshi T., Andoh K., Asaga T., Ohyasu S., Matsuura H.: *Mammography with a computer radiography system*, Radiology 173(P), 461, 1989.

[41] Yamada T., Murasmatsu Y.: *Computed radiography for breast cancer*, Jpn J. Clin Oncol, 20(2), 164-167, 1990.

[42] Kimme-Smith C., Bassett L.W., Gold R. H., Garmley L.: *Digital mammography: a comparison of two digitization methods*, Investigative Radiology 24, 869-875, 1989.

[43] Kimme C., O'Loughlin B.J., Sklansky J.: *Automatic detection of suspicious abnormalities in breast radiographs*, In: **Data Structures, Computer Graphics, and Pattern Recognition**, edited by A. K. Linger, K.S. Fu, T. L. Kunii, Academic Press, New York, 427-447, 1975.

[44] Ackerman L.V., Gose E.E.: *Breast lesion classification by computer and xeroradiography*, Cancer 30:1025-1035, 1972.

[45] Spiesberger W.: *Mammogram inspection by computer*, IEEE Trans Biomed Eng, 26:213-219, 1979.

[46] Fox S.H., Pujare U.M., Wee W.G., Moskowitz M., Hutter R.V.P.: *A computer analysis of mammographic microcalcifications: global approach*, **Proc. IEEE 5th International Conf. on Pattern Recognition**, 624-631, 1980.

[47] Semmlow J.L., Shadagoppan A., Ackerman L.V., Hand W., Alcorn F.S.: *A fully automated system for screening xeromammograms*, Computer Biod Res, 13:350-362, 1980.

[48] Hand W., Semmlow J.L., Ackerman L.V., Alcorn F.S.: *Computer Screening of xeromammograms: A technique for defining suspicious areas of the breast*, Computers Biomed Res, 12:445-460, 1979.

[49] Ackerman L.V., Mucciardi A.N., Gose E.E., Alcorn F.S.: *Classification of benign and malignant breast tumors on the basis of 36 radiographic properties*, Cancer 31:342-352, 1973.

[50] Wee W.G., Moskowitz M., Chang N-C, Ting Y-C, Pemmeraju S.: *Evaluation of mammographic calcifications using a computer program*, Radiology 116:717-720, 1975.

[51] Cook L.T., Giger M.L., Batnitzky S., Wetzel L. H., Murphy M.D.: *Digitized film radiography*, Investigative Radiology, 24:910-916, 1989.

[52] Jain A.K.: *Fundamentals of digital image processing*, Prentice Hall, Englewood Cliffs, NJ, 1989.

[53] Chan H.P., Doi K., Vyborny C. J., Lam K.L., Schmidt R.A.: *Computer-aided detection of microcalcifications in mammograms: methodology and preliminary clinical study*, Investigative Radiology 23:664-671, 1988.

[54] Chan H.P., Doi K., Vyborny C.J., Schmidt R.A., Metz C.D., Lam K.L., Ogura T., Wu Y., MacMahon H.: *Improvement in radiologists' detection of clustered microcalcifications on mammograms: the potential of computer-aided diagnosis*, Investigative Radiology 25:1102-1110, 1990.

[55] Nishikawa R.M., Giger M.L., Doi K., Vyborny C.JK., Schmidt R.A.: *Computer-aided detection of microcalcifications in digital mammograms*, Image Technology and Information Display, 23:1092-1096, 1991.

[56] Fam B.W., Olson S.L., Winter P.F., Scholz F.J.: *Algorithm for the detection of fine clustered calcifications on film mammograms*, Radiology 169:333-337, 1988.

[57] Davies D.H., Dance D.R.: *Automatic computer detection of clustered calcification in digital mammograms*, Phys Med Biol, 35:1111-1118, 1990.

[58] Astley S.M.,Taylor C.J.: *Combining cues for mammographic abnormalities*, **Proc. 1st British Machine Vision Conference**, September, 1990.

[59] Karssemeijer N.: *A stochastic method for automated detection of microcalcifications in digital mammograms*, Information Processing in Medical Imaging, Springer-Verlag, New York, 1991, 227-238.

[60] Yin F-F., Giger M.L., Doi K., Metz C.E., Vyborny C.J., Schmidt R.A.: *Computerized detection of masses in digital mammograms: analysis of bilateral-subtraction images*, Med Phys, 18:955-963, 1991.

[61] Yin F-F, Giger M.L., Metz C.E., Doi K., Vyborny C. J., Shmidt R.A.: *Computerized detection of masses in digital mammograms: investigation of feature-extraction techniques*, Med Phys, 1992.

[62] Glatt A., Longbotham H., Arnow T., Shelton D., Ravdin P.: *An application of weighted majority minimum range filters in the detection and sizing of tumors in mammograms*, **Proc. SPIE**, 1652, 1992.

[63] Lai S.M., Li X., Bischof W.F.: *On techniques for detecting circumscribed masses in mammograms*, **IEEE Trans on Med Imaging**, 8:377-386, 1989.

[64] Brzakovic D., Luo X.M., Brzakovic P.: *An approach to automated detection of tumors in mammograms*, **IEEE Trans. on Med Imaging**, 9:233-241, 1990.

[65] Giger M.L., Yin F-F, Doi K., Metz C.E., Schmidt R.A., Vyborny C.J.: *Investigation of methods for the computerized detection and analysis of mammographic masses*, **Proc. SPIE**, 1233:183-184, 1990.

[66] Patrick E.A., Moskowitz M., Mansukhani V.T., Gruenstein E.I.: *Expert learning system network for diagnosis of breast calcifications*, Investigative Radiology, 16:534-539, 1991.

[67] Magnin I.E., El Alaoui M., Bremond A: *Automatic microcalcifications pattern recognition from x-ray mammographies*, **Proc. SPIE**, 1137:170-175, 1989.

[68] Swets J.A., Getty D.J., Pickett R.M., D'Orsi C.J., Seltzer S.E., McNeil B.J.: *Enhancing and evaluating diagnostic accuracy*, Med Decis Making, 11:9-18, 1991.

[69] Gale A.G., Roebuck A.J., Riley P., Worthington B.S.: *Computer aids to mammographic diagnosis*, Br J. Radiology, 60:887-891, 1987.

[70] Getty D.J., Pickett R.M., D'Orsi C.J., Swets J.A.: *Enhanced interpretation of diagnostic images*, Investigative Radiology, 23:240-252, 1988.

[71] Puff D., Cromartie R., Pisano E.: *Evaluation and optimization of contrast enhancement methods for medical images*, **Proceedings of Visualization in Biomedical Computing Conference, SPIE**, 1808:336-346, 1992.